Needs and Assessment Strategies for Health Education and Health Promotion

FOURTH EDITION

Gary D. Gilmore, MPH, PhD, MCHES

Professor and Director
Graduate Community Health/Public Health Programs
University of Wisconsin–La Crosse and
University of Wisconsin–Extension

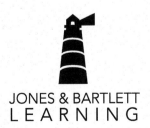

JONES & BARTLETT
LEARNING

World Headquarters

Jones & Bartlett Learning	Jones & Bartlett Learning	Jones & Bartlett Learning
5 Wall Street	Canada	International
Burlington, MA 01803	6339 Ormindale Way	Barb House, Barb Mews
978-443-5000	Mississauga, Ontario L5V 1J2	London W6 7PA
info@jblearning.com	Canada	United Kingdom
www.jblearning.com		

Jones & Bartlett Learning books and products are available through most bookstores and online booksellers. To contact Jones & Bartlett Learning directly, call 800-832-0034, fax 978-443-8000, or visit our website, www.jblearning.com.

Substantial discounts on bulk quantities of Jones & Bartlett Learning publications are available to corporations, professional associations, and other qualified organizations. For details and specific discount information, contact the special sales department at Jones & Bartlett Learning via the above contact information or send an email to specialsales@jblearning.com.

Production Credits

Publisher, Higher Education: Cathleen Sether
Senior Acquisitions Editor: Shoshanna Goldberg
Senior Associate Editor: Amy L. Bloom
Editorial Assistant: Prima Bartlett
Production Manager: Julie Champagne Bolduc
Production Editor: Jessica Steele Newfell
Associate Marketing Manager: Jody Sullivan
VP, Manufacturing and Inventory Control: Therese Connell
Composition: Laserwords Private Limited, Chennai, India
Cover Design: Scott Moden
Photo Researcher: Sarah Cebulski
Cover Images: (background) © chudo-yudo/ShutterStock, Inc.; (left) © Andresr/ShutterStock, Inc.; (middle) © Mikhail Olykainen/ShutterStock, Inc.; (right) © goodluz/Fotolia.com
Printing and Binding: Malloy, Inc.
Cover Printing: Malloy, Inc.

Photo Credits
Figure 9-1 (top, bottom left) Courtesy of Terry Wirkus and Pamela Mukaire, MPH; **(bottom right)** Courtesy of Pamela Mukaire, MPH
Unless otherwise indicated, all photographs and illustrations are under copyright of Jones & Bartlett Learning, or have been provided by the author.
Some images in this book feature models. These models do not necessarily endorse, represent, or participate in the activities represented in the images.

To order this product, use ISBN: 978-1-4496-4644-8

Library of Congress Cataloging-in-Publication Data
Gilmore, Gary D., 1943–
  Needs and capacity assessment strategies for health education and health
  promotion / Gary D. Gilmore.— 4th ed.
      p. ; cm.
  Includes bibliographical references and index.
  ISBN-13: 978-1-4496-0210-9 (pbk.)
  ISBN-10: 1-4496-0210-X (pbk.)
  1. Health education—Evaluation. 2. Health promotion—Evaluation.
  3. Medical personnel—Supply and demand. 4. Public health personnel—Supply and
    demand. I. Title.
  [DNLM: 1. Health Services Research—methods. 2. Health Education—organization & administration.
  3. Health Promotion—organization & administration. 4. Health Services Needs and Demand. W 84.3
    RA440.4.G55 2012
    362.1072'—dc22
                              2011011422
6048

Printed in the United States of America
22 21   10 9 8 7 6

To John and Ruth;
Elizabeth, Scott, Todd, and Merrily;
for your enduring support throughout the years.

Brief Contents

Contents

Part II Assessments with Individuals   59

Chapter 3 Single-Step Surveys   60

Chapter 7 Group Participation Process: Focus Group   118

Chapter 8 Community-Based Needs and Capacity Assessment Processes   127

Chapter 9 Technology-Supported Assessments   153

Chapter 10 Large-Scale Community Assessment Strategies   165

Part IV Self-Directed Assessments   179

Chapter 11 Self-Directed Assessment Inventories   180

Chapter 12 Observational Self-Directed Assessments   192

Part V Case Studies and a Needs Assessment Simulation   205

Case Study 1 Up in Smoke: A Recent History of Iowa Smokefree Legislation and Public Health Outcomes   207

Case Study 2 Public Health Needs Assessment in Waupaca County, Wisconsin: A Guide for Community Health Programs   216

Appendices

Index   345

Foreword

Since the previous editions of this well-received text, the economic crises of most nations—as well as states, communities, and their health agencies—have worsened. As economic pressures mount on local, state, federal, and voluntary agencies funding programs in health, pressures will continue to grow also for how well they are meeting the most critical needs of the community and how well they are applying "evidence-based practices" to justify expenditures. Old programs and services that had been taken for granted as community entitlements will be called into question and put to the test of how well they address community needs. Assessment of needs, therefore, will become an even more compelling imperative than it has been in the past. Similarly, community capacities to meet the needs will be weighed with increasing skepticism.

Professor Gilmore has felt these growing economic pressures as he worked on this *Fourth Edition* and has given attention to offering the best, the most practical, and the most up-to-date methods and processes of measuring needs and capacities for health education and health promotion. I am pleased that the PRECEDE-PROCEED model continues to serve as one of these resources, linking needs and capacity assessment to program planning and evaluation. The previous edition of this book came out in the same year as the *Fourth Edition* of our book on the PRECEDE-PROCEED model with its expanded scope to health program planning in general, so Dr. Gilmore is able to reflect in this edition the enhancements and the central elements of that model, which has survived continued and repeated use in over 1000 published applications. These can be searched in an online bibliography (http://www. lgreen.net). The alternative models such as APEX-PH, COMPASS, MAPP, and PATCH for broad community health education and health promotion planning are reflected in this edition of Dr. Gilmore's book, as are the many specific techniques and procedures for gathering and processing various types of needs and capacity data.

One particularly important addition to this edition, among others, is attention to "Health Impact Assessment." This is a politically charged strategy for assessing proposed policy or program initiatives in other sectors such as transportation, agriculture, and city planning, not just relative to the needs they will serve in the sector proposing them, but also relative to the impact they will have on health. Health Impact Assessments have become more extensively developed and applied in Europe and Canada than in the United States, but some jurisdictions in the United States are developing their commitment and their approach to this method of controlling the inevitable spill-over effects of initiatives across sectors of community life.

This text provides a compass and a primer for the plethora of methods and processes of needs and capacity assessment. It offers a springboard and direction for accessing the growing literature and resources for assessing the health education and health promotion needs and capacities of communities, groups, and individuals. And, it provides links to the use of needs assessments and capacity assessments in the planning and evaluation of programs and policies.

Lawrence W. Green, DrPH, DSc(Hon), FAAHB
Department of Epidemiology and Biostatistics
University of California at San Francisco

Preface

More recently, it has become abundantly clear that in addition to our being immersed in the "information age," we have become ever more accountable for our actions as professionals. By-and-large, the actions we take with others require a rationale, clear purpose, reasonable context, resourcefulness, efficiency, effectiveness, and sustainability. In the health and human service disciplines, we accomplish this responsibility with level or dwindling fiscal support each year. However, far from being dispirited, our challenge is to work within the boundaries of our resources in order to accomplish our goals. Realistic assessments contribute to that end.

Needs and Capacity Assessment Strategies for Health Education and Health Promotion was first written during the 1980s with the same purpose in mind as today: to provide professionals with the best advice and clearest processes possible for the assessment of health-related needs and capacities of groups and individuals more fully informing decision-making and eventual action steps. While the focus of this book is primarily on health education and health promotion, the principles and practices are germane to a wide array of disciplines.

Readers who have tracked the progression of this book will note that the chapters in this *Fourth Edition* have been updated, several extensively. The additional commentary related to specific assessments (e.g., motivational interviewing, photovoice), foundational principles (e.g., social determinants of health, World Health Organization [WHO] Millennium Development Goals, Community-Based Participatory Research [CBPR]), and policy-related forces (e.g., health impact assessment) offers an even greater sense of awareness regarding the complexity of preparing for and conducting needs and capacity assessments. Additionally, having a clearer sense of the contributions of the social determinants of health enables the reader to prepare more comprehensively.

The majority of the case studies in the *Fourth Edition* are new or updated so that the reader can access in-depth examples of how others developed, implemented, and derived insights from their needs and capacity assessments.

All of these case studies were written explicitly for this book by experienced practitioners. In addition, an original article addressing deconstruction and metaphoric considerations in health promotion assessments by Richard Hovey from the University of Calgary appears as one of the final thought pieces in the book.

It is important to point out that the *Fourth Edition* marks the departure of Donald Campbell who retired in 2010. He was a proponent of clear, logical, and precise communications across disciplines. He also joined me in the belief that our book made a difference because of its practical value to those engaged in the professional preparation and professional development phases of their careers. I want to wish him a fulfilling retirement after dedicating three decades of service to the University of Wisconsin–La Crosse.

Throughout this book, the reader will detect the continuing theme regarding our global engagement in health enhancement. Today, our responsibility for accurate assessments is not limited nor delimited to geographic boundaries, particularly given the ever-advancing technology for global communication and distance education, coupled with cross-cultural experiences and expanded international travel options. We have opportunities almost on a daily basis to make a decided difference as we work with those of distinct cultures, social strata, professions, and personal perspectives for the improvement of health and well-being.

Given the complexity of a writing project of this nature, it is essential to recognize the important contributions of others. Gratitude is extended to Lawrence W. Green for his most thoughtful and gracious Foreword to the *Fourth Edition*, which marks his third sage introduction to the text. Others who have made important contributions to the *Fourth Edition* are Connie Abert, Terri Ades, Palo Almond, Linda Behm, Linda Bobroff, Becky Campbell, Jennifer Gamberini, Robert Gorsky, Tabitha Hackett, Marilyn Herman, Richard Hovey, Elaine Jones, Jim Jorstad, Donell Kerns, Bethany Kies, Eleanor Long, Alyson Luchini, Brittany McIlquham, Keely Rees, Jay Schindler, Megan Sheffer, Larry Sleznikow, Robert Smith, Christopher Squier, Terry Wirkus, Arla Wojahn, and Gail Yest.

In addition, the editorial and production team at Jones & Bartlett Learning deserve special recognition for their unwavering commitment to this writing project: Shoshanna Goldberg, Senior Acquisitions Editor; Amy Bloom, Senior Associate Editor; Prima Bartlett, Editorial Assistant; Rachel Isaacs, Editorial Assistant; Jessica Newfell, Production Editor; Sarah Cebulski, Photo Researcher; and Jody Sullivan, Associate Marketing Manager.

Finally, thank you to those who provided thoughtful reviews of the *Third Edition*: Susan Butler, EdD, CHES, Emory University, Rollins School of Public Health; Gregg M. Gascon, PhD, The Ohio State University; and Dawn M. Weiler, PhD, APRN-ANP, BC, Boise State University.

About the Author

Since 1974, Dr. Gilmore has held a joint appointment with the University of Wisconsin–La Crosse and the University of Wisconsin–Extension. He is Professor and Director of Graduate Community Health/Public Health Programs. His prior experiences were in public health and preventive medicine at the Bergen County (New Jersey) Health Department and at the Preventive Medicine Unit, General Leonard Wood Hospital, U.S. Army (where he received the Army Commendation Medal in Preventive Medicine). His training in epidemiology and public health is through the School of Public Health at the University of Minnesota, with additional training in epidemiology at the New England Epidemiology Institute, Tufts University.

He is the founding and continuing Director of the first Master of Public Health Program (CEPH accredited) offered in the University of Wisconsin System. The program was ranked sixth in the nation by the 2004 *U.S. News and World Report* rankings of the Best Graduate Programs in Community Health. As an inherent part of his appointment, he also directs Community Health Programming in Continuing Education and Extension (University of Wisconsin–La Crosse and University of Wisconsin–Extension). He has served on the American Cancer Society National Board of Directors during 1986–1996 and 1999–2002, and he is the recipient of the St. George Medal. He received the 2001 Regents Teaching Excellence Award bestowed by the Board of Regents, University of Wisconsin System. He also received the 1998 Award for Excellence from the University of Wisconsin–Extension.

During 1999–2000, Dr. Gilmore served as the first Fulbright Senior Scholar at the All India Institute of Hygiene and Public Health, Kolkata (Calcutta), India. In that capacity, he taught graduate students and medical practitioners in the principles of public health and conducted population-based research in West Bengal.

His publications span more than four decades of professional activity and include peer-reviewed journal articles, books, and technical reports. He chaired the six-year *National Health Educator Competencies Update Project*, which sought to validate the entry and advanced-level competencies for health education specialists.

Dr. Gilmore was appointed in 2004, and reappointed in 2008, by the Governor of Wisconsin to serve on the Public Health Council for the State. The Council advises the Department of Health Services, the Governor, the Legislature, and Wisconsin citizens on the progress in implementing the State health plan and the coordination of responses to public health emergencies. He serves as Chair of the Council.

Introduction and Overview

In Chapters 1 and 2, emerging and established key issues related to needs, resources, and needs and capacity assessments are presented, along with consideration of how they fit into the larger framework of planning for health education and health promotion. In addition, a variety of preliminary considerations for health and human service professionals, including a review of capacity-focused assessments, advisory and planning committees, community coalitions, selected data collection considerations, and prioritization processes, are examined. All of these elements, including statements of basic premises, form a context within which the selected needs and capacity assessment strategies are employed. Throughout the text, readers will find an emphasis on practicality and time-honored methods.

Gaining a Needs and Capacity Assessment Perspective

Introduction

Trends

Needs and capacity assessments do not take place in isolation, nor are they confined solely to a phase in program-planning endeavors. They occur because, as health professionals, we are attempting to better understand the impactors on the health and well-being of individuals and population groups so that the appropriate health-enhancing next steps can take place. In this way, informed decisions can be made.

The impactors can be quite diverse and elusive, thus requiring our very best assessment efforts. We also must prepare comprehensively within the boundaries of limited resources. Although no single model assures a completely comprehensive approach, two major considerations can complement our efforts: taking an interdisciplinary approach when appropriate and being mindful of the social determinants of health. Former U.S. Surgeon General David Satcher (2010) has stated that:

> . . . we need a new way of thinking, one where, as public health professionals, we lead by taking an interdisciplinary approach and collaborating across a wide range of disciplines, developing our own workforce to effectively address social determinants of health, and insisting health and non-health policies incorporate a social-determinants approach (p. 7).

To address the influence of the social determinants of health, the World Health Organization established the Commission on Social Determinants of Health in 2005, resulting in their landmark final report in 2008, *Closing the Gap in a Generation* (Commission on Social Determinants of Health [CSDH], 2008). Of note, the Commission (CSDH, 2008) addressed the social determinants of health through a health-equity lens, stating:

> Traditionally, societies have looked to the health sector to deal with its concerns about health and disease. Certainly, maldistribution of health care—not

delivering care to those who most need it—is one of the social determinants of health. But the high burden of illness responsible for appalling premature loss of life arises in large part because of the conditions in which people are born, grow, live, work, and age—conditions that together provide the freedom people need to live lives they value (p. 26).

In the United States, the *Robert Wood Johnson Foundation Commission to Build a Healthier America* received the charge to specify strategies that would address health disparities in the country particularly as related to social and economic disadvantage. The Commission came up with approaches that address the social determinants of health, many of which have not been fully established within the realms of medicine and public health (Braveman, Egerter, Woolf, & Marks, 2011). Emphasis is placed on those social policy factors that can be addressed early rather than later by a society. The essence of this perspective resonates throughout this text.

Coupled with the social determinants of health are the Millennium Development Goals (MDGs) that have been developed by the World Health Organization. They are part of the United Nations Millennium Declaration and were approved by 189 nations in September 2000. The list, as of January 15, 2008, includes the following goals (World Health Organization [WHO], 2011):

1. Eradicate extreme poverty and hunger.
2. Achieve universal primary education.
3. Promote gender equality and empower women.
4. Reduce child mortality.
5. Improve maternal health.
6. Combat HIV/AIDS, malaria, and other diseases.
7. Ensure environmental sustainability.
8. Develop a global partnership for development.

Targets and indicators for monitoring progress are included with each goal. The World Health Organization states that the "eight goals provide a roadmap for development, setting out targets to be achieved by 2015, with 1990 data as a baseline for comparison. Although ambitious, the MDGs are feasible as well as mutually reinforcing" (WHO, 2011). The essence of the goals and social determinants of health are conveyed throughout this text as current and emerging health needs are addressed throughout the world. A compelling review of the determinants with reference to the Millennium Development Goals (MDG) occurs in a dedicated issue of *Global Health Promotion* (Supplement 1, 2009), the official journal of the International Union for Health Promotion and Education. As but one example, Lewis (2009) reflects on the burden of illness on developing countries while reminding the reader that three of the eight MDG goals are particularly health related: "The challenge for us all is to move from a report to an implementation that makes a real difference, in our case, to the poorest people of the world" (p. 35).

Although numerous professional entities develop specialties and subspecialties to delve more deeply into the focus areas of their disciplines, today it is becoming more desirable to complement that approach by working in partnership across disciplines. Similarly, the insights that health professionals can derive from the perspective of the social determinants of health begin to open up and clarify the discoveries related to actual health-related risk factors and protective factors.

During instances of almost any magnitude of impact, having health-related assessments in place promotes the systematic and timely review of requisite resources. Toward the end of the last century, and continuing into the twenty-first century, needs and capacity assessments have become more prominent procedures within health education and health promotion planning, as well as other planning endeavors. This amplification is happening with good reason. Insights into health-related impacts on a society are ever expanding in terms of their nature (e.g., the interactivity of physical, psychological, and behavioral factors related to disease risk), degree (e.g., poverty's impact on health outcomes), and setting (e.g., the global impacts of violent behavior), thus necessitating consistent, systematic assessment principles and practices. Additionally, accountability issues increase as resources become scarcer, leading to calls for more evidence-based endeavors. Furthermore, within the rubric of "workforce development," professional competencies need to be ascertained and periodically validated in health education, health promotion, and even the broader context of public health, requiring greater specificity of professional skill sets.

Specifically for health education, one of the key areas of responsibility for entry- and advanced-level health educators is the assessment of individual and community needs for health education (National Commission for Health Education Credentialing, Society for Public Health Education, & American Association for Health Education [NCHEC, SOPHE, & AAHE], 2010). Included in this responsibility area are the aspects of obtaining health-related data, distinguishing between behaviors that enhance well-being and those that impede it, and inferring needs for health education. National competency validation research (Gilmore, Olsen, Taub, & Connell, 2005; Gilmore, Olsen, & Taub, 2001) demonstrates the importance of revalidating established competencies and verifying the existence of additional competencies that have emerged in the profession.

In similar fashion, practitioners in other disciplines are recognizing the value of needs and capacity assessments as integral parts of the planning process. As one example, some business professionals involved in worksite health promotion are recommending frameworks that incorporate clearly identified needs and capacity assessments so that objective information can be collected to guide the next steps in the planning process. Bensky and Hietbrink (1994) have described a health promotion planning framework for business settings (to be discussed in greater detail in Chapter 2) in which they state that "most health promotion programs that fail to reach their goals are built upon invalid assumptions about what people need, want and will do about it" (p. 26). They then detail the first step in their planning framework, which is assessing the situation. Assessments at the worksite setting can also be quite comprehensive, as described by Oldenburg and colleagues (2002) through their 112-item checklist of workplace environmental factors that affect health both negatively and positively. Their assessment categories include a building assessment, the information environment (e.g., signs, bulletin boards), fitness facilities, grounds and neighborhood assessments, and assessments of various individual-choice practices related to nutrition, smoking, and alcohol activities at the worksite.

To track some of the patterns regarding needs and capacity assessments that have emerged during the last decade, we must recognize the eight changes noted here.

First, needs and capacity assessments are being incorporated into various professional responsibilities to a greater extent. More professionals are using these assessments as inherent parts of their work in public health departments, hospitals, clinics, schools, voluntary and other private agencies, and business sites. This shift appears to be due to a greater emphasis on documentation to justify programs and initiatives and their costs as well as the increased use of marketing strategies to address target population needs and resources in school, community, and business settings. Also, cost-conscious consumers are becoming more selective in their health-related choices, based to a large extent on a desire to have specific needs met at a reasonable cost. From a capacity perspective, community-based groups appreciate being recognized as resources that can be drawn upon during the planning, implementation, and evaluation of health education and health promotional activities. In response, health program and service providers have shown a renewed interest in ascertaining the needs and capacities, as revealed by the consumers. All of these aspects—documentation, marketing strategies, and program and service offerings—typically drive the use of needs assessments as a starting point for determining specific population needs. The results can guide more effective planning and implementation strategies. Additionally, capacity assessment procedures have been expanded in the planning process to explore existing and needed resources in school, community, and business settings.

A **second** change has to do with the broader context of the "needs" being assessed. Here reference is made to factors that influence health status, including risk factors, protective factors (assets), and a wide range of determinants that constitute a context of influence on the health status of individuals and communities. These determinants include biological, behavioral, and social influences, as detailed in the Commission on Social Determinants of Health report (2008, p. 2) and captured in that report's three principles of action:

1. Improve the conditions of daily life—the circumstances in which people are born, grow, live, work, and age.

2. Tackle the inequitable distribution of power, money, and resources—the structural drivers of those conditions of daily life—globally, nationally, and locally.
3. Measure the problem, evaluate action, expand the knowledge base, develop a workforce that is trained in the social determinants of health, and raise public awareness about the social determinants of health.

Throughout this text, although specific examples of needs will be provided, it is most important for health and human service professionals to keep this more comprehensive perspective in mind.

Third, the emergence of individualized assessment strategies is noted. These personal approaches can be quite valuable in health maintenance and health promotional efforts (see Chapters 11 and 12). They can enable a person to detect specific risk factors that may negatively affect his or her own health. Individualized capacity assessment strategies also can help a person identify other factors and resources that are quite positive and that can enhance good health in the individual's life.

A **fourth** change is the wide variance in what is meant by *needs assessment* and *capacity assessment*, and how these terms are used. Regarding needs assessments, there is much discussion as to what a "need" is, and whether we assess actual or perceived needs. Health and human service professionals have different reasons for using this process. Some professionals use needs assessments as starting points for program planning. Others use them on a continuing basis with the same populations to detect changing needs over a certain period of time, with the objective of adjusting the services based on those needs. Similarly, in addressing capacity assessment, ascertaining actual and potential resources can contribute to more efficient planning, in preparing to use available and emerging population-based resources to complement external wherewithal. This approach also can result in meta-benefits, such as the involved individuals having a greater sense of feeling valued as contributors, thereby resulting in increased commitment to a project or initiative.

Fifth, community-based participatory approaches to research and practice have emerged to address the social determinants of health in particular (Schulz, Krieger, & Galea, 2002). As Schulz et al. (2002) point out, risk factors explain only a portion of outcomes, such as coronary heart disease, because the risks themselves can be affected by more contextual factors such as poverty, discrimination, education, and housing policies (CSDH, 2008). To address these complexities, collaborative and innovative research and intervention strategies are required, necessitating the awareness and involvement of community members in organized research and intervention strategies.

This awareness by health and human service professionals and community members has led to the emergence of community-based participatory approaches in which community members become involved in the essential phases of project planning, implementation, and evaluation. As an inherent part of community-based assessment activity, it is increasingly important to work in partnership with the community, rather than viewing it as a setting in which professionals conduct investigations known only to them.

The Office of Disease Prevention and Health Promotion (2001), which is part of the U.S. Public Health Service, has called for more of a collaborative endeavor, viewing communities as cornerstones of public health action, and offering a planning guide to be discussed in more detail in Chapter 10. Corroborating this perspective, the 2003 Institute of Medicine report *Who Will Keep the Public Healthy?* has addressed the value and importance of community-based research, in which key community representatives become engaged in the development and implementation of such investigations. Israel and colleagues (2001) have defined *community-based participatory research* as a "partnership approach to research that equitably involves community members, organizational representatives, and researchers in all aspects of the research process" (p. 2).

Miller, Bedney, and Guenther-Grey (2003) have emphasized the degree to which collaborative efforts can facilitate community-wide change. As they point out, "collaborative work highlights the role of community systems and the interdependence among community sectors in affecting health outcomes" (p. 583). To collaborate effectively, they point to the importance of all partners sharing a clear mission with planning centered on mutual goals. The importance of community involvement is conveyed in community-based participatory research (CBPR), and, as pointed out by Faridi, Grunbaum, Gray, Franks, and Simoes (2007), it "is gaining increasing credence among public health researchers and practitioners" (p. 1).

In their extensive publication on the topic of health-related CBPR, Israel, Eng, Schulz, and Parker (2005, pp. 6–9) have detailed nine principles of CBPR that convey the importance of seeking the active participation of all partners involved in a given investigation. These include the tenets that CPBR:

- Facilitates a collaborative, equitable partnership in all phases of research, involving an empowering and power-sharing process that attends to social inequalities
- Fosters co-learning and capacity building among all partners
- Involves a long-term process and commitment to sustainability

Sixth, there is a continuing emphasis on capacity analysis to complement the needs assessment process. As Kretzmann and McKnight (1993) have pointed out, a capacity-focused approach addresses the capacities, skills, and assets of a community. Through this approach, which will be covered in more detail in Chapters 2 and 8, the assets of a community are mapped by examining the potential contributions of individuals, organizations, associations, and institutions. In the years following the insights first provided by Kretzmann and McKnight (1993), capacity-building approaches to community health promotion have been more widely embraced and incorporated into systematic planning efforts, including school health promotion efforts (Bond, Glover, Godfrey, Butler, & Patton, 2001). Of note, the Centers for Disease Control and Prevention (CDC) offers capacity-building support in areas like HIV prevention through technology transfer, technical assistance, training, and information dissemination (http://www.cdc.gov/hiv/topics/cba/cba.htm). Complementing these types of efforts are social environmental strategies that focus upstream in directly modifying social environmental conditions (Barnett, Anderson, Blosnich, Menard, Halverson, & Casper, 2007).

Seventh, large-scale community assessment formats have appeared on the scene, providing comprehensive direction to planners seeking organizational and community assessments. These frameworks use a variety of assessment approaches that draw upon previously gathered information (secondary data), while preparing to collect additional information from the target population (primary data). Some of the formats (as discussed in more detail in Chapter 10) provide ongoing assessments for comparison over time.

Eighth, needs and capacity assessments are being incorporated into emergency circumstances where there is an urgency in assessing human needs and the capacity to assure health and well-being. Global examples include the assessment measures taken following the March 2011 earthquake and tsunami that impacted much of Japan leading to radiation emergencies and emergency communications and assessments through social media ("Protecting Public Health After Major Radiation Emergencies," 2011; "Social Media, Texting Play New Role in Response to Disasters," 2011) and the major earthquake that struck Turkey in 1999 (Daley, Karpati, & Sheik, 2002). Preparation for future emergency circumstances is an imperative for community planning measures regarding the roles of health care, public health, and human service professionals, along with the needed communication technology and content appropriate for both professionals and the public (Taintor, 2003).

Key Questions About Assessment

Whether one is a health or human service professional just beginning employment or someone with considerable experience, the meaning and processes of needs and capacity assessment can appear to be quite confounding. The following questions represent those heard most frequently. For the sake of clarification, preliminary responses are offered.

What Is a Need?

A *need* is the difference between the present situation and a more desirable one. The present situation may have some undesirable characteristics that motivate a person to consider a more desirable situation. For example, we might realize that we are overweight and "need" to identify the causes and ways to resolve the problem. But needs are not solely related to undesirable situations; a very positive situation can be further enhanced. For example, you might jog 2 miles every other day to keep fit, and now you want to increase the distance. Or, you might have learned to avoid some of the risk factors related to cancer (e.g., smoking), and now you want to learn more about protective factors against cancer (e.g., adding more fiber to your diet).

What Is a Needs Assessment?

A *needs assessment* is a planned process that identifies the reported needs of an individual or a group. Individuals can conduct needs assessments that reveal reported areas of personal needs. A person can review these needs, consider their relative importance and practicality, and then take steps to address them. With groups, a subgroup that is representative of the larger group can work through the needs assessment process. Health professionals can use the reported needs from this representative group for planning purposes.

Are the Reported Needs Actual or Perceived?

It is difficult for the health or human service professional, and even for the target audience, to know whether the needs identified by an individual or group are the actual needs (the *true needs*). These actual needs are difficult to identify and measure because they continually change. Perceived needs are those envisioned and reported by the participants in a needs assessment process (the *reported needs*). As professionals involved in a needs assessment, we rely on people as primary sources of information. These people draw from their experiences, observations, ideas, opinions, and feelings to guide them toward conclusions about needs—*perceived needs*. Perceived needs are important because they represent the experiences and perceptions of the individuals or groups involved. It is inefficient to expend a great deal of energy trying to determine whether perceived needs are actual needs. Because individuals and groups are continually changing and growing, their needs are changing as well. The strategies presented in this book do not attempt to determine true needs beyond any shadow of a doubt. Rather, the purpose is to describe workable processes that assess perceived needs of individual and group importance.

Why Conduct a Needs Assessment?

A needs assessment provides a logical starting point for individual action and program development, as well as a continuing process for keeping activities on track. As described later in this book, a needs assessment can be repeated to monitor program impacts. This process enables our educational and promotional efforts to be guided by a realistic database. Overall, a needs assessment process can assist practitioners in a variety of ways: Program development efforts can be based on reported needs, changes and trends assessed over a period of time, individuals and target audiences can be involved in purposeful activities, and the target audience can be more accurately characterized.

What Does Capacity Mean?

Capacity refers to both individual and collective resources that can be brought to bear for health enhancement. It includes assets in individuals that can provide certain protective influences that affect whether people engage in certain risk-related behaviors, such as tobacco use (Atkins, Oman, Vesely, Aspy, & McLeroy, 2002). Clark (2000) has made reference to a matrix of needs and responses that ensure quality of life, referring to individual and collective responses in relation to personal and societal needs. Reference is also made to the importance of developing community capacity and power, which are integral to the enhancement of personal capacity and power needed to ensure quality of life. As Clark (2000) points out, "individuals must develop the perspectives, values, and skills necessary to maintain the quality of their lives as appropriate and desired in their particular community and culture, and they must be enveloped by a society that is socially integrated, is cohesive, and provides moral and material support when needed" (p. 704).

What Is a Capacity Assessment?

A *capacity assessment* is a measure of actual and potential individual, group, and community resources that can be inherent to and/or brought to bear for health maintenance and enhancement. From an individual perspective, capacity can be measured in terms of assets or protective factors (Atkins et al., 2002); at the group or community level, capacity can be considered as unique histories, cultures, structures, personalities, politics, and systems, all brought together for health enhancement (Bond et al., 2001; Cheadle, Sullivan, Krieger, Ciske, Shaw, Schier, & Eisinger, 2002). Included in the capacity assessment approach is the process of mapping community assets (Parks & Straker, 1996; Kretzmann & McKnight, 1993).

Why Conduct a Capacity Assessment?

From a community-based perspective, capacity assessment provides an opportunity to engage multiple stakeholders and others in a review of actual and potential resources that can influence current and future partnership efforts. Capacity assessment also enables individuals to review sources of support in their lives (e.g., individual protective factors, significant others, educational and worksite settings). It is essential to review the actual and potential availability of resources for the sake of establishing realistic project starting points and ascertaining project sustainability.

Balancing Science and Art

Qualitative and Quantitative Issues

Human needs and capacities are diverse and changing. No single approach to assessing them would always be appropriate. Instead, a variety of approaches usually is necessary. One way to expand the approach is to consider the use of both quantitative and qualitative information. Health and human service professionals are familiar with quantitative data. Newspapers are full of statistics describing increases in health care costs, changes in the incidence of specific diseases, and various lifestyle trends. Professional journals rely heavily on quantitative data to report the results of scientific and applied research. Most people usually have a greater familiarity, and perhaps security, with numbers. Our society has been conditioned to focus on something ranked number one, rather than number ten.

However, numbers do not always tell the full story. In fact, they can oversimplify matters. For this reason, they need to be balanced with qualitative data. Narrative information is necessary to elaborate on statistical data and to contribute insights. A narrative format can capture variations and exceptions and portray the needs and available resources as completely as possible. As has been pointed out by Creswell (2003), the qualitative approach is basically an interpretive process, with a reliance on text and image data. More specifically, several reasons for collecting visual data are offered by Banks (2007, pp. 3–4):

- Images are ubiquitous in society, and because of this some consideration of visual representation can potentially be included in all studies of society.
- Images . . . might be able to reveal some sociological insight that is not accessible by any other means.
- There is also the caveat . . . that to restrict oneself to a single methodology or area of investigation is as sociologically limiting as willfully ignoring a methodology or area.

As one example, in a given community there could be a relatively high incidence of teenage deaths, in comparison with state statistics. Recent local statistics regarding the causes of teenage deaths might show that motor vehicle accidents represent the leading cause of death. However, other sources of information could include one's coworkers, representatives from local and state organizations, and key individuals in the community. Discussions with these people might reveal contributing factors that are associated with motor vehicle accidents, such as an awareness of increasing alcohol consumption among teens, observed high-speed travel on secondary roads, and a sense of increased stress in the family. This qualitative information yields a more complete picture of teenage deaths and suggests possible contributing factors for the professional to address.

Intuition's Contributions

Instincts and feelings count in needs and capacity assessments. In addition to gathering quantitative and qualitative information, these more intuitive responses of health and human service professionals and community members also are important and should not be ignored. At the core, intuition refers to direct insight that is not initially inferred through facts.

Another, more focused approach to comprehending intuition is based on personality type theory, where intuition is described as one of two key constructs within the psychological realm of perception (i.e., all the ways we become aware of things, people, happenings, or ideas). In this context, intuition focuses on possibilities and what "might be," rather than specifics and "what is," which is more of a sensing perspective (Allen & Brock, 2000; Hirsh & Kummerow, 1997). Further, while the perceiving process of *sensing* means that we are becoming aware of things directly through our five senses, *intuition* means that we are indirectly becoming aware of things through considerations of meanings, relationships, and possibilities. Using our intuition typically means reading between and beyond the lines. Allen and Brock (2000) have used the personality type approach effectively in reviewing the distinctions that occur in health care communications. To become more cognizant of differences, the preferences of both the practitioner and the client/patient are assessed, eventually leading to the development of improved written and interactive communications.

Drawing on this orientation, an early study by Agor (1984) examined the value of intuition for making practical management decisions. He cited examples, as well as data from his own research, that demonstrated how some successful managers made major decisions based on intuition. In some cases, intuition took precedence over conflicting or inadequate information. In a national study involving 1679 managers, Agor found use of intuition to be more prevalent with those advanced in management rank. Top managers in every sample group tested used intuition in decision making to a greater extent than middle- and lower-level managers. This type of finding has been documented by others as well (Roach, 1986; Reynierse, 1991).

When later studies were conducted at the international level, such clear-cut distinctions did not emerge. For example, Reynierse (1995) compared the preference data from a sample of 3688 Japanese managers, executives, and CEOs with data he had collected on 1952 American managers and executives. Although the data for the American executives revealed increasing intuitive preferences at the higher management levels (as predicted), the Japanese data showed a notable intuitive preference at all management levels. This finding may reflect the decision-making distinction between American and Japanese companies: Japanese decision making is highly participatory, in contrast to American approaches in which decision making and final authority are detailed through job descriptions and organizational frameworks.

In a more recent Finnish study by Jarlstrom and Valkealahti (2010) using psychological type assessments to compare managers with business students, feeling and intuition emerged to a greater extent in the students. The authors speculate that this may be due to the people-orientation of the students. They continue by stating, "Intuitive managers are good at having a vision, selling their visions, and negotiating with the environment. As a consequence, Intuitive managers might be better at living with and managing change and at creative thinking at the strategic level of management in a changing environment" (p. 48). The authors indicate that these qualities appeared to be more aligned with transformational leadership that exhibits "vision, proactive thinking, novelty, creativity, flexibility" (p. 49), as contrasted with a transactional approach, more so maintaining the status quo. Overall, it is important to point out that the findings from one cultural context cannot automatically be applied to others.

In a general sense, however, one's intuition increases with experience. New health and human service professionals may not have a wealth of experience from which to draw. There may be a hesitation in trusting individual feelings about needs and priorities and a desire to rely more extensively on quantitative data. With increasing experience, however, individual insights take on a greater significance in the planning process.

Assumptions and Assessments

Two types of groups are involved in needs and capacity assessments. One group comprises the professionals directly involved in the planning, coordinating, or facilitating of the assessments. They bring to the process health-related expertise and often previous assessment experience. The other group consists of the target audience or target group. These individuals bring their expectations and life experiences, which help them identify a range of needs, wants, interests, and capacities. They also should be engaged from the outset so that their contributions can be made during the planning, implementation, and evaluation phases, as appropriate.

When the two groups enter into the assessment processes, individuals in both groups bring some assumptions about the needs and resources at hand. These assumptions are intuitive in nature, influenced by the previous experiences, opinions, feelings, and ideas of each individual. Practitioners develop assumptions based on ongoing interaction with community members and other professionals; examination of demographic data and vital statistics; comprehension of the various political and socioeconomic forces influencing the community; and personal insights, awareness, and experience. Members of the target group draw on their own insights and experiences in making their own assumptions.

If accurate, these assumptions can be very helpful in identifying a starting point. They can help to narrow the focus of a too-broad or too-generalized approach to a needs or capacity assessment. Collective assumptions from practitioners and community representatives can be discussed to help guide the assessment process in the right direction.

However, assumptions are not meant to take the place of assessments. In a sense, they act as precursors to sets of reported needs and resources. It is through the assessment process that these assumptions become more clearly defined and are possibly revised, resulting in some specifically identified needs and capacities.

Once specific needs and capacities have been assessed, it is important for the practitioner to offer a summary of the preliminary results to the community representatives. This approach provides all stakeholders with the opportunity to clarify and acknowledge the extent to which the identified needs and resources accurately reflect those of the involved groups. At that point, practitioners and representatives can reach a joint agreement regarding which needs to address and how best to address them with the resources at hand.

Some Basic Premises

The overall approach to needs and capacity assessment in this text is based on certain premises. Prior to your review of the individual and group needs and capacity assessment processes in the following chapters, consider these grounding points:

1. *People* are important to needs and capacity assessments. Individuals have the capacity to reflect on their health-related needs and to report these needs. Practitioners also can draw from their education and experience to reflect and report on the health-related needs and capacities of the people with whom they work. Not only do the assessments provide necessary insights and information, but involvement in their planning and implementation can also contribute to the development of meaningful working relationships.

2. The *needs* that people report are realistic issues to consider, particularly when a trend is apparent. We can view reported needs as one source of information. (Other sources will be addressed in the forthcoming chapters.)

3. A *needs assessment* is an applied process for gathering useful information for individual and group planning purposes. Its basic purpose is not to construct or test a scientific hypothesis, although good research techniques often are used in data collection and analysis. Throughout the book, you will note the focus on better preparing the practitioner to address key needs and capacity assessment issues that have a high potential for being experienced.

4. *Capacity assessments* can be quite varied because they assess individual and group resources over an array of parameters. They can cover distinct time dimensions (past, present, future), settings (local, state, regional, national, international), and contexts (social, cultural, political, and the like). Importantly, such resources need to be considered in as comprehensive a manner as time, fiscal, and human resources will allow.

5. *Planning and advisory committees* are important to the needs and capacity assessment processes. Often, such committees are established after the needs have been determined and the program is about to be planned. Alternatively, planning and advisory committees made up of practitioners and stakeholders (i.e., those involved in and affected by the issues being addressed) can help to plan and conduct the assessments. A committee can determine which kinds of needs and resources to consider, from whom to gather information, and which strategies to use. Committee members also can assist with data collection and analysis. Involving such committees at this early stage can ensure that the program is based on the perceived needs and the available and potential resources of the intended participants.

6. Needs and capacity assessments are *integral parts of the project/ program planning process.* These assessments represent key steps in planning effective health education and health promotion activities.

Summary

This chapter has addressed the value of an increased focus on needs and capacity assessments, questions regarding their nature, some of the basic principles, and our own premises. Human needs and capacities, although complex, are able to be assessed within the context of target group settings and situations that affect those needs and resources. Practitioners also have a context from which to draw preliminary needs- and capacity-related inferences based on their experiences and impressions. However, these are merely starting points for the professional; they offer clues to possible target group needs and capacities. Practitioners must consider the value of determining the prioritized needs and capacities of groups in a structured, collaborative fashion so that effective health education and health promotion efforts can be continued, adjusted, or developed, as appropriate.

Online Resources

Visit go.jblearning.com/gilmore4 for links to these Web sites.

Centers for Disease Control and Prevention
This Web site is the Capacity-Building Assistance (CBA) Branch of the CDC.

Office of Environmental Health Assessments
This Web site is from the Washington State Department of Health and includes definitions of health assessments and health education.

Minnesota Department of Health
This site describes needs assessments and questions to ask before preparing a needs assessment.

Supercourse: Epidemiology, the Internet, and Global Health

This site features a PowerPoint presentation that describes needs assessments.

Laboratory for Community and Economic Development

This site discusses why assessments should be done, who should be involved, what the steps of an assessment are, and where communities can go for help on conducting a needs assessment.

Ohio State University

This site discusses why and how a needs assessment should be used, what the benefits and challenges are to using one, how to plan a needs assessment, and how to report and use the information retrieved.

References

Agor, W. (1984). *Intuitive management.* Englewood Cliffs, NJ: Prentice Hall.

Allen, J., and Brock, S. (2000). *Health care communication using personality type.* Philadelphia: Routledge Publishing.

Atkins, L., Oman, R., Vesely, S., Aspy, C., and McLeroy, K. (2002). Adolescent tobacco use: The protective effects of developmental assets. *American Journal of Health Promotion, 16,* 198–205.

Banks, M. (2007). *Using visual data in qualitative research.* Los Angeles: Sage Publications.

Barnett, E., Anderson, T., Blosnich, J., Menard, J., Halverson, J., and Casper, M. (2007). *Heart healthy and stroke free: A social environment handbook.* Atlanta: U.S. Department of Health and Human Services, Centers for Disease Control and Prevention.

Becker, S. M. (2011). Protecting public health after major radiation emergencies. *British Medical Journal, 342,* d1968.

Bensky, J., and Hietbrink, R. (1994). Getting down to business. *Worksite Health, 1,* 25–28.

Bond, L., Glover, S., Godfrey, C., Butler, H., and Patton, G. (2001). Building capacity for system-level change in schools: Lessons from the gatehouse project. *Health Education and Behavior, 28,* 368–383.

Braveman, P., Egerter, S., Woolf, S., and Marks, J. (2011). When do we know enough to recommend action on the social determinants of health? *American Journal of Preventive Medicine, 40,* Supplement 1, S58–S66.

Cheadle, A., Sullivan, M., Krieger, J., Ciske, S., Shaw, M., Schier, J., and Eisinger, A. (2002). Using a participatory approach to provide assistance to community-based organizations: The Seattle Partners Community Research Center. *Health Education and Behavior, 29,* 383–394.

Clark, N. (2000). Understanding individual and collective capacity to enhance quality of life. *Health Education and Behavior, 27,* 699–707.

Commission on Social Determinants of Health (CSDH). (2008). *Closing the gap in a generation: Health equity through action on the social determinants of health.*

Final report of the Commission on Social Determinants of Health. Geneva: World Health Organization.

Creswell, J. (2003). *Research design: Qualitative, quantitative, and mixed methods approaches.* Thousand Oaks, CA: Sage Publications.

Daley, W., Karpati, A., and Sheik, M. (2002). Needs assessment of the displaced population following the August 1999 earthquake in Turkey. *Disasters, 25,* 67–75.

Faridi, Z., Grunbaum, J., Gray, B., Franks, A., and Simoes, E. (2007). Community-based participatory research: Necessary next steps. *Preventing Chronic Disease, 4,* 1–5. Available at: http://www.cdc.gov/pcd/issues/2007/jul/06_0182.htm. Accessed April 20, 2011.

Gilmore, G., Olsen, L., and Taub, A. (2001). *Competencies Update Project: Promoting quality assurance in health education.* Bethesda, MD: Bureau of Health Professions, Health Resources and Services Administration, USDHHS, No. 00-257(P).

Gilmore, G., Olsen, L., Taub, A., and Connell, D. (2005). Overview of the National Health Educator Competencies Update Project, 1998–2004. *Health Education and Behavior, 32,* 725–737. Co-published in the *American Journal of Health Education (2005), 36,* 363–370.

Hirsh, S., and Kummerow, J. (1997). *Lifetypes.* New York: Warner Books.

Institute of Medicine (IOM). (2001). *Health and behavior: The interplay of biological, behavioral, and social influences.* Washington, DC: National Academies Press.

Institute of Medicine (IOM). (2003). *Who will keep the public healthy? Educating public health professionals for the 21st century.* Washington, DC: National Academies Press.

International Union for Health Promotion and Education. (2009). Closing the gap in a generation: Health equity through action on the social determinants of health. *Global Health Promotion, Supplement 1,* 1–120.

Israel, B., Eng, E., Schulz, A., and Parker, E. (Eds.). (2005). *Methods in community-based participatory research for health.* San Francisco: Jossey-Bass.

Israel, B., Lichtenstein, R., Lantz, P., McGranaghan, R., Allen, A., Guzman, J., Softley, D., and Maciak, B. (2001). The Detroit Community Academic Urban Research Center: Development, implementation, and evaluation. *Journal of Public Health Management and Practice, 7,* 1–19.

Jarlstrom, M., and Valkealahti, K. (2010). Person–job fit related to psychological type of Finnish business students and managers: Implications for change in the management environment. *Journal of Psychological Type, 70,* 41–52.

Kretzmann, J., and McKnight, J. (1993). *Building communities from the inside out.* Chicago: ACTA Publications.

Lewis, I. (2009). Global partners: Addressing the social determinants of health through international development. *Global Health Promotion, Supplement 1,* 33–35.

Miller, R., Bedney, B., and Guenther-Grey, C. (2003). Assessing organizational capacity to deliver HIV prevention services collaboratively: Tales from the field. *Health Education and Behavior, 30,* 582–600.

National Commission for Health Education Credentialing (NCHEC), Society for Public Health Education (SOPHE), and American Association for Health Education (AAHE). (2010). *A competency-based framework for health education specialists—2010.* Allentown, PA: Authors.

Office of Disease Prevention and Health Promotion. (2001). *Healthy people in healthy communities: A community planning guide using Healthy People 2010.* Rockville, MD: Office of Public Health and Science, U.S. Public Health Service.

Oldenburg, B., Sallis, J., Harris, D., and Owen, N. (2002). Checklist of health promotion environments at worksites (CHEW): Development and measurement characteristics. *American Journal of Health Promotion, 16,* 288–299.

Parks, C., and Straker, H. (1996). Community assets mapping: Community health assessment with a different twist. *Journal of Health Education, 27,* 321–323.

Reynierse, J. (1995). A comparative analysis of Japanese and American management types through organizational levels in business and industry. *Journal of Psychological Type, 33,* 19–32.

Reynierse, J. (1991). The psychological types of outplaced executives. *Journal of Psychological Type, 25,* 11–23.

Roach, B. (1986). Organizational decision-makers: Different types for different levels. *Journal of Psychological Type, 12,* 16–24.

Satcher, D. (2010). Include a social determinants of health approach to reduce health inequities. *Public Health Reports, 125,* Supplement 4, 6–7.

Schulz, A., Krieger, J., and Galea, S. (2002). Addressing social determinants of health: Community-based participatory approaches to research and practice. *Health Education and Behavior, 29,* 287–295.

"Social Media, Texting Play New Role in Response to Disasters." (2011 May/June). *The Nation's Health, 41,* 1 and 18.

Taintor, Z. (2003). Addressing mental health needs. In Levy, B., and Sidel, V. (Eds.), *Terrorism and public health: A balanced approach to strengthening systems and protecting people* (pp. 49–68). New York: Oxford University Press.

World Health Organization (WHO). (2011). What are Millennium Development Goals? Available at: http://www.wpro.who.int/sites/mdg/home.htm. Accessed April 19, 2011.

Needs and Capacity Assessments Within the Bigger Picture

Introduction

Needs and capacity assessments for health education and health promotion do not stand alone. Rather, they are part of a bigger picture—namely, the development, implementation, and evaluation of health education strategies for health promotional purposes. This chapter reviews key contexts for the assessment strategies detailed in later chapters. These include the meanings of health as related to health promotion and health education; how needs and capacity assessments fit into program development; the roles of advisory groups, planning committees, and community coalitions; key data collection considerations; and needs prioritization.

The Context of Health, Health Promotion, and Health Education

The terms *health promotion* and *health education* encompass broad dimensions in addressing health, a term that also has a variety of definitions. The World Health Organization's (WHO) definition of *health* in 1948 moved us from a static, singular depiction of one's physical status into a more multidimensional perspective of "a state of complete physical, mental and social well-being—not merely the absence of disease, or infirmity" (U.S. Department of Health and Human Services [USDHHS], November 2000, p. 4; World Health Organization [WHO], 1985). In the past, that definition was critiqued by some as more of an ideal than a reality that could feasibly be obtained. In 1987, Noack offered a definition of health that was more process and systems oriented, and more of an operational definition of health: "a state of dynamic balance—or more appropriately as a process maintaining such a state—within any given subsystem, such as an organ, an individual, a social group, or a community" (p. 14). He added that health has two key dimensions: *health balance* (a dynamic equilibrium) and *health potential* (capacity for balance between person and environment), at the individual and community levels in both instances. Examples of health balance at the individual and community levels would be a relaxed state and a sense of family well-being in the community, respectively. Examples of health potential at the same levels would be nutritional status and the proportion of a health agency's budget aligned with health promotion activities, respectively.

Whereas the WHO preliminary perspective is considered to offer a broad definition of health, others have taken a more limited approach to the measurement of health in the United States by focusing on ill health in its severe manifestations as diagnosed through clinical tests (USDHHS, November 2000). As pointed out by the Centers for Disease Control and Prevention (CDC), other important aspects of individual or community health, such as disease-related dysfunction and disability, injuries, and other health problems, may be missed in taking such a measurement. The public health community currently views health status as a multidimensional construct, which includes "premature mortality and life expectancy, various symptoms and physiologic states, physical functions, emotional and cognitive functions, and perceptions about present and future health" (USDHHS, November 2000, p. 5). Taking such a perspective of health moves it into the realm of *quality of life*, which refers to "an overall sense of well-being, including aspects of happiness and satisfaction with life as a whole" (USDHHS, November 2000, p. 5). In addition to health, other domains are embodied within quality of life—for example, jobs, housing, schools, and one's neighborhood. Importantly, the WHO has stated through its Commission on Social Determinants of Health (CSDH) that it is essential to "reaffirm the central importance of health, the need for social and participatory action on health, and the core human value of equity in health" (Commission on Social Determinants of Health [CSDH], 2008, p. 34).

For this more inclusive perspective, a health-related quality of life (HRQOL) metric has been developed. It includes "those aspects of overall quality of life that can be clearly shown to affect health—either physical or mental" (USDHHS, November 2000, p. 6). Numerous reports have used this measurement approach to quantify HRQOL in a variety of public health issues (USDHHS, January 2001; May 2000; April 2000; Campbell, Crews, Moriarty, Zack, & Blackman, 1999; Hennessy, Moriarty, Zack, Scherr, & Brackbill, 1994).

Contributing to this broader approach, the Institute of Medicine's 2001 report *Health and Behavior: The Interplay of Biological, Behavioral, and Social Influences* views health from a perspective in which any health problems fall along a continuum based on the influence of various risk factors that can range from bio-behavioral (e.g., stress response, coping patterns), to behavioral (e.g., tobacco use, diet, physical activity), to social (e.g., positive relationship pathways, social networking, socioeconomic status) (Pellmar, Brandt, & Baird, 2002). Additionally, interactions among risk factors can influence health (Mokdad, Marks, Stroup, & Gerberding, 2004). These interactions become particularly apparent in the realm of socioeconomic factors. For instance, among the socioeconomically advantaged, lower mortality, morbidity, and disability rates have been observed over time. Individuals who are poor are more likely to engage in risk-related behaviors and are less likely to engage in health-promotional behaviors (Pellmar et al., 2002). As has been pointed out by Green (1999), "a balanced portfolio of factors under greater control of individuals and more distal risk conditions controlled by others, as determinants of health, is needed to correct the poor penetration by health programs in poor and marginalized populations" (p. 81). Key reports and frameworks for the twenty-first century are being grounded in the more comprehensive approach to health impacts offered by our better understanding of the determinants of health (Mokdad et al., 2004; Committee on Assuring the Health of the Public in the 21st Century, 2003; Gebbie, Rosenstock, & Hernandez, 2003). Gebbie and colleagues (2003) have emphasized that practitioners "must be aware of not only the biological risk factors affecting health; they must also understand the environmental, social, and behavioral contexts within which individuals and populations operate in order to identify factors that may hinder or promote the success of their interventions" (p. 34).

As emphasized by Cromley and McLafferty (2002), an essential consideration for our understanding of health is the person within an environmental context who is "connected to natural, social, and economic processes that operate on the local, regional, and global scales" (p. 2). They note that not all factors affecting our state of health are under our control because "how people behave contributes to their health status, but we cannot divorce behavior from the environmental and social contexts in which it occurs" (p. 2).

The Committee on Assuring the Health of the Public in the 21st Century (2003), in reviewing the major trends influencing the health of the United States, cited three in particular (pp. 34–41):

1. Population growth and demographic change, with the "population growing larger, older, and more racially and ethnically diverse, with a higher incidence of chronic disease"
2. Technical and scientific advances, which "create new channels for information and communication, as well as novel ways of preventing and treating disease"
3. Globalization and health, to include the "geopolitical and economic challenge of globalization, including international terrorism"

These contexts are viewed as both opportunities and threats.

Clearly, defining *health* involves numerous dimensions that are not easily quantifiable. This complexity heightens even further as we advance into a more specific review into the contexts of health promotion and health education. *Health promotion* can be viewed as a collective effort in health enhancement. The process has been defined by the Joint Committee on Health Education and Promotion Terminology as "any planned combination of educational, political, environmental, regulatory, or organizational mechanisms that supports actions and conditions of living conducive to the health of individuals, groups, and communities" (2001, p. 101). This definition expands upon the definition offered by Green and Kreuter (1999) by including the environmental dimension. Importantly, Breslow (1999) refers to *health promotion* as a "more recent and elusive concept that has appeared prominently in the health lexicon only during the latter part of the 20th century" (p. 1030). He differentiates health promotion from disease prevention in that the former "means facilitating at least the maintenance of a person's current position on the continuum (degree of health) and, ideally, advancing toward its positive end (health). Disease prevention, on the other hand, means avoiding specific diseases that carry one toward the negative end (infirmity)" (p. 1032). Additionally, he calls for not only a maintenance of balance in one's life, but also attempts to maximize one's enjoyment potential. From a more global perspective, *health promotion* was defined by the WHO's Working Group on Concepts and Principles of Health Promotion (1987, p. 654) as the process of enabling people to increase control over, and to improve, their health. This promotional perspective is derived from a conception of health as the extent to which an individual or group is able to realize aspirations and satisfy needs, and to change or cope with the environment. Health in this context is seen as a "resource of everyday life, not the objective of living; it is a positive concept emphasizing social and personal resources as well as physical capacities" (p. 654). The Working Group on Concepts and Principles (1987, p. 654) identified the following basic characteristics of health promotion:

1. Enabling people to take control over, and responsibility for, their health as an important component of everyday life—both as spontaneous and as organized action for health
2. Requiring the close cooperation of sectors beyond the health services, reflecting the diversity of conditions that influence health
3. Combining diverse, but complementary, methods or approaches, including communication, education, legislation, fiscal measures, organizational changes, community development, and spontaneous local activities against health hazards
4. Encouraging effective and concrete public participation encompassing the development of individual and collective problem-solving and decision-making skills, and involving health professionals in education and health advocacy, particularly those in primary care

In attempting to achieve these aspects of health promotion, recommendations were advanced that focused on equitable health policies, work and home environments conducive to health, establishment of social networks, social support, coping strategies, and health-related lifestyles. Additionally, there was a call for increases in knowledge as drawn from epidemiology, social, and other sciences. With this as background, the Working Group on Concepts and

Principles (1987, p. 657) cited a series of selected considerations for prioritiz-ing health promotion policy development:

- Indicators of health and their population distributions
- Current population knowledge, skills, and health practices
- Current policies in government and other sectors
- Expected impact on health
- Economic constraints and benefits
- Social and cultural acceptability
- Political feasibility

Realistically, to address the health-related focus, properly supported popula-tion health approaches that incorporate health care and public health systems working together need to be in place (Nash, Reifsnyder, Fabius, & Pracilio, 2011; Hemenway, 2010). As an inherent part of this process, health outcomes need to be measured over time (Maki, Qualls, White, Kleefield, & Crone, 2008). In reviewing health promotion in a community context, Green and Raeburn (1990) refer to its major purpose being the "increasing transfer of control of impor-tant resources in health, notably knowledge, skills, authority, and money, to the community" (p. 37). They expand on this perspective by calling for an enabling approach in which the people of a community establish their own activities for improved health in accordance with their understanding of needs. In addition to the potential health benefits for the community using this self-help approach, there are the benefits of an increased sense of social support from peers and a sense of control in their own lives. Pellmar and colleagues (2002) refer to several lessons learned from community intervention experiences as including the importance of the community itself in defining needs and priorities, rather than an outside organizer, and the need for community diagnosis and assessment to be conducted in an ongoing manner. Health education is an educational context within health promotion. Although numerous definitions of health education exist, much of what is practiced relates to the blending of two widely recognized definitions. The Joint Committee on Health Education and Promotion Terminology (2001) defines *health education* as "any combination of planned learning experiences based on sound theories that provide individuals, groups, and communities the opportunity to acquire information and the skills needed to make quality health decisions" (p. 99). Notably, the theoretical basis for the learning, coupled with information and skills acquisition for health-related decision making, repre-sent key ingredients. Green and Kreuter (2005) define *health education* as "any planned combination of learning experiences designed to predispose, enable, and reinforce voluntary behavior conducive to health in individuals, groups, or communities" (p. G4). In doing so, they incorporate the three key factors hav-ing the potential to influence voluntary health behavior: predisposing factors, as "any characteristic of a person or population that motivates behavior prior to the occurrence of the behavior;" enabling factors, as "Any characteristic of the environment that facilitates action and any skill or resource required to attain a specific behavior;" and reinforcing factors, as "Any reward or punishment following or anticipated as a consequence of a behavior, serving to strengthen the motivation for the behavior after it occurs" (pp. G3–G7). A blending of these seminal definitions can best guide the health educator's efforts. The view of the health educator as planning educational experiences guided by theory that voluntarily foster health enhancement is a key grounding point in this book.

How Needs and Capacity Assessments Fit into Program Planning

Many distinctive approaches to health education planning are utilized, usually focusing on many or all of the generic phases of assessing needs, stating the issues or problems to be addressed, developing goals and objectives, reviewing resources (capacities) and barriers, determining methods, implementing, and evaluating. A specific example includes the PRECEDE-PROCEED approach (Green & Kreuter, 2005), which emphasizes problem-aligned deductive diagnoses. The process comprises the phases depicted in **Figure 2-1**.

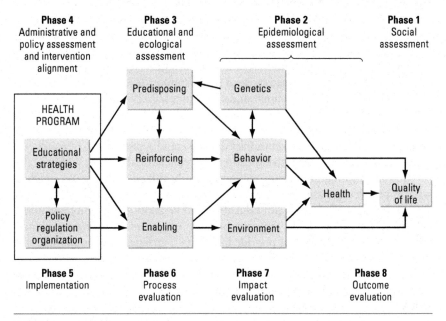

FIGURE 2-1

This generic representation of the PRECEDE-PROCEED model for health program planning and evaluation shows the main lines of causation, from program inputs and determinants of health to outcomes by the direction of arrows. It shows the opposite sequence of analysis in planning and development for implementation and evaluation in the first four phases. This rendition of the model does not show the feedback processes inherent in the systems theory or the specific social science theories underlying the model.

Source: Green, L., and Kreuter, M. (2005). *Health program planning: An educational and ecological approach,* 4th ed. Boston: McGraw-Hill. © The McGraw-Hill Companies.

PRECEDE is an acronym for Predisposing, Reinforcing, and Enabling Constructs in Educational/ecological Diagnosis and Evaluation, with the goal of assuring comprehensive assessment and planning phases. Working in tandem with these phases is the PROCEED approach, which is an acronym for Policy, Regulatory, and Organizational Constructs in Educational and Environmental Development; here the goal is to address the implementation and evaluation components of health education and health promotion endeavors. As Green and Kreuter (2005) have pointed out, "As one turns the corner from PRECEDE to PROCEED in Phase 5 and moves into implementation, the principal evaluation task is one of *using* the information gained from monitoring those indicators to make program adjustments and to inform stakeholders of program progress" (p. 16, 190–254). Needs and capacity assessments are particularly aligned with the PRECEDE portion of the model (Green & Kreuter, 2005, pp. 7–23, 29–60, 147–178). Phases 1–4 of PRECEDE address individual and group needs through the social, epidemiological, behavioral, environmental, educational, and ecological needs assessments. Helpful examples of the types of outputs from the assessments conducted in Phases 1 and 2 of the model are depicted in **Figure 2-2**. Phase 5 addresses the administrative and policy assessments related to organizational and community capacity (e.g., the resources and policies in place).

Given the wide acceptance of the PRECEDE-PROCEED model for health promotion planning, we believe there is value for the professional to give strong consideration to its utility in program development. Green and Kreuter (1999; 2005) emphasize that it is not to be considered the only approach for health promotional efforts, but it does appropriately address both health promotion and health education through a comprehensive planning approach. The model is one of the more complete planning approaches because of this comprehensive focus.

Their fourth edition (2005) merges the epidemiological, behavioral, and environmental assessment phases (to include genetics) into one phase. Realizing that individuals become engaged with the model at different phases of their professional activities, an algorithm is provided to recognize their previous project endeavors as they connect with different points in the model. Green and Kreuter are moving in this direction to enable professionals to focus on those phases that will have value to them depending on the project stage in which they are currently engaged. To their credit, Green and Kreuter's revision is based to a large extent on the continuing feedback they seek from the field to assure that their model remains practical and up-to-date. Current information and endnote updates regarding the PRECEDE-PROCEED model can be accessed through their Web site (http://www.lgreen.net). Another helpful planning perspective offered as an outgrowth of the national health initiative, *Healthy People 2010: Healthy People in Healthy Communities*, is entitled MAP-IT (USDHHS, February 2001). This easy-to-use format is aligned with the two major goals of (1) increasing the quality of years of healthy life

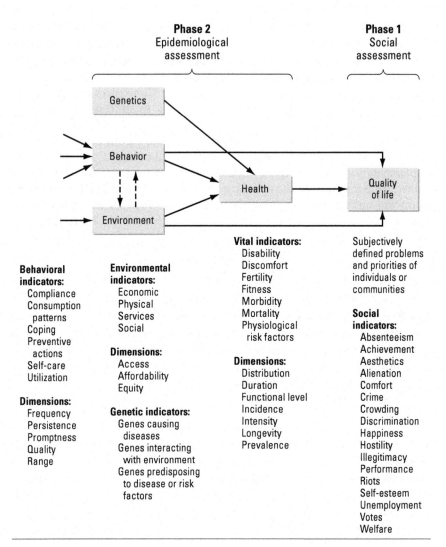

Phase 2
Epidemiological
assessment

Phase 1
Social
assessment

Behavioral indicators:
Compliance
Consumption patterns
Coping
Preventive actions
Self-care
Utilization

Dimensions:
Frequency
Persistence
Promptness
Quality
Range

Environmental indicators:
Economic
Physical
Services
Social

Dimensions:
Access
Affordability
Equity

Genetic indicators:
Genes causing diseases
Genes interacting with environment
Genes predisposing to disease or risk factors

Vital indicators:
Disability
Discomfort
Fertility
Fitness
Morbidity
Mortality
Physiological risk factors

Dimensions:
Distribution
Duration
Functional level
Incidence
Intensity
Longevity
Prevalence

Subjectively defined problems and priorities of individuals or communities

Social indicators:
Absenteeism
Achievement
Aesthetics
Alienation
Comfort
Crime
Crowding
Discrimination
Happiness
Hostility
Illegitimacy
Performance
Riots
Self-esteem
Unemployment
Votes
Welfare

FIGURE 2-2
This more detailed representation of the output model suggests relationships, indicators, and dimensions of factors that might be identified in phases 1 and 2 of the PRECEDE assessment process or evaluated as outcomes in PROCEED phases 6, 7, and 8.
Source: Green, L., and Kreuter, M. (2005). *Health program planning: An educational and ecological approach,* 4th ed. Boston: McGraw-Hill. © The McGraw-Hill Companies.

and (2) eliminating health disparities. Whereas *healthy life* refers to both qualitative and quantitative dimensions, as described earlier in Chapter 1 (USDHHS, January 2000), *health disparities* is defined as the "differences in the burden and impact of disease among different populations, defined, for example, by sex, race or ethnicity, education or income, disability, place of residence, or sexual orientation" (USDHHS, 2003, p. A3). Coupled with the two overarching goals are 10 priorities (10 Leading Health Indicators): physical activity; overweight and obesity; tobacco use; substance abuse; responsible sexual behavior; mental health; injury and violence; environmental quality; immunization; and access to health care. Within the context of these key elements in the national framework for health enhancement, the MAP-IT model (USDHHS, February 2001, p. 7) provides the following actions:

- Mobilize individuals and organizations that care about the health of your community into a coalition
- Assess the areas of greatest need in your community as well as the resources and other strengths that you can tap into to address those areas
- Plan your approach—start with a vision of where you want to be as a community, and then add strategies and action steps to help you achieve that vision
- Implement your plan using concrete action steps that can be monitored and will make a difference
- Track your progress over time

Mobilizing refers to the development of a community coalition, as appropriate, by bringing together committed individuals and organizations gathered around a vision of how the coalition would like the community to be.

Assessing refers to the process of determining the health issues of greatest importance in the community and ascertaining the available strengths and resources. Both primary and secondary data should be compiled into baseline information prior to the initiation of any action or program.

Planning includes the development of objectives that have specific targets for change (criteria) in comparison to the baseline data; action steps, which are concrete actions in alignment with the objectives; assigned responsibilities to facilitate the action plan; and a proposed time line. Implementing involves taking the concrete actions specified in the action plan, along with monitoring the events as they transpire.

Tracking entails a two-part evaluation phase that includes progress reviews and the assurance of continuing support. As a part of this phase, the recommendation is made to celebrate small successes en route to the larger goal (overall direction). Within the context of planning for worksite health promotion, Bensky and Hietbrink (1994) have suggested starting with an STP team, which focuses on the current Situation, the Target outcome for health promotional activity, and the proposed Plan. This team is then guided by considerations of issues that influence the decisions to be made, information that will clarify any assumptions about the issues, interpretation of what the information means, implications about how the program will be affected if the interpretation is accurate, and initiative regarding which actions to take.

Bensky and Hietbrink's (1994) rather straightforward planning framework addresses the following points: (1) assessment of the situation from a who, what, when, where, and why perspective (this incorporates a *SWOT* analysis, which reviews any current program's Strengths and Weaknesses as well as Opportunities and Threats to programming in the next year); (2) setting the goals; (3) developing appropriate strategies; and (4) writing a plan that can achieve buy-in by those most directly affected by the initiative.

There is no shortage of quality planning approaches available with which to expand on traditional and nontraditional planning models. The reader is encouraged to review texts that take a more health promotional perspective (i.e., overall health enhancement), such as McKenzie, Neiger, and Thackeray (2009) and Timmreck (2003). The generic planning model described by McKenzie and colleagues (2009) can be a helpful starting point for the practitioner. This more traditional approach to planning offers the following components:

- Assessing *needs*
- Setting *goals* and objectives
- Developing an *intervention*
- *Implementing* the intervention
- *Evaluating* the results

Overall, in developing the objectives four elements need to be addressed in terms of "*who* will attain *how much* of *what* by *when?*" (Green & Kreuter, 2005, p. 100). Additionally, it is recommended to develop *SMART* objectives—those that are Specific, Measurable, Achievable, Realistic, and Time related (Centers for Disease Control and Prevention [CDC], 2003).

Initially, it will be helpful to the practitioner to track these procedures by using the highlighted entities as prompts while health education and health promotion strategies are being developed. Other aspects of planning, such as assessing the capacity of an organization or community to support change, eventually will need to be taken into consideration as well. Readers who have aligned themselves successfully with a particular health education planning process are advised to continue with that approach. The needs and capacity assessment strategies described in this book will provide a starting point for issue and resource identification for a wide array of planning models.

Capacity-Focused Assessments

As pointed out earlier, capacity assessments can be included in other planning models under different names (e.g., the Administrative and Policy assessment in the PRECEDE-PROCEED model). Capacity assessments can be conducted at the organizational and community-based levels to assess actual and potential resources, policies, and support entities that will fortify and sustain project and program endeavors. As pointed out by Bartholomew, Parcel, Kok, and Gottlieb (2001), at the outset of program planning, assessing community-based competencies and resources focuses attention on the importance of capacity enhancement during the development and implementation phases of planning.

Along these lines, Kretzmann and McKnight (1993) pioneered capacity-focused, or asset-based, approaches to community planning. The driving force behind this approach initially was the focus on rebuilding troubled communities by undertaking asset-based community development, rather than by focusing on the needs, deficiencies, and problems of a community. The latter approach is believed to foster client neighborhoods in which there is little or no empowerment for the residents due to reliance on outside experts; fragmented attempts at solutions that focus on isolated clients rather than the community as a whole; funding that is basically directed toward service providers; and, consequently, a deepening sense of dependence and hopelessness among the residents. As an alternative, capacity-focused community development seeks to build on the "capacities, skills, and assets of lower income people and their neighborhoods" (Kretzmann & McKnight, 1993, p. 5). The assets are established based on the assessment of contributions that can be made by individuals, citizens' associations (e.g., churches, cultural groups), and local institutions (e.g., businesses, schools, libraries, health care facilities). This approach is designed to foster an internal focus for problem solving and relationship building that emphasizes "the primacy of local definition, investment, creativity, hope and control" (Kretzmann & McKnight, 1993, p. 9).

The primary capacity-focused assessment process advanced by Kretzmann and McKnight (1993), known as the *Capacity Inventory*, comprises four parts seeking the following information: skills learned at home, in the community, or in the workplace; experience in community activities and future participation possibilities; business interests and experiences; and personal information. For the most part, this assessment has been implemented as a face-to-face interview, but it can also be modified for use as a survey instrument that individuals complete on their own. The Capacity Inventory is designed to assess how a particular individual can contribute to the community development process. An array of helpful Capacity Inventory examples are provided in workbooks by Kretzmann, McKnight, and Puntenney (1998); Kretzmann, McKnight, and Sheehan (1997); and Dewar (1997).

Using today's technology, the results of such capacity and needs assessments can be plotted using printed maps as well as geographic information systems (GIS), which are computer-based systems for integrating and analyzing geographic information, thereby enabling spatial relationships between objects to be displayed (e.g., concentrations of certain community-based services in selected census tracks). The convenience and timeliness of a GIS approach facilitates the development of "databases of health events located on the earth's surface that can be processed and stored by computers, keeping track of changes by adding and deleting events from those databases, and editing the location and public health attributes of these events" (Cromley & McLafferty, 2002, p. 19).

Because of the influence of environmental factors on health, GIS tracking will have increasing value in health-related assessments. As pointed out by Cromley and McLafferty (2002, p. 2):

> [The] environment is connected to natural, social, and economic processes that operate on the local, regional, and global scales. How people behave contributes to their health status, but we cannot divorce behavior from the environmental and social contexts in which it occurs. Not all of the factors that affect our well-being are under the immediate direct control of the individual. The environment of the person is one starting point for public health GIS.

The use of a capacity-based approach to assessment and information plotting aligns with the focus on the empowerment of the community to be involved in actions for improvement. This view of empowerment has been defined by Wallerstein (1992) as "a social-action process that promotes participation of people, organizations, and communities towards the goals of increased individual and community control, political efficacy, improved quality of community life, and social justice" (p. 198). From this perspective, community empowerment could potentially address the effects of powerlessness (lack of control, which is considered to be a broad risk factor for disease).

These perspectives serve to expand one's understanding of health issues and potential directions for health enhancement. As summarized by Robertson and Minkler (1994), prominent features of such a perspective include the following (p. 296):

1. Broadening the definition of health and its determination to include the social and economic context within which health—or, more precisely, nonhealth—is produced
2. Going beyond the earlier emphasis on individual lifestyle strategies to apply health to broader social and political strategies
3. Embracing the concept of empowerment—individual and collective—as a key health promotion strategy (also see Wallerstein, 1992)
4. Advocating the participation of the community in identifying health problems and strategies for addressing those problems

Within this context, Robertson and Minkler (1994) caution that communities are not homogeneous; many diverse areas of interest may exist. It is possible that conflict, rather than consensus, can be generated when using a community-driven process, where "communities may assess social problems and propose solutions that reflect racism, sexism, ageism, or other problematic and divisive approaches" (p. 307).

With these cautions and considerations in mind, we view the capacity-focused approach to resource, policy, and support entity assessment as complementing needs assessment activities and as aligning with the planning models described previously.

Health Impact Assessments

On an international basis, *health impact assessment (HIA)* is defined as "an approach that aims to support public policies by providing more information on the potential health consequences of decisions that government authorities are about to make" (National Collaborating Centre for Healthy Public Policy [NCCHPP], 2008, p. 4). It is quite similar to the environmental impact assessments that are required when environmental changes are projected. Standard procedures have been developed for HIA in Europe, Canada, and other nations for guidance purposes.

As has been emphasized by Cohen (2010), HIA aligns with community-based primary prevention efforts within the context of health; that is, "to include the promotion of equity; physical, mental, and social well-being; and the prevention of illness, injury, and violence." He continues (2010, p. 1) that the:

> ... primary prevention approach—calling for comprehensive community level changes—aligns perfectly with HIA which seeks to document the potential health impacts of a project or policy *before* it is carried out. HIA's dual emphasis on community participation and community outcomes makes this tool a significant contributor in advancing primary prevention and equity.

Cohen further details a major strength of HIA, which is that, for the most part, it addresses issues that are not medically related, but that nonetheless have health-related impacts.

Key examples of the foundation for HIA in Canada have been provided in the provinces of British Columbia (1993) and Quebec (2001) through its Public Health Act. However, some cautions have been issued not to have HIA become solely aligned with public health, thus limiting its intent and effectiveness (NCCHPP, 2008). Needs and capacity assessments go to the heart of the HIA process, as demonstrated by several key initiatives at the local level in Canada.

As just one example, in Nova Scotia, using support from Health Canada to review the potential effects of decentralized health services in that province's eastern health region, communities identified those factors influencing their health. In this example, findings from the overall adult education and community development approach included: (1) change related to the determinants of health (aligned with decentralized health services) needed to not only involve individuals and groups but also systems; (2) resource needs (to include time and financing) had to be an inherent part of the process of planning and change; and (3) citizens needed to be participants in the decision-making process (NCCHPP, 2008).

Logic Models

Another planning approach in which both needs and capacity assessments are undertaken is through the application of the logic model. The *logic model approach* (also termed the *model of change* or *causal chain approach*) to program planning enables the professional to link program inputs and activities to program outcomes. The process also can be of value in generating planner and stakeholder buy-in through a concise review of how the program design will make a difference for program participants and the overall community (Harvard Family Research Project, 2002). **Figure** 2-3 depicts basic logic model considerations (MacDonald, Starr, Schooley, Yee, Klimowski, & Turner, 2001).

Usually initiated following the assessment of needs, the inputs phase encompasses the assessment of capacity, which can include direct and in-kind funding, staffing, partner organizations, equipment, and materials. Activities are the events that take place as a part of the program, such as developing a media plan and forming coalitions. Outputs are the direct products of the activities of the program, such as a written plan for a population-specific media plan and quantification of the actions taken (e.g., the number of smokers enrolled in a cessation program). Outcomes refer to the intended program effects (expected changes). Short-term outcomes entail the immediate effects on the target audience, usually in terms of knowledge, attitudes, and skills (e.g., a more positive attitude toward smoke-free policies among business owners). Intermediate outcomes refer primarily to behavior and policy changes (e.g., an increase in the percentage of adults who implement household smoking restrictions, and the adoption of clean indoor-air policies). Long-term outcomes are changes that occur over much longer periods of time, such as years (e.g., decreases in the prevalence of tobacco use, and reduced tobacco-related morbidity and mortality among the target populations). Logic model development moves from right to left. A detailed example of a smoking cessation promotion effort for youth and adults is presented in **Figure 2-4.**

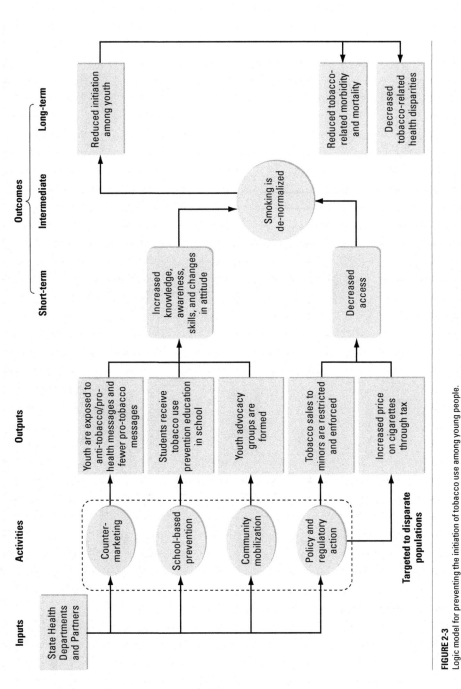

FIGURE 2-3

Logic model for preventing the initiation of tobacco use among young people.

Source: Macdonald, G., Starr, G., Schooley, M., Yee, S., Klimowski, K., and Turner, K. (2001). *Introduction to Program Evaluation for Comprehensive Tobacco Control Programs.* Atlanta: Centers for Disease Control and Prevention, Office on Smoking and Health.

33

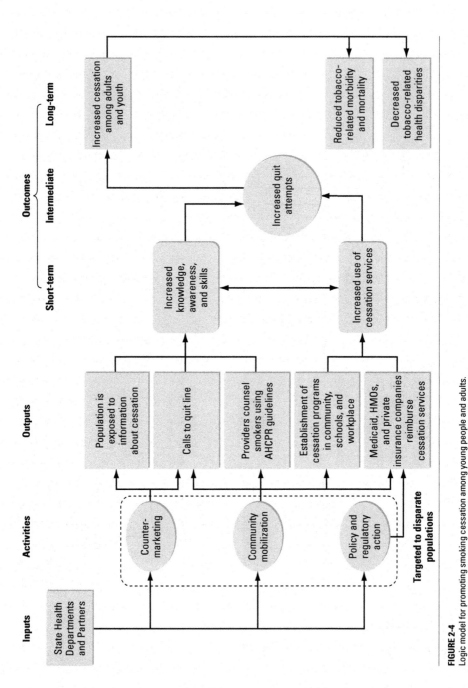

FIGURE 2-4

Logic model for promoting smoking cessation among young people and adults.

Source: Macdonald, G., Starr, G., Schooley, M., Yee, S., Klimowski, K., and Turner, K. (2001). *Introduction to Program Evaluation for Comprehensive Tobacco Control Programs.* Atlanta: Centers for Disease Control and Prevention, Office on Smoking and Health.

Advisory and Planning Committees

One very helpful method to develop a clearer and more comprehensive planning approach is to establish a committee. Two types of committees can be organized: advisory and planning committees. An advisory committee usually consists of individuals who are in a position to periodically report on their actual experiences related to some common issue. Members of this committee are then able to offer their advice to a key individual who is bringing them together, or to another group that will be making programmatic decisions. A planning committee may be made up of advisory committee members, experts, and agency staff. Its lifespan may be episodic (with limited duration) or continuing (ongoing). In some instances, advisory committees have been transformed into planning committees, with the addition of key people, so that a particular program can be developed.

Both types of committees usually share one common denominator: They are task oriented. In addition, both types of committees are important to the long-term assessment processes. They enable firsthand insights and experiences to be offered, they encourage brainstorming, and, particularly in the planning committee process, their members can make an early commitment to undertake key program planning responsibilities at appropriate times. In addressing community involvement through the elements of community-based participatory research (CBPR), McKenzie and colleagues (2009) have cited a helpful series of at least four factors that come into play: "(1) community empowerment (i.e., community members control decision making); (2) collaboration; (3) acquisition of knowledge through hands-on participation; and (4) a focus on social change" (p. 101).

One can find many examples of advisory and planning groups that have a needs and capacity assessment responsibility. For instance, in the city of Penrith, Australia, a 10-year project focusing on improving a community's food system so as to enhance overall nutrition status is guided by a Food Policy Committee. The committee consists of city councilors as well as representatives from public health and agricultural departments, health-related university departments, food processing and grocery retailers, banks, and the chamber of commerce, among others. The committee operates with a rather high degree of formality guided by a multiyear strategic plan. Included in the committee's numerous responsibilities are the assessment of needs, capacities, opportunities, and relationship development for the furtherance of improved nutritional practices. It has not been an easy task for either the committee or other partners in the project. As Webb, Hawe, and Noort (2001) point out, "the challenge remains to document the impact of the project on the local food system and on the capacity of community organizations to reform and implement food policies consistent with improved nutrition" (p. 317). Importantly, this type of committee structure has fostered the institutionalization of the project into the activities of local government.

As another example, a Community Advisory Board was established as part of a community-wide campaign to reduce the cigarette-smoking levels in a predominantly African American community in Richmond, California (Hunkeler, Davis, McNeil, Powell, & Polen, 1990). The effort was based on the assumption that "changing the health norms and beliefs of an entire community will change the health habits of individuals" (p. 278). The 30-member board met monthly for 3 years, advising the campaign workers on almost every aspect of the project. Of interest, rather than setting up ongoing task forces, board members chose instead to establish small working groups with specific assignments addressed through one or two meetings. Organizers believed that the incorporation of the Community Advisory Board legitimized the effort and assured community ownership.

Community-Based Coalitions

On a larger planning scale, community coalitions can be formed as interorganizational and cooperative groups that establish formal, multipurpose, and long-term alliances (Butterfoss, Goodman, & Wandersman, 1993). The following characteristics more fully describe the uniqueness of coalitions and their purposes:

1. Coalitions enable organizations to become involved in new and broader issues without assuming the sole responsibility for managing or developing those issues.
2. Coalitions can demonstrate and develop widespread public support for issues, actions, or unmet needs.
3. Coalitions can maximize the power of individuals and groups through joint action.
4. Coalitions can minimize the duplication of effort and services.
5. Coalitions can help mobilize more talents, resources, and approaches to influence an issue than any single organization could achieve alone.
6. Coalitions can provide an avenue for recruiting participants from diverse constituencies, such as political, business, human service, social, and religious groups, as well as less organized grassroots groups and individuals.
7. The flexible nature of coalitions allows them to exploit new resources in changing situations (Butterfoss et al., 1993, p. 315).

Florin, Mitchell, and Stevenson (1993) detail seven stages of coalition development:

1. Initial mobilization, which involves participant recruitment and community constituency engagement
2. Establishing an organizational structure for the working group

3. Building a capacity for action, which involves member skills development and networking
4. Planning for action, which includes the assessment of perceived needs of community constituencies, goal and objective setting, and planning intervention strategies
5. Implementing activities based on a sequential work plan
6. Refining the program based upon evaluation data
7. Institutionalizing the membership process and organizational buy-in

These authors have described the activities of 35 community coalitions that were organized to address alcohol and other drug abuse prevention, particularly from the perspective of their training and technical assistance needs. Among the various needs assessments employed by the coalitions, they noted the use of surveys, focus groups, and town meetings. Plans of action were developed from the assessment data. The relationship between the assessments and the resulting plans could not be evaluated, however, because insufficient information regarding the needs assessment processes was provided in the plans. Overall, the coalition process facilitates collaborative efforts in addressing health-related issues in the community. Due to the usual large-scale nature of a coalition, as well as the ability of organizations to freely enter or leave the structure, considerable effort needs to be directed toward the establishment of committed leadership and interorganizational communication (Bracht & Gleason, 1990). As emphasized by Rooney and Thompson (2009), there needs to be a sense of ownership by the members, and that becomes stronger with community-based representation "since most community members understand how a health concern affects their neighbors, schools, coworkers, and the community" (p. 403).

Key Informant Insights

Additional insights can be gained from contact with individuals, or key informants, who are able to express their perceptions of the needs of others. Such individuals can include community leaders, health and human service professionals, leaders of religious organizations, public officials, educators, and the like. Oftentimes, the information and insights provided by these sources can help to frame key areas of need, which then can be followed up through more definitive needs assessment strategies.

Such a process was employed by the author in his needs and capacity assessment work in Dubna, Russia (Gilmore & Hartigan, 1998). Key questions were developed for use during each interview session with health and human service professionals in that city. The overall focus of the assessment and questions had to do with key health-related risk and protective factors affecting the public in Dubna. The key informant information provided a basis for more involved follow-up assessments (e.g., questionnaire, group interviews), eventually leading to a citywide program development and evaluation. The key informant information assisted the project staff in properly delimiting the objectives and educational methods eventually employed.

Bond and colleagues (2001), as part of their Gateway Project, incorporated several data-gathering approaches in their mental health promotion capacity assessments in secondary schools, including key informant interviews. The key informants were individuals who held various coordinating positions in the intervention schools, such as assistant principals, curriculum coordinators, and student welfare coordinators. The resulting key informant insights were then combined with other sources of information, such as field notes, surveys, background audits, and student and teacher assessments. Bond et al.'s report specifies how this multiyear project has resulted in system-level changes (e.g., through networks of support and school-based health enhancement teams) based on their capacity-building endeavors.

The process of interviewing key informants is discussed further in Chapter 5, including a key informant approach with a Native American population in South Dakota involving the efforts of a public health team (Gilmore, Kies, McIlquham, Nogle, Whitty, & Xie, 2010). Several preliminary considerations must be taken into account when preparing to collect data, particularly through a key informant approach, due to it usually being one of the very first information-gathering procedures. First, it is important to state (in writing) the purpose of the assessment (this usually will lead to the development of assessment objectives). The following operational framework (see **Figure 2-5**) developed by the author is one way to ensure that the information gathering is in alignment with the stated and agreed upon purpose and that all appropriate sources of information are considered during the planning stages.

Note that in addition to in-person interviews with leaders and family representatives, the verification phase (final column) includes cross-checking the information with other teams, going back to discuss information summaries with previous respondents, and the use of evidence such as artifacts and observational cues. Helpful insights in going through the visual processes are offered by Angrosino (2007) and Banks (2007).

Another important consideration during the planning phase for key informant interviews and beyond has to do with the type of relationship with others that will be established. Rowitz (2006) has depicted the matrix of strategies for relationship building as conceived by Himmelman (2002), as presented in **Table 2-1**.

The increased degree of connectivity and commitment among those who will be involved in the assessment and follow-up processes is depicted in the table as one reviews each column to the right. From the outset, it is important for all parties to understand the degree of investment and commitment

| Health Indices/Impactors | Additional Information Needed | | Sources | | Verification |
	Needs	Capacity			(across teams, respondent validation, and evidence)
Education					
Village	Challenges	Opportunities	Leaders	Families	
Neighborhoods		Support provided	Leaders		
Employment		Do they exist?	Leaders		
Worker influx	Challenges	Opportunities	Leaders	Families	
Family units:	Challenges	Opportunities	Leaders	Families	
• Gender		Support provided		Families	
• Ages					
• Culture					
Vital Statistics					
Mortality	Challenges				
Natality					
Morbidity					
Natural Environment					
Water availability/quality	Challenges	Opportunities			
Land contaminants					
Air contaminants					
Weather patterns					

(continues)

FIGURE 2-5
Community-based operational assessment framework.

39

Health Indices/Impactors	Additional Information Needed		Sources		Verification (across teams, respondent validation, and evidence)
	Needs	Capacity			
Built Environment Housing Home setting Transportation Energy • Availability • Consistency of electricity Recreational facilities Other physical structures Safety issues	Challenges	Opportunities			
Education Ministry of Education Grade levels: • Elementary • High school • College Literacy levels Parents' education Community education	Challenges	Opportunities	Leaders	Families	
Diseases Infectious (communicable) Chronic	Challenges			Ministry of Health/local health department/local health professionals	

	Challenges	Opportunities	Leaders	Families Ministry of Health/local health department/local health professionals
Lifestyle Nutrition Physical Activity Tobacco use Drug and Alcohol use Faith-based actions				
Resources (capacity and assets) Official organizations Non-governmental organizations Medical care/public health: • Ministry of Health • Regional medical care • District public health clinic • Village clinic • Other (e.g., local healers) Village schools Higher level education Telecommunications Financial contributions Consumer purchases • Food purchases • Food security • Area commerce		Opportunities	All sources	

FIGURE 2-5
Continued

41

TABLE 2-1
Matrix of Strategies for Working Together

	Networking	Coordinating	Cooperating	Collaborating
Definition	Exchanging information for mutual benefit	Exchanging information for mutual benefit, and altering activities to achieve a common purpose	Exchanging information for mutual benefit, and altering activities to achieve a common purpose	Exchanging information for mutual benefit, altering activities, and sharing resources to achieve a common purpose
Relationship Characteristics	Informal	Formal	Formal	Formal
	Minimal time commitments, limited levels of trust, and no necessity to share turf; information exchange is the primary focus	Moderate time commitments, moderate levels of trust, and no necessity to share turf; making access to services or resources more user-friendly is the primary focus	Substantial time commitments, high levels of trust, and significant access to each other's turf; sharing of resources to achieve a common purpose is the primary focus	Extensive time commitments, very high levels of trust and extensive areas of common turf; enhancing each other's capacity to achieve a common purpose is the primary focus
Resources	No mutual sharing of resources necessary	No or minimal mutual sharing of resources necessary	Moderate to extensive mutual sharing of resources and some sharing of risks, responsibilities, and rewards	Full sharing of resources, and full sharing of risks, responsibilities, and rewards

Source: Rowitz, L. (2006). Based on a relationship model conceived by Himmelman (2002). Used with permission.

to the overall project. For example, this type of understanding needs to be established by coalition members their constituents, and the resource people who are brought into the process of relationship development.

Secondary Information

As practitioners, we gain insights from a variety of sources. In Chapter 1, we referred to insights as being derived from experience and intuition— understandings that have arisen through our collective professional involvement in health-related matters, rather than as specific results of preplanned assessments. These insights are important in our work and form a backdrop against which we can analyze the findings of our intentional assessment efforts. In a more structured fashion, additional background and supplemental information can be garnered through a review of secondary information, which offers social and health indicators for inferential purposes.

Important insights can be derived from analyzing raw data and published data summaries. These data are termed *secondary information sources* because the analyst did not collect and compile the original data. Sources of these data compilations include libraries, reports of experts and authorities, agency and organizational reports, and commercial information services. Compiled health-related information abounds, as exemplified by reports from the U.S. Census, *Morbidity and Mortality Weekly Report* (MMWR) from the Massachusetts Medical Society, and the *Monthly Vital Statistics Report* (MVSR) from the National Center for Health Statistics (NCHS) at the Centers for Disease Control and Prevention (CDC).

Secondary information can be derived from local, state, national, and international sources. It can be obtained directly from the publisher (in many instances free of charge and in an ongoing manner from public agencies) or indirectly through a library. In some instances, specific documents will be on hand or easily obtainable. In other circumstances, one will have a general idea about the type of information required, but will not be able to cite a specific reference. In these cases, guides and directories are most beneficial.

Examples of data sources at the local level include those maintained by a vital statistics section of a local health department, economic and human resource information available from a human services office, and regional health-related data collected by a health planning agency. Particularly in more rural settings, helpful morbidity and mortality insights can be gained through hospital and coroner records. A particularly helpful example of a regional source of health-related data is available through the Health Scorecard of the La Crosse Medical Health Science Consortium in Wisconsin (Rooney & Thompson, 2009). It first became available in 2007 via the Web site http://www.communityscorecard.com, and it enables a user to access county, state, and national information. Of note, the Web site provides a consolidation of the data, and in the future it will provide in-depth reports about selected health topics.

At the national level, valuable data and informational updates are provided by the MMWR, MVSR, and NCHS reports as well as the *Guide to Federal Statistics: A Selected List* published by the Bureau of the U.S. Census and the *Guide to U.S. Government Statistics*. The NCHS provides important U.S. trend data over time, such as the 1960–2006 overweight and obesity data for adults and youths (see **Figure 2-6**). Distinct, consistent increases over the years in both overweight and obesity levels signal the high-priority need for key lifestyle-change intervention strategies. Additional resources include the

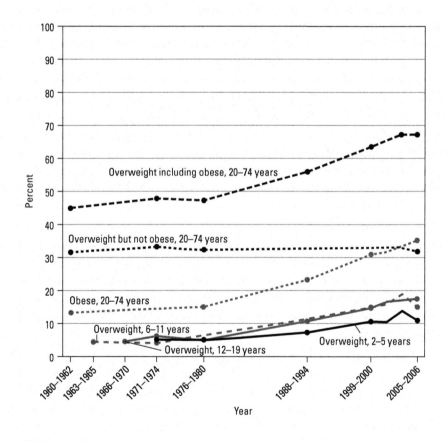

FIGURE 2-6
Overweight and obesity data for adults and youths, United States, 1960–2006.
Source: National Center for Health Statistics (NCHS). (2010). *Health, United States, 2009: With Special Feature on Medical Technology*, Figure 7. Hyattsville, MD: U.S. Department of Health and Human Services. Available at: http://www.cdc.gov/nchs/data/hus/hus09.pdf. Accessed April 20, 2011.

Statistical Abstract of the United States and special reports incorporating data from Standard Metropolitan Statistical Areas (SMSAs), with each SMSA being a single county or cluster of contiguous counties that has at least one city with a minimum of 50,000 people. The Measure of America 2010–2011 report (2010) provides mappings of health risks and risk reduction throughout the United States (Lewis & Burd-Sharps, 2010). A comprehensive overview of sources of electronic and print-related surveillance systems is provided in Teutsch and Churchill (2000). Of note, this source provides a comprehensive review of measures and determinants (direct, indirect, remote, and underlying) of health status, in addition to addressing the strategies and capacities for health improvement (Parrish & McDonnell, 2000). Highly regarded international resources include those provided by the World Health Organization, such as *World Health Statistics* and *Weekly Epidemiological Record*. An overview of available international data sources is provided by the *Directory of United Nations Information Systems and Services.*

These types of sources provide health-related statistical data. Additionally, one can examine demographic data on population patterns, absenteeism records for work and school, income distribution, and political preferences. When we examine this broader context of statistical and demographic data across a population, we are reviewing social indicators (see Shi, 1997; Doyle & Ward, 2001). These data can be subjective or objective, direct (data with direct implications, such as achievement test scores) or indirect measures (data used to proxy possible effects, such as the number in a given school receiving AFDC assistance), or descriptive (descriptions of social characteristics) or analytic (relationships among characteristics). Examination of such social indicators can provide the health professional with an understanding of the community context in which he or she is working. Questions may arise that will, in turn, lead to potential clarification through the structured needs and capacity assessment strategies. Social indicators also may support and supplement the results derived from the structured strategies.

Primary Data Collection

Primary needs and capacity assessment data are observations that the practitioner collects to make informed decisions regarding the next steps. Usually, these data complement and expand upon any secondary data collected from the work of others. Prior to the collection of primary data, human subjects' review should proceed through one's own organization or a partner organization (e.g., academic institution, medical center). The protection of human subjects is the key consideration. This assurance should apply to individuals of all ages who will be offering information. The National Institutes of Health (NIH) has established very clear guidelines for those engaged in needs assessments (see the NIH training Web site, Human Participant Protections Education for Research Teams at http://phrp.nihtraining.com). It usually will be necessary to have a proposal reviewed by an Institutional Review Board (IRB), which follows the NIH guidelines in analyzing the proposal. Although the IRB process is important for the protection of all human subjects, it is even more imperative for those who are younger than 18 years of age or who have particular impairments. Researchers who are working with organizations that do not have their own IRB processes can check with local postsecondary education, medical, and/or human service institutions regarding the IRB processes they may have in place. This approach is particularly a reasonable one to follow when such agencies are involved in the assessment/planning process in a collaborative manner.

The strategies presented in the following chapters provide methods for the collection of primary data. Underlying all data collection procedures is the idea that observations must be collected in an accurate and consistent fashion. To accomplish this goal, the following need to be addressed when planning the assessment process.

Validity and Reliability

Validity refers to measuring what one purports to be measuring. It deals with the accuracy of the assessment process in detecting observations based on the principles and concepts underlying the measurement intent. Another measurement consideration closely aligned with validity is *reliability*, which refers to the consistency of the assessment process. Excellent extended discussions regarding validity and reliability in health education/health promotion contexts are provided by Baumgartner, Strong, and Hensley (2002), Green and Kreuter (2005), and Green and Lewis (1986).

Typically, validation procedures are used in developing measurement instruments for accurate data collection in research and evaluation efforts. Additionally, one can conduct a review of internal validity (i.e., observed program effects are based on an intervention) and external validity (i.e., ability to generalize the observed effects to similar populations). Research and evaluation procedures for assuring reliability relate primarily to the internal consistency (i.e., intercorrelations of all instrument items) or the stability (i.e., measurement association over time) of a measurement instrument. The resulting instruments then can be used in formative evaluation efforts (measurements before or during an intervention) and summative evaluation efforts (measurements regarding intervention impact). Because of the measurement's use with summative evaluation, "the stakes are higher for measurement error" (Green & Lewis, 1986, p. 121). For this reason, greater precision in validity and reliability determinations is required.

Needs assessments are used to detect and depict the perceived and actual needs of a given population so that realistic health education/health promotion objectives can be formulated. Capacity assessments typically are system-related resource review endeavors. Both types of assessments are more formative in nature. When instruments (e.g., surveys, wellness inventories, health-risk appraisals) are to be used in needs and capacity assessments, validity and reliability concerns should be addressed. Chapter 3 discusses validity and reliability as they relate to survey development. For noninstrument formats (e.g., group assessments such as the nominal group and focus group processes), validity is the only factor of the two that can realistically be addressed.

Remember that needs and capacity assessment formats are used for the determination of needs and resources, not primarily for the research and evaluation of intervention impacts. For these purposes, we would recommend a validation procedure that incorporates the review of an advisory and/or expert group. Here individuals who are most familiar with the target population and some of its basic characteristics and issues can respond to the proposed process and make suggestions for improvement. This approach to validation then could be considered similar to the content validation process, in which experts are used in the development of research and evaluation instruments.

Sampling

Because it usually will be impossible to involve everyone from a given group in a needs and capacity assessment process, establishing a population sample is generally a more realistic approach. Samples are classified as *probability samples*, in which all individuals have an equal probability of being selected for the sample (e.g., simple random sample), or *nonprobability samples*, in which subject selection is based on key characteristics in a population (e.g., heterogeneous sample). An excellent in-depth discussion of these sample categories is provided by Green and Lewis (1986), including the justifications for using a given sampling approach. In addition, Creswell (2003) presents a very practical research design overview that differentiates among qualitative, quantitative, and mixed methods (i.e., combining qualitative and quantitative approaches) for the collection and analysis of data. For many locally based needs and capacity assessment efforts that are not meant to have the results projected widely, the nonprobability sampling approach should be sufficient. In instances where it is imperative that the sample be truly representative of a larger population, probability sampling would be the approach of choice.

Needs and Capacity Analysis and Prioritization

Once data are collected through the secondary sources and/or through the structured strategies (to be detailed in forthcoming chapters), analyses of the meaning of the data must take place. It is strongly recommended that these procedures be established prior to the collection of the data, as part of the overall needs and capacity assessment plan. Because much of the information collected may be qualitative in nature, it is helpful to review in advance data analysis procedures for qualitative research methods. A succinct and practical overview is provided by Morse and Field (1995), who discuss the four cognitive processes of qualitative research: *comprehending* (clearer understanding of the circumstances being studied), *synthesizing* (aggregation of information), *theorizing* (finding the "best fit" explanation for the collected information), and *recontextualizing* (theory generalized into different settings). In concert, theoretical frameworks in qualitative research are addressed in good depth and with practicality by Anfara and Mertz (2006). In terms of the collection, coordination, and analyses of qualitative data, Flick (2007) and Gibbs (2007) offer clear procedures for drawing reasonable insights from the data. In each of the subsequent chapters, specific analytic procedures are addressed in the sections entitled "Using the Results."

Another important process in analyzing the collected information is prioritization. This analysis should be based on the needs and resources of the target group, as well as those of the population's service providers. The simplest method of prioritizing is to have the assessed needs and necessary resources ranked by target group members and representatives. In this process, individuals are asked to rank the top five (or some other predetermined number) needs and/or needed resources, out of all of those presented. In analyzing the group results, each need and/or resource has the potential of receiving a series of rankings, which can subsequently be averaged for a mean rank, or weighted. For example, on a 1–5 scale, a rank of 1 will have a weighting of 5; a rank of 2 will have a weighting of 4; and so forth. The weights are then added together for each need, with the highest-valued need being top ranked.

Due to the complexity of needs and capacities that can be assessed through various strategies, no one analytic process can serve all purposes. Thus, for more in-depth discussions regarding selected procedures, one may wish to review McKenzie et al. (2009, pp. 103–105), Doyle and Ward (2001, pp. 147–149), Dever (1991, pp. 45–73), McKillip (1987, pp. 105–119), and Witkin (1984, pp. 206–240).

A helpful model developed by Sork (1982) at the University of British Columbia is reviewed by Witkin (1984, pp. 230–232). This model offers a systematic process for determining priorities with a certain degree of built-in flexibility. The basic steps include the following:

1. *Select appropriate criteria.* Two general categories of importance and feasibility are suggested. Examples of importance are the number of people affected, the magnitude of the difference between present and future status, and the alignment with organizational goals. Examples of feasibility are efficacy levels of health education and promotion interventions (i.e., degree of benefit for those receiving the intervention), resource availability, and perceived ability to change.

2. *Assign a relative importance to each criterion.* Criteria are weighted equally or by degree on a scale of 1 to 10. The criterion of least weight

(1) is identified first, and each subsequent criterion compared against it, so that the criterion weighted 10 is 10 times the weight of 1.

3. *Apply each criterion to each need.* A separate list of priorities is established for each criterion used, with priority values expressed numerically or through descriptors such as high, medium, and low.

4. *Combine individual values to yield a total priority value for each need.* One approach here is to add weighted ranks and establish mean ranks for each identified need.

5. *Arrange needs from highest to lowest total priority.* Value and indicate how priorities will be used. Resource alignment with the identified needs can be established in this step.

From another vantage point, some decision makers may wish to review the assessed needs and resources in a highly qualitative fashion. Using this approach, special criteria can be established as questions against which the needs and resources will be reviewed through group discussion. Examples of such questions are offered in a manual published by the Ministry of Education in Victoria, British Columbia (Lund & McGechaen, 1981, pp. 16–17), and reviewed by Witkin (1984, p. 230):

- Does the target group recognize this need?
- How many people are affected?
- What would be the consequences if this need is not met?
- Can this need be met by an educational activity?
- Does this need coincide with your department or institution's program policies? If not, what are the reasons for the present policies? What procedures are available for influencing needed change?
- Can you rely on co-sponsorship or cooperation with another agency?
- Is this a critical need that should be met before other educational needs are addressed?
- Will resources (funds, staff) be adequate to meet those needs?

Using this approach, health professionals have the opportunity to discuss multiple responses to the questions, as well as the various rationales for those responses. Although this approach typically takes more time, the complexity of the issues being addressed could well merit it.

Yet another prioritization approach has been advanced by Green and Kreuter (2005, pp. 99–100) based on a series of questions during their phase of epidemiological assessment:

- Which problems have the greatest impact in terms of death, disease, days lost from work, rehabilitation costs, disability (temporary and permanent), family disorganization, and cost to communities and agencies for damage repair or loss and cost recovery?

- Are certain subpopulations, such as children, mothers, ethnic minorities, refugees, or indigenous populations, at special risk?
- Which problems are most amenable to intervention?
- Which problem is not being addressed by other organizations in the community?
- Which problem, when appropriately addressed, has the greatest potential for yielding measurable improvements in health status, economic savings, or other benefits?
- Are any of the health problems also highly ranked as a regional or national priority? (State health agencies develop priorities among health problems, often based on local epidemiological data.)
- To what extent does the problem(s) as manifested in the community constitute a disproportionately high burden compared to other communities or the rest of the state?

The results of needs and capacity assessments can guide the practitioners into the planning phases of program development. Key questions should serve as a guide, and those suggested by MacDonald et al. (2001, p. 22) are particularly straightforward:

- What is the health problem and its consequences for the state or community?
- What is the size of the problem overall and in various segments of the population?
- What are the determinants of the health problem?
- Who are the target groups?
- What changes or trends are occurring?

In seeking the information needed to address these questions, MacDonald and colleagues recommend the use of secondary health status data at the national and state levels, particularly for specific groups. They encourage the assessment of capacity and infrastructure issues that can serve as indicators of issues needing to be addressed (e.g., disparities). Examples of capacity and infrastructure issues include the availability of researchers and research data and the availability of effective programs, community leadership, organizations, and networks.

Taken as a whole, these approaches assist the practitioner in keeping in mind the big picture of external forces and resources, as more delimited issues for a given target population (e.g., socioeconomic influences on youth tobacco use) are being assessed and reviewed for resolution. A national framework for such an overview perspective is provided through *Healthy People 2020* in **Figure 2-7**.

Vision

A society in which all people live long, healthy lives.

Mission

Healthy People 2020 strives to:

- Identify nationwide health improvement priorities
- Increase public awareness and understanding of the determinants of health, disease, and disability, and the opportunities for progress
- Provide measurable objectives and goals that are applicable at the national, state, and local levels
- Engage multiple sectors to take actions to strengthen policies and improve practices that are driven by the best available evidence and knowledge
- Identify critical research, evaluation, and data collection needs

Overarching Goals

- Attain high quality, longer lives free of preventable disease, disability, injury, and premature death
- Achieve health equity, eliminate disparities, and improve the health of all groups
- Create social and physical environments that promote good health for all
- Promote quality of life, healthy development, and healthy behaviors across all life stages

Foundation Health Measures

Healthy People 2020 includes broad, cross-cutting measures without targets that will be used to assess progress toward achieving the four overarching goals.

Overarching Goals of *Healthy People 2020*	Foundation Measures Category	Measures of Progress
Attain high quality, longer lives free of preventable disease, disability, injury, and premature death	General Health Status	<ul><li>Life expectancy</li><li>Healthy life expectancy</li><li>Physical and mental unhealthy days</li><li>Self-assessed health status</li><li>Limitation of activity</li><li>Chronic disease prevalence</li><li>International comparisons (*where available*)</li></ul>
Achieve health equity, eliminate disparities, and improve the health of all groups	Disparities and Inequity	Disparities/inequity to be assessed by:<ul><li>Race/ethnicity</li><li>Gender</li><li>Socioeconomic status</li><li>Disability status</li><li>Lesbian, gay, bisexual, and transgender status</li><li>Geography</li></ul>
Create social and physical environments that promote good health for all	Social Determinants of Health	Determinants can include:<ul><li>Social and economic factors</li><li>Natural and built environments</li><li>Policies and programs</li></ul>
Promote quality of life, healthy development, and healthy behaviors across all life stages	Health-Related Quality of Life and Well-Being	<ul><li>Well-being/satisfaction</li><li>Physical, mental, and social health-related quality of life</li><li>Participation in common activities</li></ul>

FIGURE 2-7

The mission, vision, and goals of *Healthy People 2020.*

Source: Centers for Disease Control and Prevention. *Healthy People 2020.* Available at: http://www.healthypeople .gov/2020/topicsobjectives2020/pdfs/hp2020_brochure.pdf. Accessed April 20, 2011.

Summary

The context of a practitioner's program planning experiences, observations, and secondary information sources provides a valuable framework for active involvement in health education and health promotion. This context also enables the professional to make decisions about more appropriate next steps for structured needs and capacity assessment strategies. Chapters 3 through 12 will detail these strategies by addressing selection considerations, along with preparation, implementation, and follow-up procedures.

Online Resources

Visit go.jblearning.com/gilmore4 for links to these Web sites.

American Journal of Health Promotion

Defines health promotion and the dimensions of health.

La Crosse Medical Health Science Consortium—Health Scorecard Project

Regional vital statistics are provided for Western Wisconsin with an opportunity to track health risk and disease trends over time.

Public Health in America

Explains public health and the services and responsibilities of the profession, which include assessments, policy development, and assurance.

World Health Organization

Provides a definition of *health*. Describes the strategic approach methodology, the first step of which is the strategic assessment.

The Urban Institute

Describes capacity and needs assessments of youth services in the District of Columbia.

Healthy People 2000

Healthy People 2000 publications broken down into documents and sections.

Western Rural Development Center

Outlines community assessment techniques. This site includes participant observation, social network analysis, the Delphi survey, the nominal group process, advisory groups, community forums, and application of these techniques.

Wisconsin Department of Public Instruction

Provides guidance through the Safe and Drug-Free Schools program, which includes the importance of needs assessments.

National Academies Press
Provides reference material regarding public health recommendations for the twenty-first century by the Institute of Medicine.

Community Tool Box
The Community Tool Box, sponsored by the University of Kansas, is designed to provide examples of assessment tools and guidance frameworks (e.g., logic model) to practitioners and community groups involved in planning, implementing, and evaluating health enhancement opportunities. A Tool Box search engine also is provided to assist in locating specific assessments within the Web site.

References

Anafara, V., and Mertz, N. (2006). *Theoretical frameworks in qualitative research.* Thousand Oaks, CA: Sage Publications.

Angrosino, M. (2007). *Doing ethnographic and observational research.* Los Angeles: Sage Publications.

Banks, M. (2007). *Using visual data in qualitative research.* Los Angeles: Sage Publications.

Bartholomew, L., Parcel, G., Kok, G., and Gottlieb, N. (2001). *Intervention mapping.* Mountain View, CA: Mayfield Publishing.

Baumgartner, T., Strong, C., and Hensley, L. (2002). *Conducting and reading research in health and human performance.* New York: McGraw-Hill.

Bensky, J., and Hietbrink, R. (1994). Getting down to business. *Worksite Health, 1,* 25–28.

Bond, L., Glover, S., Godfrey, C., Butler, H., and Patton, G. (2001). Building capacity for system-level change in schools: Lessons from the Gatehouse Project. *Health Education and Behavior, 28,* 368–383.

Bracht, N., and Gleason, J. (1990). Strategies and structures for citizen partnerships. In Bracht, N. (Ed.), *Health promotion at the community level* (pp. 109–124). Newbury Park, CA: Sage Publications.

Breslow, L. (1999). From disease prevention to health promotion. *JAMA, 281,* 1030–1033.

Butterfoss, F., Goodman, R., and Wandersman, A. (1993). Community coalitions for prevention and health promotion. *Health Education Research, 8,* 315–330.

Campbell, V., Crews, J., Moriarty, D., Zack, M., and Blackman, D. (1999). Surveillance for sensory impairment, activity limitation, and health-related quality of life among older adults—United States, 1993–1997. *Morbidity and Mortality Weekly Report, 48,* 131–156.

Centers for Disease Control and Prevention (CDC). (2003). *CDCynergy 3.0: Your guide to effective health communication.* Atlanta: Author.

Cohen, L. (2010). *What role can health impact assessment play in the national health reform initiative?* Oakland, CA: Prevention Institute.

Commission on Social Determinants of Health (CSDH). (2008). *Closing the gap in a generation: Health equity through action on the social determinants of health. Final report of the Commission on Social Determinants of Health.* Geneva: World Health Organization.

Committee on Assuring the Health of the Public in the 21st Century, Board on Health Promotion and Disease Prevention. (2003). *The future of the public's health in the 21st century.* Washington, DC: National Academies Press.

Creswell, J. (2003). *Research design: Qualitative, quantitative, and mixed methods approaches.* Thousand Oaks, CA: Sage Publications.

Cromley, E., and McLafferty, S. (2002). *GIS and public health.* New York: Guilford Press.

Dever, G. (1991). *Community health analysis: Global awareness at the local level.* Gaithersburg, MD: Aspen Publishers.

Dewar, T. (1997). *A guide to evaluating asset-based community development: Lessons, challenges, and opportunities.* Chicago: ACTA Publications.

Doyle, E., and Ward, S. (2001). *The process of community health education and promotion.* Mountain View, CA: Mayfield Publishing.

Flick, U. (2007). *Managing quality in qualitative research.* Los Angeles: Sage Publications.

Florin, P., Mitchell, R., and Stevenson, J. (1993). Identifying training and technical assistance needs in community coalitions: A developmental approach. *Health Education Research, 8,* 417–432.

Gebbie, K., Rosenstock, L., and Hernandez, L. (Eds.) (2003). *Who will keep the public healthy? Educating public health professionals for the 21st century.* Washington, DC: National Academies Press.

Gibbs, G. (2007). *Analyzing qualitative data.* Los Angeles: Sage Publications.

Gilmore, G., Kies, B., McIlquham, B., Nogle, A., Whitty, J., and Xie, H. (2010). *Pine Ridge Reservation public health needs and capacity assessment, July 18–23, 2010: Process and summary.* La Crosse, WI: University of Wisconsin-La Crosse.

Gilmore, G., and Hartigan, J. (1998). *Results of the April 1998 Rotary 3-H health planning assessment in Dubna, Russia.* La Crosse, WI: Gundersen Lutheran Medical Center.

Green, L. (1999). Health education's contributions to public health in the twentieth century: A glimpse through health promotion's rearview mirror. *Annual Review of Public Health, 20,* 67–88.

Green, L., and Kreuter, M. (1999). *Health promotion planning: An educational and ecological approach,* 3rd ed. Mountain View, CA: Mayfield Publishing.

Green, L., and Kreuter, M. (2005). *Health program planning: An educational and ecological approach,* 4th ed. Boston: McGraw-Hill.

Green, L., and Lewis, F. (1986). *Measurement and evaluation in health education and health promotion.* Palo Alto, CA: Mayfield Publishing.

Green, L., and Raeburn, J. (1990). Contemporary developments in health promotion. In Bracht, N. (Ed.), *Health promotion at the community level* (pp. 29–44). Newbury Park, CA: Sage Publications.

Harvard Family Research Project. (2002). *Learning from logic models in out-of-school time.* Cambridge, MA: Author.

Hemenway, D. (2010). Why we don't spend enough on public health. *New England Journal of Medicine, 362,* 1657–1658.

Hennessy, C., Moriarty, D., Zack, M., Scherr, P., and Brackbill, R. (1994). Measuring health-related quality of life for public health surveillance. *Public Health Reports, 109,* 665–672.

Himmelman, A. (2002). *Collaboration for change.* Minneapolis: Himmelman Consulting.

Hunkeler, E., Davis, E., McNeil, B., Powell, J., and Polen, M. (1990). Richmond quits smoking: A minority community fights for health. In Bracht, N. (Ed.), *Health promotion at the community level* (pp. 278–303). Newbury Park, CA: Sage Publications.

Joint Committee on Health Education and Promotion Terminology. (2001). Report of the 2000 Joint Committee on Health Education and Promotion Terminology. *American Journal of Health Education, 32,* 90–103.

Kretzmann, J., and McKnight, J. (1993). *Building communities from the inside out.* Chicago: ACTA Publications.

Kretzmann, J., McKnight, J., and Puntenney, D. (1998). *A guide to creating a neighborhood information exchange: Building communities by connecting local skills and knowledge.* Chicago: ACTA Publications.

Kretzmann, J., McKnight, J., and Sheehan, G. (1997). *A guide to capacity inventories: Mobilizing the community skills of local residents.* Chicago: ACTA Publications.

Lewis, K., and Burd-Sharps, S. (2010). *The Measure of America 2010–2011: Mapping risks and resilience.* New York: New York University Press.

Lund, B., and McGechaen. (1981). *Continuing education programmer's manual.* Victoria, British Columbia: Continuing Education Division, Ministry of Education.

MacDonald, G., Starr, G., Schooley, M., Yee, S., Klimowski, K., and Turner, K. (2001). *Introduction to program evaluation for comprehensive tobacco control programs.* Atlanta, GA: USDHHS, CDC.

Maki, J., Qualls, M., White, B., Kleefield, S., and Crone, R. (2008). Health impact assessment and short-term medical missions: A methods study to evaluate quality of care. *BMC Health Services Research, 8,* 121–129.

McKenzie, J., Neiger, B., and Thackeray, R. (2009). *Planning, implementing, and evaluating health promotion programs: A primer.* San Francisco: Pearson/ Benjamin Cummings.

McKillip, J. (1987). *Need analysis: Tools for the human services and education.* Beverly Hills, CA: Sage Publications.

Mokdad, A., Marks, J., Stroup, D., and Gerberding, J. (2004). Actual causes of death in the United States, 2000. *Journal of the American Medical Association, 291,* 1238–1245.

Morse, J., and Field, P. (1995). *Qualitative research methods for health professionals.* Thousand Oaks, CA: Sage Publications.

Nash, D., Reifsnyder, J., Fabius, R., and Pracilio, V. (2011). *Population health: Creating a culture of wellness*. Sudbury, MA: Jones & Bartlett Learning.

National Collaborating Centre for Healthy Public Policy (NCCHPP). (2008). *Canadian roundtable on health impact assessment (HIA)*. Montreal: Author.

Noack, H. (1987). Concepts of health and health promotion. In Abeline, T., Brzezinski, Z., and Carstairs, V. (Eds.), *Measurement in health promotion and protection*. Geneva: World Health Organization.

Parrish, R., and McDonnell, S. (2000). Sources of health-related information. In Teutsch, S., and Churchill, R. (Eds.), *Principles and practice of public health surveillance*. New York: Oxford University Press.

Pellmar, T., Brandt, E., and Baird, M. (2002). Health and behavior: The interplay of biological, behavioral, and social influences: Summary of an Institute of Medicine Report. *American Journal of Health Promotion, 16,* 206–219.

Robertson, A., and Minkler, M. (1994). New health promotion movement: A critical examination. *Health Education Quarterly, 21,* 295–312.

Rooney, B., and Thompson, J. (2009). The value of a Web-based interactive regional health scorecard in setting public health priorities. *Wisconsin Medical Journal, 108,* 403–406.

Rowitz, L. (2006). *Public health for the 21st century: The prepared leader*. Sudbury, MA: Jones and Bartlett Publishers.

Shi, L. (1997). *Health services research methods*. New York: Delmar Publishers.

Sork, T. (1982). *Determining priorities*. Vancouver, British Columbia: University of British Columbia.

Teutsch, S., and Churchill, R. (2000). *Principles and practice of public health surveillance*. New York: Oxford University Press.

Timmreck, T. (2003). *Planning, program development, and evaluation: A handbook for health promotion, aging, and health services*, 2nd ed. Sudbury, MA: Jones and Bartlett Publishers.

U.S. Department of Health and Human Services (USDHHS). (2003). *A public health action plan to prevent heart disease and stroke*. Atlanta, GA: USDHHS, CDC.

U.S. Department of Health and Human Services (USDHHS). (February 2001). *Healthy people in healthy communities: A community planning guide using Healthy People 2010*. Washington, DC: USDHHS, Office of Disease Prevention and Health Promotion.

U.S. Department of Health and Human Services (USDHSS). (January 2001). Health-related quality of life among persons with epilepsy. *Morbidity and Mortality Weekly Report, 50,* 24–35.

U.S. Department of Health and Human Services (USDHHS). (November 2000). *Measuring healthy days: Population assessment of health-related quality of life*. Atlanta, GA: USDHHS, CDC.

U.S. Department of Health and Human Services (USDHHS). (May 2000). Health-related quality of life among adults with arthritis—behavioral risk factor surveillance system, 11 states, 1996–1998. *Morbidity and Mortality Weekly Report, 49,* 366–369.

U.S. Department of Health and Human Services (USDHHS). (April 2000). Community indicators of health-related quality of life—United States, 1993–1997. *Morbidity and Mortality Weekly Report, 49,* 281–285.

U.S. Department of Health and Human Services (USDHHS). (January 2000). *Healthy People 2010: Understanding and improving health.* Washington, DC: Author.

Wallerstein, N. (1992). Powerlessness, empowerment, and health: Implications for health promotion programs. *American Journal of Health Promotion, 6,* 197–205.

Webb, K., Hawe, P., and Noort, M. (2001). Collaborative intersectoral approaches to nutrition in a community on the urban fringe. *Health Education and Behavior, 8,* 306–319.

Witkin, B. (1984). *Assessing needs in educational and social programs.* San Francisco: Jossey-Bass Publishers.

Working Group on Concepts and Principles of Health Promotion. (1987). Health promotion: Concepts and principles. In Abeline, T., Brzezinski, Z., and Carstairs, V. (Eds.), *Measurement in health promotion and protection.* Geneva: World Health Organization.

World Health Organization (WHO). (1985). *Basic documents.* Geneva: Author.

Assessments with Individuals

The three chapters in this section address the needs and capacity assessment strategies that can be used with individuals. The strategies presented incorporate the use of surveys and interviews. Many survey approaches involve just one contact with the participants. In addition to these approaches, the Delphi Technique also will be discussed, which involves multiple contacts with the same participants on an individual basis over time. After reviewing each strategy, suggestions are offered for preparing and conducting the needs and capacity assessment processes and then using the results in the planning process.

3

Single-Step Surveys

Introduction

Surveys are one of the oldest methods for gathering information. At first, face-to-face surveys were preferred, because they could include a more representative cross-section of the population (Fowler, 2002, p. 75). Telephone surveys initially were considered unreliable. Because not all homes had phones, telephone surveys tended to include primarily educated and at least middle-income people.

Today's phone surveys have the potential to provide more reliable information and may be a more preferred method (Fowler, 2002). Although unlisted numbers are increasing, "no call" lists are emerging, and more than half the phones in the world are now cellular, random-digit dialing and similar techniques can enable surveyors to reach individuals who opt out of directory listings.

The rapid growth of the Internet in recent years has opened a new way of conducting surveys. A brief survey can be conducted using e-mail, or a longer survey can be posted on the World Wide Web for participants to complete. Internet surveys may become the preferred method of data collection in the years ahead, especially given that people are becoming more and more reluctant to participate in telephone surveys.

A survey is a structured process for collecting primarily quantitative data directly from individuals by asking questions. It can show the distribution of certain characteristics within a population, usually by surveying only a small portion of that population (Fowler, 2002, pp. 1–2).

Surveys have been widely used to assess educational needs. Mailing a questionnaire is probably the most frequently used strategy, and telephone surveys are also popular for this purpose. Face-to-face surveys have continuing importance for community health education, and Internet surveys are increasingly used as well. In this chapter, we will discuss all four strategies.

You can learn to conduct good surveys, and you do not have to be an expert researcher to do so. You can follow the steps outlined in this chapter and obtain good results.

Reviewing and Selecting a Strategy

MAIL SURVEYS

Advantages

Mail surveys have the following advantages:

- *Low cost.* Surveys have similar basic costs, which include developing and producing the questionnaire, analyzing the data, and communicating the results. The cost of collecting data is the primary way costs differ among the various ways of conducting surveys. For mail surveys, the major data collection expense is postage. For many needs assessments, one person with a few basic research skills can conduct an entire mail survey from start to finish. Larger projects may require assistance from staff members with expertise in questionnaire design and data analysis, but one central office can handle the entire project.
- *Wide distribution.* Mail surveys can reach anyone who receives mail from a country's postal service, making it relatively easy to access diverse groups of people.
- *Reasonably valid information.* Mail surveys usually offer better chances of obtaining truthful answers than telephone or face-to-face surveys, especially when asking potentially sensitive questions (Fowler, 2002, p. 64). People can respond in the privacy of their homes or workplaces and they can feel that the process is a bit more confidential.

  Mail surveys provide opportunities to obtain thoughtful replies (Fowler, 2002, pp. 64, 73). Respondents can complete a survey when they have the time and perspective to give the best answers, rather than responding on the spot to an interviewer's questions. Mail surveys also eliminate the bias and influence that interviewers bring to telephone or face-to-face surveys.

Disadvantages

Mail surveys have the following disadvantages:

- *Lengthy process.* Although mail surveys save money and personnel, time is lost while waiting for the return of the questionnaires. Data collection alone typically takes 2 months to complete (Fowler, 2002, p. 68), waiting for the returns from an initial mailing and subsequent follow-up efforts.
- *Limited number and type of questions.* A lengthy questionnaire can discourage recipients from completing it. Simple and straightforward questions are most desirable. Complex questions are difficult to include, because you cannot follow up to clarify the meaning of responses.

- *No control over answers.* You cannot control who answers your questionnaire. You may send it with explicit instructions for a teenager to complete, but you do not know whether that person completed the survey or the parent did. You cannot keep a respondent from consulting with another person before giving an answer. Nor can you encourage the respondent to answer all questions instead of skipping some.
- *Mailing list required.* Complete mailing lists for a group you want to survey may not always be readily available. If they are available, they may not be accurate. The more accurate lists may be expensive to obtain. Suddenly, what seemed to be an inexpensive survey becomes more costly.

INTERNET SURVEYS

Advantages

Internet surveys have the following advantages:

- *Lower cost.* Internet surveys are even cheaper to conduct than mail surveys, because they eliminate the cost of postage. Assuming that you have access to an Internet connection, distributing the survey is free. Some additional costs are possible for a Web survey, though, depending on your computer expertise. You may need assistance with posting the survey on the Web and retrieving the data received.
- *Shorter process.* Communication between you and your participants is instantaneous. Compared to a mail survey, you save the time that the postal service needs to deliver your questionnaire to the respondents and then return the completed questionnaire to you. All follow-up contacts are delivered instantly as well. As with mail surveys, though, you still have to wait for respondents to take the time to complete the survey. People who actually complete an Internet survey may not wait as long as they would with a mail survey. Either they complete it relatively soon, or they forget about it (Dillman, 2000, pp. 366, 370).
- *Reasonably valid information.* Internet surveys offer the same opportunity for obtaining truthful answers as mail surveys.
- *Higher response rate possible.* Today, people may be more inclined to complete an Internet survey than a mail survey. It may be shorter and much quicker to fill out than a typical mail survey. It should be noted that this is not always the case, particularly with longer surveys (Gilmore, Olsen, Taub, & Connell, 2005). Internet surveys also are a bit more novel. People who resist completing yet another mail survey may be willing to complete an Internet survey, simply because it is a different format and usually more easily completed and returned.

Disadvantages

Internet surveys have the following disadvantages:

- *Limited distribution.* Although the number of people in the United States with Internet access is growing rapidly, you simply cannot reach as many people as you would by regular mail.
- *Mailing list required.* As with mail surveys, you need a list of e-mail addresses of people who fit the population you wish to sample. These days, we change our e-mail addresses more frequently than we change residences, so ensuring accuracy of the e-mail list is a major challenge. When possible, obtain a list of individuals who are likely to respond favorably to receiving an e-mail from you—for example, past participants or people who have had some previous contact with your organization.
- *Potential sample bias.* Involvement in the survey would be limited to people with Internet access. Some people may use the Internet at public libraries or community agencies, but they would not have their own e-mail addresses so that you could invite them to participate in the survey.
- *Even more limited number and type of questions.* An Internet survey generally needs to be shorter than a mail survey. A long computer document is more difficult for people to work with than a document they can handle physically (Gilmore et al., 2005). A well-designed Web survey can ask a number of questions, but you will need technical assistance to design it in a way that keeps respondents engaged, which could add to the cost of your survey.
- *No control over answers.* The same lack of control you have with mail surveys applies to Internet surveys as well.

TELEPHONE SURVEYS

Advantages

Telephone surveys have the following advantages:

- *More and different questions possible.* Because talking is easier than writing, participants are typically willing to answer more questions for phone surveys than for mail or Internet surveys. For the general public, a survey lasting 10 to 20 minutes is reasonable. Participants usually will tolerate open-ended questions much better over the phone than by mail. If needed, complex questions are easier to ask, because follow-up questions are possible.
- *Better control over answers.* Unlike mail or Internet surveys, which are out of your hands once you drop them in the mail or hit the send button, with telephone surveys you can make sure you are

questioning the appropriate person. You can also discourage consultation with other people and encourage responses to all questions.

- *Shorter process.* Preparation time for telephone surveys is slightly longer than for mail and Internet surveys, but data collection is quicker (Fowler, 2002, p. 68). You can call participants and have your information immediately. You do not have to wait weeks or months for mail returns.
- *Good access to respondents.* Although you can reach slightly fewer people by phone than by regular mail, a very high percentage of American households have access to a telephone. Random-digit dialing techniques can be used to reach people with unlisted numbers (Fowler, 2002, pp. 23–25).
- *Immediate data entry.* If computer-assisted telephone interviewing (CATI) is used, data are available in an electronic format immediately following the interview. Although more costly to set up, this approach reduces transcription errors and turnaround time.

Disadvantages

Telephone surveys have the following disadvantages:

- *Response rate declining.* People are becoming increasingly reluctant to participate in telephone surveys. Aided by caller identification features, they are hesitating to even answer their phones when they do not recognize the caller. When they do answer, they may quickly hang up if a pause occurs before the surveyor responds or decline to participate when they realize the purpose of the call. This behavior is partly a reaction to the increasing number of telemarketing calls at inconvenient times and partly a reflection of the increasing desire for privacy in our culture. Some people do not want to be bothered when they are at home.

    Many states and the federal government have passed legislation creating "no-call" lists, prohibiting telemarketers from calling individuals who request not to be contacted. In many cases, this legislation applies to for-profit businesses and not to nonprofit organizations. Even if your organization is not restrained from contacting people on a "no-call" list, these individuals may not respond favorably to your call.
- *More costly.* Collecting data typically is more expensive than for mail or Internet surveys. If long-distance calls are necessary, the calls may cost more than the postage needed to mail questionnaires. Conducting telephone interviews also is much more time consuming than tracking mail or Internet surveys. For some telephone surveys, one person might conduct all of the interviews, but extra help often is needed. Additional interviewers may require payment for their training and for the time spent conducting interviews. For a large

project involving several interviewers, supervisory help is needed as well.

- *Socially desirable responses.* There is a greater likelihood of receiving socially desirable responses to potentially threatening or sensitive questions by phone than by mail or Internet (Fowler, 2002, p. 72). Candid answers are more easily written than stated to interviewers.

FACE-TO-FACE SURVEYS

Advantages

Face-to-face surveys have the following advantages:

- *Best opportunity for questioning.* A face-to-face survey is the best way to administer a lengthy questionnaire (Fowler, 2002, p. 71). Open-ended and complex questions are best handled in face-to-face surveys, because follow-up questions are more easily asked.
- *Most control over answers.* Compared to telephone surveys, you have even more assurance that the appropriate person is answering your questions and is not consulting with other people. Using both verbal and nonverbal expressions, you can also strongly encourage the respondent to answer all of the questions.

Disadvantages

Face-to-face surveys have the following disadvantages:

- *Most costly.* Because interviewers must travel, often from house to house, to collect data, travel time and transportation expenses are significant. The interview itself typically takes longer to conduct in person than by phone. Although one person can carry out an entire mail or telephone survey, a face-to-face survey will require at least one other person to assist with interviews. Large projects require several interviewers as well as supervisory help. Training is more extensive, because interviewers must make judgments in the field without the benefit of consulting with a supervisor.
- *Socially desirable responses.* Potentially threatening questions are the most difficult to ask in face-to-face surveys. Participants are most tempted to give a socially desirable answer when they have to face another person (Dillman, 2000, p. 226).
- *Difficulty in gaining access to participants.* Historically, face-to-face surveys have offered good access to the public. However, because many people are busier than in the past and concerns about privacy and security have increased, face-to-face surveys have become more difficult to conduct. In many cases, both spouses work outside of the

home, leaving fewer people at home during the day. Families often have evening activities as well. In addition, some surveyors have concerns about their personal safety in some metropolitan neighborhoods, especially during evening hours, and many apartment buildings have installed security systems (Fowler, 2002, p. 66). Public places are also difficult for conducting surveys, because people are often in a hurry.

Criteria for Selection

As you consider the advantages and disadvantages of mail, Internet, telephone, and face-to-face surveys, it is suggested that you keep five criteria in mind: (1) the type of information needed, (2) from whom it is needed, (3) the money available to conduct the survey, (4) the time available, and (5) the personnel who can assist you.

1. *Type of information.* If the information you need is potentially threatening or sensitive for the participants, especially details about behavior patterns, a mail or Internet survey typically will yield more accurate data. If you need to ask complex questions that require follow-up questions for clarification, a face-to-face survey offers the best opportunity. Open-ended questions are also best handled face-to-face. If you have many questions to ask, a face-to-face survey usually is best, followed by a telephone survey.

2. *Audience.* A face-to-face survey is usually best if your objective is to survey people from low-income groups or groups with low literacy levels. In addition, a face-to-face survey usually is best when surveying people for whom English is a second language (Fowler, 2002, p. 61). Individuals from these groups may be unable to complete a mail survey and may not feel comfortable talking to a stranger on the phone. For a professional audience, however, a telephone survey may be more feasible. Professionals tend to be comfortable using the phone and may resist completing yet another mail survey. The Internet survey is an increasingly appropriate way to reach a professional audience. E-mail addresses for professionals at their place of employment are often relatively easy to obtain. Professionals make frequent use of their computer and the Internet and can complete the survey at times convenient for them.

3. *Money.* If financial resources are limited, mail and brief Internet surveys are your best options. A simple telephone survey, however, can be inexpensive, as long as many long-distance calls are not required.

4. *Time.* If you need the survey done quickly, use the telephone or develop a brief e-mail survey. Note that if you use the phone you will need time to recruit and train interviewers.

5. *Personnel.* A mail or brief e-mail survey requires the smallest number of personnel, whereas a face-to-face survey requires the largest number. A face-to-face survey also requires the most-qualified interviewers because they are basically on their own when conducting the survey.

Finally, keep two other important considerations in mind no matter which survey method you use to assess needs and capacities. First, remember that people respond based on how they feel at the time of the survey. They will not necessarily take action to meet their perceived needs at a later time. Second, remember that surveys have been widely used to assess needs. What once was novel is now potentially overused.

Preparing for the Assessment

Because the preparation phase is similar for mail, Internet, telephone, and face-to-face surveys, we will discuss the steps that apply generally to all four strategies. For some steps we will suggest considerations applicable to a particular survey method.

Decide What You Want to Know

Determine exactly what you need to learn from the individuals you plan to survey. Having a clear idea of the purpose for the assessment before you begin can direct the development of your questions and save valuable time for both you and your participants.

Decide whether you need to ask people what they know, what their attitudes are about a certain subject, or how they would describe certain behaviors. If you plan to ask about behavior, consider whether describing this behavior will be threatening to the individual. With this in mind, plan for an Institutional Review Board (IRB) review to determine the need to address consent considerations (Schiff, 2003). Also determine if an informed consent form will be necessary (see Chapter 5 for an example).

Develop a Budget

Before you begin to develop a survey, be aware of budgetary constraints. You will already have an approximate budget in mind, which helped you select which survey method to use. Now you will put the budget in final form, including personnel costs for developing the questionnaire and collecting and analyzing the data, printing of the survey and final report, postage, long-distance telephone calls, travel expenses, and computer analysis. Having a detailed budget will help you decide, for example, how many people to employ, how many people to survey, and how much data analysis can be performed.

Prepare Your Questions

Before rushing ahead to develop your own questions, consider whether someone else has previously developed questions you could use. For a needs or capacity assessment, existing questions that fit your situation exactly may be difficult to find. With some modification, however, preexisting questions might be suitable. Alternatively, they might suggest other questions you can develop yourself.

When developing questions, keep in mind the purpose for the assessment, which type of survey you plan to use, who you will survey, and how you will analyze the data you collect. Align your questions directly with the survey objectives. Remember that a mail survey should include primarily "closed" questions, which give the respondent a choice of answers from which to select. Examples include responding yes or no, indicating how frequently a certain situation applies, or rank ordering several possibilities.

Open-ended questions require participants to generate answers themselves. For a mail survey, limit the number of open-ended questions. Usually, the shorter the answer required, the better. An Internet survey offers more potential for open-ended questions, because using a computer to generate narrative responses is faster and easier than putting pen to paper. Telephone and face-to-face surveys can handle more plentiful and less focused open-ended questions.

The sample group you plan to survey will affect the types of questions you will develop. If you plan to survey a sample of the general public, remember that many potential respondents will not be highly motivated to participate. Usually, they will respond better to closed questions than to open-ended ones. They may also refuse to answer what appear to be threatening or sensitive questions about their behavior.

If you plan to survey people who are highly motivated to participate, perhaps because they identify with your efforts or have a stake in the outcome, open-ended questions are more appropriate (see, for example, the Delphi Technique in the next chapter). These individuals will take more time to respond in a thoughtful manner.

How you plan to analyze your data should also influence the questions you develop. Open-ended questions may yield excellent information, but they take much more time and skill to analyze. If you are short on time, money, or skilled personnel, limit the number of open-ended questions.

Test and Modify Your Questions

After spending time and energy on developing questions, we all have a tendency to think we are finally ready to proceed with the survey. We may have some very good questions, but we need to submit them to careful scrutiny to make them even better. Taking time to revise your questions is the best way to decrease measurement error in responses, thereby increasing the reliability and validity of your survey.

When developing your questions, seek to establish content validity by sharing them with colleagues who have experience with or expertise in the subject area of the survey. Inform these people about the scope and purpose of your assessment and have them use a consistent format in providing written feedback.

At this stage, your colleagues may be better able than you to spot ambiguities or suggest alternate wording. In addition, you should solicit the opinions of people who will analyze the data. Ask them to critique the questions and suggest ways to improve the wording. Ask them to tell you what they think the questions mean. Do not be afraid of criticism! Think of your initial questions as first efforts, rather than polished masterpieces. Small changes in wording can influence how people respond. Revise your questions as many as 10 times, if necessary. You want the intended meaning of the questions to be as direct as possible.

Develop a Draft of Your Survey

Keep your respondents in mind as you develop your questionnaire. Remember that they may not be very motivated to participate. Once they begin answering your questions, you want to ensure that they continue doing so. You do not want them to give up in the middle out of fatigue or frustration.

Start with questions that build interest in your survey and are relatively easy to answer. The first question is very important. It should apply to everyone, interest the respondent, and be easy to answer (Dillman, 2000, p. 92). Like a long-distance runner, the respondent needs to warm up and get into the flow of your survey. Use closed questions at this early stage, if possible.

Order your questions in a way that will seem logical to the respondent (Dillman, 2000, p. 88). Place difficult or potentially threatening or sensitive questions near the middle. Open-ended questions also work best in the middle of the survey. You want the respondents to answer these questions after they are warmed up, but before they become tired.

Ask demographic or potentially objectionable questions at the end (Dillman, 2000, p. 87). Questions about the respondent's age, income, and family status can scare off some respondents. Demographic questions are also answered quickly. When the finish line is in sight, having just a few quick questions left can help.

Continually remind yourself about the purpose of the assessment. Develop your questions while keeping this purpose ever-present in your mind. Also, if research questions are guiding your assessment, make sure the survey questions (also called items) are in alignment with the research questions. Survey questions assist in addressing the assessment purpose and in answering the research questions you developed.

If you have no specific use for the answer, or are not sure, omit the question. Do your participants a favor. They have to answer all your questions. The more questions you ask, the more fatigued they will become, and the more you risk having an incomplete survey or invalid information. Do yourself a favor, too. The more data you collect, the more you will have to summarize and analyze. You have only so much time and money to devote to this project, so use both wisely. Aim to have a few good questions.

Draft Coding and Data Analysis Procedures

Before pilot testing the survey, think through how you will analyze the data. Plan for statistical analysis, if appropriate. Consult with staff members who will handle the data analysis. They can suggest the best way to format the survey to make the data as easy to understand and categorize as possible.

Planning the data analysis procedures at this stage also ensures that it is done promptly. You could get so caught up in collecting data that they could sit on the shelf too long before being used.

Pilot Test Your Survey

Be sure to allow enough time to conduct a pilot test. The time invested in this important preliminary activity should result in an appropriate format and increased response rate.

For a large research project, a rigorous regimen of pilot testing is strongly recommended to increase readability, reliability, and validity. Sudman and Bradburn (1983, p. 282) recommend several steps, including peer critique of a draft questionnaire, revision and testing with friends and colleagues, pilot testing with a small sample of respondents, written comments from interviewers and respondents, and pilot testing again.

If you cannot afford extensive pilot testing, at least find a group of people to practice taking your survey. Try to simulate the conditions to be used for the final version. Select a small sample of people, typically no more than 20, who are similar to those who will participate in the survey. Administer the practice survey, using the same directions you will use later. Include an extra page at the end for these pilot testers to comment about the questionnaire. Have them identify confusing questions and state the reasoning they used to answer them. Using consistent questions for the pilot testers, ask them to critique the survey questions and suggest any improvements. Comments on the layout and format of the questionnaire also are useful.

This feedback about the questions themselves is important for large or small pilot-testing efforts. Determining what the questions mean to the respondents and ensuring that the questions elicit the responses you intend are important ways to increase validity. For more information about these cognitive-debriefing approaches, see Tanur (1992).

Once you have received the completed pilot surveys, analyze the data just as you would with the final version. Determine as best you can whether the questions are providing the information you need and whether the coding and data analysis procedures are clear and effective.

Design the Final Survey

Consider three groups of people when designing the final questionnaire: the respondents, the interviewers (if used), and the data analysts.

For a mail survey, give the respondents primary consideration. Remember that length is important, especially for the general public. Generally, the shorter the survey and the simpler the questions, the better the responses. For the general public, try to limit your questionnaire to approximately four pages. For relatively homogeneous groups who identify with your project, however, longer surveys are feasible. Use only a few open-ended questions, if any.

It is important that your survey is easy to read. Use a relatively large and legible typeface. Do not try to shorten the survey by reducing the type size. What you gain by having fewer pages, you will lose by having difficult-to-read type. A slightly longer survey, if you really need to ask all those questions, is better than a survey with type that is too small. Also, make sure you include good directions. If respondents must skip certain questions based on how other questions are answered, make sure these directions are clearly identified. Feedback from the preliminary review and pilot will help you here. Design your mail survey to look as professional as possible, without being slick. Everything you do to design the questionnaire should be geared toward obtaining the best response for the resources available. Use different fonts, variable type size, boldface, shading, and other word-processing and desktop-publishing enhancements to create an attractive, easy-to-follow, low-cost survey. If the budget allows, an attractive booklet with a cover page, preferably printed on legal-size paper folded to become an 8.5-by-7-inch booklet, can increase responses (Dillman, 2000, pp. 81–83, 102–108).

An e-mail survey typically consists of a brief set of questions included in the e-mail message. Participants insert their responses into the message and return it to the sender. Some people are more comfortable working with paper and pen, so offer them the option of printing a copy, marking their responses on the hard copy, and returning it via regular mail.

Simplicity is key for an e-mail survey. If reasonable, limit the number of questions to as few as three to five (Dillman, 2000, p. 372). Because many people tend to delete e-mail messages after reading just a few lines, make sure the first question is especially interesting to the respondents. Use the first question to pique their interest and encourage completion of the survey. Use bracket symbols ([ ]) to indicate where they should place their responses. Brackets are not frequently used in narrative writing and will tend to stand out for the respondent (Dillman, 2000, pp. 370–371).

Because respondents will have different computers and e-mail programs, an e-mail questionnaire can appear differently on their computer screens than it does on yours. A question that fits on one line on your screen may extend to two lines on a respondent's screen, making the questionnaire less attractive and more confusing to complete. Keep lines as short as possible to avoid this "wraparound" effect (Dillman, 2000, pp. 369–370).

A Web survey offers several opportunities not available with an e-mail survey. You can dress up the questionnaire with color, attractive graphics, or pictures. These features enable you to include questions that require respondents to view a picture or diagram and answer questions about it. A Web survey also offers a better opportunity to use open-ended questions than a mail or e-mail survey. People are more inclined to generate narrative responses to open-ended questions when using their computer than when using handwriting. A Web survey can also be longer than an e-mail survey, because it offers various ways to sustain interest.

Keep the survey on continuous scrolling, rather than using a method that requires exiting from one page to another. Continuous scrolling allows respondents to mark their progress in completing the survey (Dillman, 2000, pp. 395–396). Allow respondents to skip questions they do not wish to answer, rather than forcing them to answer each question before proceeding to the next. Clarify this approach in the directions. If respondents are forced to answer all questions, they may stop working on the survey if they are asked a question they do not wish to answer. Forcing respondents to answer all questions can also introduce bias, because mail, e-mail, telephone, and face-to-face surveys all allow respondents to skip questions (Dillman, 2000, p. 394).

Although a Web survey offers many attractive possibilities, exercising restraint is key. Respondents may not have computers as powerful or Internet connections as fast as you do, especially if they are completing their surveys at home. Try not to make extensive use of color, graphics, and pictures, since some of the respondents' computers may be unable to load them or their computers may take so long to load that respondents stop working on the survey. It is better to design a Web survey that will load quickly and completely on less powerful computers and slower Internet connections (Dillman, 2000, pp. 385–389).

The more elaborate the Web survey, the more likely you will need to pay for assistance in developing it. Thus, the size of your budget will influence the number of features that are included.

For telephone and face-to-face surveys, give the interviewers primary consideration. A good design can help alleviate some of the pressure that is a normal part of conducting a survey. The length of the questionnaire is no longer as important. Instead, make sure you include clear directions and enough space to record answers. Design the booklet to be easy to use during the survey. Use extra white space to set the questions apart from one another.

As much as possible, design the survey to enhance good data analysis. Place the answers in a consistent location for easy reading. If the survey will be scored by a computer, include the appropriate field numbers. If the budget allows, consider using a software program that enables interviewers to enter data directly into a computer while conducting the survey.

Conducting the Assessment

Although the preparation phase is similar for mail, Internet, telephone, and face-to-face surveys, the conducting phase varies significantly. Appropriate steps for each type are discussed below.

MAIL SURVEY

Select a Sample of Respondents

Unless you have a very small group of people to survey, you will have to sample from a larger population. A probability sample (defined in Chapter 2) is usually the best option in this case. A mail survey enables you to obtain information about educational needs from a comparatively large and potentially diverse group of people. Selecting a probability sample ensures that this information is representative of the population you want to serve.

Basic discussions regarding the sample size determination and simple random sampling for quantitative and qualitative research are provided by Orcher (2005) and Baumgartner and Hensley (2006). Web sites also are available for determining the sample size (a good example is http://www.surveysystem .com/sscalc.htm). Additionally, pure forms of random selection are not always used in practice. Instead, one could use a systematic sample, which in most cases provides a good estimate of the population being studied. It is created by selecting names at regular intervals from a mailing list (Baumgartner & Hensley, 2006; Orcher, 2005).

To obtain a systematic sample, first decide how many respondents you want to survey, and then make sure your budget can handle this number. Then divide the number of names on the list by the size of the sample needed to determine the size of the interval between names to be selected. Pick a number at random between one and the size of the interval, inclusive. Draw this number from a hat or select it from a table of random numbers; it is the number of the first name selected from your mailing list. Skip as many names as the size of the interval and select that name. Proceed through the entire list to complete your sample, selecting names at each interval.

For example, if you want to select 50 participants from a mailing list of 500 people, the interval size is 10. Randomly select a number between 1 and 10, inclusive. If that number is seven, choose the seventh person on the list. Then choose the 17th person, the 27th person, and so on, through the entire list.

When conducting a survey, you may want to make sure that certain groups of people are adequately represented in the sample. For a survey of the health education needs of a particular community, for example, you will want to understand the needs of all age groups. If you rely exclusively on a telephone directory, voter registration records, or a list of motor vehicle licenses, your sample will include primarily working adults. To ensure representation from young people and older adults, seek other sources of information, such as school registration records and lists of individuals currently served by programs for seniors. In some instances, structured list acquisition procedures will need to be developed specifically for the assessment endeavor. Gilmore and colleagues (2005; 2004) provide a detailed discussion of their list acquisition process on a national basis.

Once you have obtained appropriate lists that represent these different age groups, select a stratified sample. Divide the young people, working adults, and older people into three discrete groups, called *strata*, using the different mailing lists. Make sure that no one appears on more than one list. Then proceed to select systematic samples from each of these lists using the procedure described earlier. For each age group, try to make the sample size proportional to the population of that age group in the community.

Cluster sampling is another way to select representative groups using naturally occurring groups or clusters, such as schools, clinics, worksites, or census tracks. All, or a random selection of some, of the individuals in a cluster can be used, depending on the intent of the assessment. In most instances, even though individuals are in close proximity in a cluster, there is sufficient variability or heterogeneity. Cluster sampling is particularly helpful when a list of group members is not available, when the population is spread over a large area, or when it is not convenient to remove selected individuals from their group to conduct the assessment. Keep in mind that conclusions and inferences drawn from the data need to include reference to the particular cluster sampled (Baumgartner, Strong, & Hensley, 2002).

Mail the Questionnaires

Include a brief cover letter that explains who is conducting the survey, why it is important, and what benefits will result from it. Explain how the respondents were selected, and note that their responses will be kept confidential. Code the questionnaires with a number in an inconspicuous place. That way you can tell who has and who has not responded. Assure the respondents that this number is just for coding purposes.

Indicate a date by which the respondents should return the questionnaire, typically two weeks. Busy people may not complete the survey right away, but you do not want it sitting around for so long that they forget about it. Include a stamped, self-addressed, or business-reply envelope for return of the survey.

You also may want to consider sending a letter to your sample a few days to a week in advance of mailing the survey. This letter alerts the sample members to the coming survey and seeks their cooperation in completing it.

If the project budget and organization policy allow, consider a small financial incentive to encourage participation in the survey. To counter growing resistance to surveys, especially from younger adults, including a small monetary payment in the original mailing can increase response rate (Dillman, 2000, p. 168). If you are especially concerned about a low response rate, consider offering a small gift certificate for a major bookstore or franchise restaurant. While conducting a national survey, the author and colleagues had a good response by entering respondents into a drawing for savings bonds and donated professional memberships and books (Gilmore et al., 2005, 2004).

Follow Up the Initial Mailing

Three additional contacts with potential respondents are recommended to increase the response rate (Dillman, 2000, pp. 156–188). Send a reminder postcard one week after mailing the survey. Two weeks later, mail a letter and another copy of the questionnaire to those people who have not responded. Wait another 4 weeks to contact individuals who still have not responded, perhaps using the telephone. If resources permit, offer to conduct the survey by phone for these nonrespondents. For all follow-ups, include investigator contact information for respondents to raise questions, if desired.

At this point, your response rate may not be as high as you would like it to be. It is tempting to continue contacting people in an effort to increase the response. Always, however, maintain a balance between trying to increase the response rate as much as possible and bothering people to the point that they will not complete your survey (Dillman, 2000, pp. 29, 187).

INTERNET SURVEY

In many ways, conducting an Internet survey is similar to conducting a mail survey. You need to develop an instrument, pretest it, obtain a mailing list, distribute the survey, and have follow-up contact. In other ways, though, an Internet survey differs from a mail survey.

Decide Who to Survey

Although the number of people in the United States with Internet access is growing rapidly, we cannot assume that it is representative of all population segments. Thus, using the Internet to select a sample that is representative of a particular population can pose a challenge. If you plan to survey a professional population, however, you have a better chance of selecting a representative sample. Many professional groups have widespread Internet access, and e-mail addresses are relatively easy to obtain.

Because distributing an e-mail or Web survey is so easy and essentially free once you have an e-mail list, you may want to survey an entire population for some surveys instead of sampling.

Distribute the Survey

For an e-mail survey, it is important to send a note before the survey is distributed. People can easily overlook or quickly delete an e-mail message. Sending a note 2 days in advance will alert the respondents to anticipate the survey and deter them from deleting it too quickly (Dillman, 2000, p. 368).

For a Web survey, you can distribute the survey with an e-mail message, embedding the Web address in the e-mail. Respondents can click on the Web address to get transferred to the survey. Alternatively, you can telephone or send a letter, directing respondents to the Web address to complete the survey. This latter approach is useful when you do not have access to an e-mail list.

Follow Up the Initial Distribution

Continue to have the same number of contacts with the e-mail/Web sample as with a mail survey, but shorten the interval of time between contacts. The first follow-up can include another copy of the questionnaire, because it is easy and inexpensive to distribute. All subsequent follow-ups can include a copy of the questionnaire as well (Dillman, 2000, pp. 367–368).

TELEPHONE SURVEY

Select a Sample of Respondents

If you plan to survey employees or members of an organization, obtain the staff directory or membership list. Then draw a systematic sample from this population.

If you plan to survey the general public, the community telephone directory is a usual source of land-line phone numbers. This directory, however, will not include unlisted numbers. Computer-assisted random-digit dialing is the best way to gain access to unlisted numbers, but a simple and effective method is to add a digit (Frey, 1989, pp. 90–104). Draw a systematic sample of telephone numbers, and then add one digit to every number. That way you are not limited to just phone numbers in the directory.

Gaining cooperation in completing the survey is a challenge when using random-digit dialing. There is often a delay after the respondent answers the phone until the interviewer begins to speak. This delay alerts the respondent that some kind of solicitation is about to occur, which typically results in a negative reaction.

Select and Train the Interviewers

Consider age and experience when recruiting interviewers. Older interviewers and interviewers with some experience may obtain better response rates than younger interviewers.

Explain the purpose of the survey, who is conducting it, why it is important, and what benefits will result from it. Give the interviewers written instructions on how to conduct the surveys. Specify how many attempts to make to reach a participant before proceeding to someone else, how to introduce the survey, how to handle ambiguous answers, and how to record the data.

Have the interviewers practice conducting telephone interviews and critique one another. If possible, have them contact people similar to the survey participants or have them practice on one another.

Collect and Record the Data

The interviewers simply proceed through the survey, following the directions on the questionnaire and the instructions they received during training. If possible, have all interviewers place calls from a central location during the same period of time. That way one supervisor can handle any problems that arise.

As noted earlier, using computer-assisted telephone interviewing (CATI) makes data available in electronic format immediately following the interview. Weekday evenings from January through March have been shown to be the best times to conduct telephone interviews (Dillman, 2000, p. 176). People tend to spend more time at home in winter.

FACE-TO-FACE SURVEY

Decide Who and Where to Survey
Various possibilities exist for conducting a face-to-face survey. You can select a systematic sample of participants from a membership list and arrange to survey them in person. You can also interview, for example, the oldest female member of every fifth household in a neighborhood, or randomly select people at a shopping mall or on a street corner.

A cluster sample is another way to obtain a probability sample for a face-to-face survey. First, divide the total population into natural groupings or clusters. To understand the health education needs of an entire community, for example, we might divide the community into neighborhoods, city blocks, or even types of nonprofit community organizations. Then randomly or systematically sample a certain number of respondents from within each cluster (Green & Lewis, 1986, p. 230).

Select and Train Interviewers
The selection of interviewers is more critical for a face-to-face survey than for a telephone survey. Interviewers need to enjoy and feel comfortable in a face-to-face situation. Because they will conduct these surveys with little or no supervision, they need to exercise good judgment. Once the interviewers are selected, training is similar to phone survey training.

Collect and Record the Data
Give the interviewers explicit instructions on who and where to survey. The data collection itself is similar to the telephone survey.

CASE STUDIES COMBINED WITH SURVEYS
Another survey approach is to combine it with a case study. This approach has been described by Yin (2003), and it is particularly useful when a variety of sources of data and information are sought. Yin defines the *case study* as "an empirical inquiry that investigates a contemporary phenomenon within its real-life context, especially when the boundaries between phenomenon and context are not clearly evident" because it "relies on multiple sources of evidence, with data needing to converge in a triangulating fashion" (pp. 13–14). A helpful example of this approach is provided by Yin for those who wish to further examine this combined process for data and information gathering (pp. 91–92).

Using the Results

After a sustained preparation and data collection effort, you may prefer to set the data aside while you catch up with other projects. However, it is important to maintain the momentum you have established to this point. If you set the data aside now, you may have difficulty returning to the project later. Planning your data analysis earlier will help you keep going now, working through any slump that might occur.

Most of the data you collect from a survey will be quantitative data. You need some way to summarize these numbers for your planning committee or other interested groups. Sophisticated statistical tests typically are not necessary for a needs assessment. As discussed in Chapter 1, a needs assessment is not the same as rigorous academic research. Although some of the same research skills are used, the data are used differently.

Simple descriptive statistics are usually sufficient for a needs assessment. You should perform the following calculations:

1. *Tabulate frequency distributions.* Count the number of times each response occurs for each item. For a small survey, count these responses manually, or use a simple software spreadsheet program to summarize frequencies. For a large survey, enter response data into a computer to obtain frequency distributions.
2. *Determine the range of responses.* Note the lowest response and the highest response for each item.
3. *Calculate the most appropriate measure of central tendency.* The *mean*—the arithmetic average of all responses to the item—is used most often. It is appropriate when you have a relatively narrow range of responses with a relatively even distribution. To calculate the mean, add the scores and divide by the number of responses.

Sometimes the median or the mode is a more helpful statistic. The *median* can best be understood as the middle score in the distribution. It is a more appropriate measure of central tendency when a few scores are skewed much higher or much lower than the rest of the scores. To determine the median, arrange all responses in ascending order from low to high. Count the scores, beginning with the lowest score, until you reach the middle score. That is the median. If you have an even number of scores, determine the point halfway between the two middle scores (i.e., the average of these two scores).

The *mode* is the response that occurs most frequently. It is an appropriate measure of central tendency when one particular response to an item is clearly more frequent than any other.

Statistically, calculating the mean is appropriate when analyzing interval or ratio data (e.g., age). Determining the median is appropriate when analyzing ordinal data (e.g., strongly agree, agree, disagree, strongly disagree). The mode is appropriate for nominal data (e.g., yes, no).

Desktop computers and laptops have simple spreadsheet programs that can analyze data and compute these statistics for even small surveys.

Although most survey data are quantitative, some data may be qualitative; that is, you will have verbal responses to analyze instead of numbers. If you have surveyed only a few people, you can handle open-ended questions by simply listing verbatim the responses received. Typically, the open-ended questions from a survey will yield responses that are relatively short and to the point. Some respondents may add comments in the margins that you may want to summarize as well.

Another way to handle verbal responses, especially when you have a large number of participants, is to combine similar responses into more of a summary statement. Indicate how many people offered each type of response. Be careful not to collapse similar statements too much, such that you lose some of the meaning. The more you summarize, the more you introduce your own interpretation into the responses. You want to present the responses as faithfully as possible in the way they were received. Later, you can add your own interpretation.

If you have a variety of responses to a particular question, you may need to do more collapsing and interpreting. First, read quickly through all responses to the item to get a sense of the range of responses. Think of possible categories as you read, and jot them down. Next, develop an initial list of categories. Reread the responses, and count the responses that fit into each category. As you make this first attempt at categorizing responses, you may think of additional categories that fit the data better. Add these categories to your list, rather than forcing a response into a category that seems to distort the meaning. After completing this second reading of the data, consider combining similar categories or rearranging them in some way. Finally, some miscellaneous responses may not fit any category, so report them separately. After this qualitative analysis, you may want to report the results in some quantitative form. Use frequency tabulations, the range, and measures of central tendency, as appropriate.

The final step in this phase is to share the results with your planning committee or other interested groups. Remember that the caution was raised earlier against collecting extraneous data. If you do collect too much data, you will spend too much time analyzing it. You might also give your planning committee too much information and confuse, rather than help, the planning process. Consider using graphics and PowerPoint presentations, which are readily available with most computer software suites (Dillman, 2000, pp. 95, 106).

Reviewing an Example

In addressing system-level change in schools in Victoria, Australia, through capacity building, Bond, Glover, Godfrey, Butler, and Patton (2001) described their multiple assessment efforts in the Gatehouse Project. In this school-based mental health promotion program, "the intervention is based on an under-standing of individual and social risk processes for adolescent depression and emotional well-being" (p. 370). The authors focused on the school's social environment (e.g., bullying, conflict, isolation, alienation), as well as individual cognitive and social skills. To gather the necessary information, Bond et al. (2001) used a battery of process evaluation assessments, including field notes, key informant interviews, school background audits, and the Gatehouse Project Adolescent Health Questionnaire for student input. This particular survey was quite comprehensive in terms of assessing students' perceptions of social connectedness (e.g., levels of social interaction, school connectedness, issues of victimization), levels of anxiety and depression symptoms, degree of deliberate self-harm, and usage of tobacco, alcohol, and illicit drugs. Based on the assessments, realistic capacity-building interventions were developed from a whole-school approach.

Online Resources

Visit go.jblearning.com/gilmore4 for links to these Web sites.

American College Health Association
Describes the National College Health Assessment, including generalizability, reliability, and validity discussions.

National Network for Child Care
An example of a needs assessment for a school-aged childcare program. An example of a nutrition assessment.

Western Rural Development Center
Outlines community assessment techniques. This site includes information on participant observation, social network analysis, the Delphi Technique, the nominal group process, advisory groups, community forums, and the application of these techniques.

Centers for Disease Control and Prevention
Description of the CDC's National Maternal and Infant Health Survey.

Wisconsin Department of Health and Family Services
Provides access to information on the Behavioral Risk Factor Survey and the Family Health Survey.

National Family Health Survey
Provides state and national information for India on fertility, infant and child mortality, family planning practices, maternal and child health, reproductive health, nutrition, anemia, and utilization and quality of health and family planning services.

Wisconsin's Information Network for Successful Schools (WINSS)

Examples of successful school surveys from the Wisconsin WINSS program.

References

Baumgartner, T., and Hensley, L. (2006). *Conducting and reading research in health and human performance*, 4th ed. Boston: McGraw-Hill.

Baumgartner, T., Strong, C., and Hensley, L. (2002). *Conducting and reading research in health and human performance*. New York: McGraw-Hill.

Bond, L., Glover, S., Godfrey, C., Butler, H., and Patton, G. (2001). Building capacity for system-level change in school: Lessons from the Gatehouse Project. *Health Education and Behavior, 28*, 368–383.

Bowling, A. (2006). *Research methods in health: Investigating health and health services*, 2nd ed. New York: Open University Press.

Dillman, D. A. (2000). *Mail and Internet surveys: The tailored design method*, 2nd ed. New York: John Wiley & Sons.

Fowler, F. J. (2002). *Survey research methods*, 3rd ed. Thousand Oaks, CA: Sage Publications.

Frey, J. H. (1989). *Survey research by telephone*, 2nd ed. Newbury Park, CA: Sage Publications.

Gilmore, G., Olsen, L., Taub, A., and Connell, D. (2005). Overview of the national health educator competencies update project, 1998–2004. *Health Education and Behavior, 32*, 725–737. Co-published in the *American Journal of Health Education, 36*, 363–370.

Gilmore, G., Olsen, L., Taub, A., and Connell, D. (2004). *The national health educator competencies update project, 1998–2004: Research process and methodological innovations/insights*. Silver Spring, MD: Agency for Healthcare Research and Quality.

Green, L. W., and Lewis, F. M. (1986). *Measurement and evaluation in health education and health promotion*. Palo Alto, CA: Mayfield Publishing.

Orcher, L. (2005). *Conducting research: Social and behavioral science methods*. Glendale, CA: Pyrczak Publishing.

Salant, P., and Dillman, D. A. (1994). *How to conduct your own survey*. New York: John Wiley & Sons.

Schiff, L. (2003). *Informed consent: Information, production, and ideology*. Lanham, MD: Scarecrow Press, Inc.

Sudman, S., and Bradburn, N. M. (1983). *Asking questions: A practical guide to questionnaire design*. San Francisco: Jossey-Bass Publishers.

Tanur, J. M. (Ed.). (1992). *Questions about questions: Inquiries into the cognitive bases of surveys*. New York: Russell Sage Foundation.

Yin, R. (2003). *Case study research: Design and methods*, 3rd ed. Thousand Oaks, CA: Sage Publications.

4

Multistep Surveys: The Delphi Technique

Introduction

The Delphi Technique had its beginnings in the 1950s in a study performed by the Rand Corporation for the United States Air Force, in which it was reasoned that one gets closer to the truth when there is the combined judgment of a large number of people (Linstone & Turoff, 2002). The name of the technique is derived from the Oracles at Delphi, who the ancient Greeks believed were able to predict the future (Moore, 1987). In addition to forecasting, the Delphi Technique can be used for the following purposes, as detailed by Moore (1987, p. 50): to identify goals and objectives, to examine possible alternatives, to establish priorities, to reveal group values, to gather information, and to educate a respondent group. Overall, Linstone and Turoff (2002) define the Delphi method as "a method for structuring group communication process so that the process is effective in allowing a group of individuals, as a whole, to deal with a complex problem" (p. 3).

The Delphi Technique is a group process that generates a consensus through a series of questionnaires. Usually, the respondents are unable to meet in one place due to geographical or time limitations. The process typically involves three groups: decision makers, staff, and respondents (Delbecq, Van de Ven, & Gustafson, 1986). In some organizations, decision makers and staff are in the same group. The size of the respondent group varies, with 10 to 15 participants recommended for each representative group. A questionnaire consisting of one or two broad questions is sent out to the respondents. Their responses are analyzed, and from these a second questionnaire is developed. The respondents are then asked to answer additional, more specific questions for further clarification. Their responses are again analyzed, and a third questionnaire is sent out asking for additional information. The process may end here or continue until a consensus is reached. Usually, three to five rounds are necessary. Many times, if there are no more than three rounds, the process is referred to as modified. The Delphi process aligns with the Social Diagnosis phase of the PRECEDE-PROCEED model (Green & Kreuter, 2005).

Reviewing the Strategy

Advantages
The following are some of the advantages of the Delphi Technique:

- *Pooled responses.* The Delphi Technique draws from subjective responses and is appropriate in situations where objective information is not available from other sources.
- *Spans distance and time.* People who are separated by geography or busy schedules can be involved. This ability to span distances and longer time frames is especially useful when trying to obtain an expert opinion.
- *High motivation and commitment.* Individuals who agree to participate in a Delphi study are usually highly motivated and committed, contributing a substantial amount of information.
- *Reduced influence by others.* The lack of face-to-face contact reduces conformity, domination, and/or conflict. Of note, participants can remain anonymous (Butler & Howell, 1996).
- *Enhanced response quality and quantity.* The written-response format encourages an increase in both the quality and the quantity of ideas.
- *Equal representation.* Participants' ideas are given equal representation through the synthesis.
- *Consistent participant contact.* The feedback process enables the participants to respond throughout the study and have a sense of closure upon completion of the study. The quality of the process has been enhanced with the advent of computer-based Delphi processes. This approach presents the opportunity for continuous feedback, rather than being locked into a circular response structure (Turoff & Hiltz, 1996).

Disadvantages
The Delphi Technique has the following disadvantages:

- *High cost and time commitment.* A large amount of administrative time and high costs are involved. A considerable time commitment is also required on the part of the participants. Responding to the questionnaires may take 10 hours or more.
- *Reduced clarification opportunities.* Fewer opportunities are available to clarify the meanings of specific responses, which then become open to interpretation by the staff. Because the participants do not meet directly, opportunities for clarification of comments or further discussion on areas of disagreement are limited. Points of disagreement are synthesized rather than addressed or resolved (Gilmore, 1977).

- *Reduced immediate reinforcement.* In comparison with needs assessment strategies that encourage direct participant interactivity, the Delphi Technique has fewer immediate rewards for the respondents. Thus, they must be more inherently motivated to participate.

Preparing for the Assessment

At least 30 to 45 days should be allocated to prepare for the Delphi Technique. During this time, the following tasks should be accomplished.

Develop a Workgroup

The workgroup, which usually has five to nine members, consists of staff and administrators. This group will develop and revise the questions, synthesize the responses, and determine the usefulness of the questionnaires.

Assign a Project Manager

This person should be experienced in the Delphi Technique and knowledgeable about the problem being explored. The project manager will guide the workgroup.

Enlist Sufficient Support Staff

You will need assistance with word processing the questionnaire, mailing it, and organizing the responses in a way that will facilitate the synthesis.

Establish a Timeline

A timeline will be very helpful in keeping the project on schedule.

Identify Potential Participants

The workgroup or other people who are knowledgeable about the particular need area can generate a list, or lists, of potential contacts who might be interested in participating in the Delphi exercise. These potential participants should be interested in and knowledgeable about the topic and be motivated to complete the series of questionnaires. Depending on the scope of your needs assessment, the list for each representative group can range from 25 to 100 or more people. In a study by Kroth and Peutz (2011), 113 Extension agents and educators from 13 Western states and 13 North Central states were invited to participate, with 46 agreeing to be involved. The purpose was to assess issues most needing attention over the next 5 to 7 years to attract, motivate, and retain those professionals. For the first round, there was a 41 percent return rate using a Zoomerang online survey.

Clarify Your Goals and Objectives

If your organization's decision makers are not directly involved in the Delphi process, it is important that you understand exactly what it is they seek to accomplish. Clarification of goals and objectives will help structure the questions and organize the results of each questionnaire.

Conducting the Assessment

Once the preliminary steps are completed, you are ready to begin the Delphi process. Conducting the Delphi process requires the following steps.

Develop the First Questionnaire and Pretest It

This step is crucial. The question(s) must be understandable to the respondents and generate the kind of information you are seeking. Have several members of the staff or representative groups review the question(s) for any needed clarity. The first questionnaire is generally broad in nature and simple in form, consisting of one or two open-ended questions, a request for a list with examples, or some other format that will generate information that is relevant and manageable for further questionnaires.

Choose the Participants

Individuals from the participant list, or lists, can be contacted and asked to nominate other respondents. Alternatively, the individuals can be randomly selected from the list(s). A total of 10 to 15 people should be selected for each representative group. More people may be selected if you are working with only one homogeneous group, although this number should not exceed 30 (Delbecq et al., 1986). Once the potential respondents have been identified, they should be contacted in person or by phone. Prior to asking for their involvement, they should be informed about the type of needs assessment, the purpose of the process, the composition of the respondent group(s), the time investment and commitment required on the part of each respondent, and the ways that the results will be shared. Depending on the complexity of the process, it may be necessary to convey detailed information in writing prior to asking for a commitment to be involved.

Send Out the Questionnaire with a Cover Letter to the Respondents

This step should be done as soon as possible after the respondents have been contacted. Both the questionnaire and the cover letter should be well constructed and well designed. Along with expressing appreciation for participating in the study, the cover letter should briefly outline the points that were presented in the initial contact with the participant. A response date of 2 weeks should be emphasized, and a stamped, self-addressed envelope should be enclosed for ease in responding. To encourage a timely response, you may want to send a letter or postcard in the second week, reminding the participants of the response date. A phone call also may be necessary for the late respondents.

Synthesize and Analyze the Responses to the First Questionnaire

As the questionnaires are returned, the responses can be recorded on a master list for ease of analysis. Once all questionnaires have been returned, call a meeting of the workgroup. Provide the members with a copy of the master list, which they can use to sort the items into similar categories. Each item can be placed on an index card and placed into a pile of similar items. Then, each pile can be labeled and the labeled categories listed and discussed until the group members reach a consensus regarding a final list. The items in the final list should next be summarized into clear and concise statements, which will make up the second questionnaire. Instead of using index cards, a computer can be used for this step and subsequent ones in the process.

Develop and Send Out the Second Questionnaire

The purpose of the second questionnaire is to get further clarification concerning the information gathered from the first questionnaire. It should provide an accurate summary of the results of the first questionnaire. Participants are asked to review, comment, clarify, and vote on each specific item listed in the summary from the first questionnaire. The process of developing the second questionnaire should follow the same steps as the first questionnaire. The format employed will depend on the kind of information obtained from the first questionnaire and the kind of additional information needed. Try to keep the new questionnaire short enough so that it can be completed in less than 30 minutes.

Synthesize and Analyze the Responses to the Second Questionnaire

The synthesis of the second questionnaire consists largely of a tally of the votes for each item. A tally sheet can be used that includes the list of items, the number of individuals voting for each item, the values of the individual votes, and the total vote. Comments should be summarized and then grouped with each item, as in the first questionnaire.

Develop and Send Out a Third Questionnaire, If Necessary

Often, when a ranking of importance of each item is desired, a third questionnaire can be developed and sent out. A third questionnaire can help reinforce the consensus and provide closure for the participants. The questionnaire should be designed to enable the participants to review a summary of previous comments and the results of the first vote for each item under consideration. A final ranking or vote plus any additional comments can be requested. The procedure for developing and sending out the questionnaire is the same as for the questionnaires discussed previously.

Synthesize and Analyze the Responses to the Third Questionnaire

The responses to the third questionnaire can be summarized by tallying the final vote and incorporating additional comments into the previous commentary.

Using the Results

Depending on the needs you are assessing, additional questionnaires may need to be developed and sent out to the respondents. The final questionnaire should provide a prioritized list of items that can help in the planning process. The ranking of the items can indicate to the planners which items need to be addressed early in the planning process.

When you have all the information you need, assemble the workgroup to review the data and develop a final report. This report should include a summary of all questionnaire results and recommendations for further planning based on the prioritization of the needs.

Reviewing an Example

Ratnapradipa and colleagues (2011) explored core curricular needs related to environmental health by using a modified Delphi assessment process involving 16 federal, state, and local experts. The authors used a consensus criterion of at least 60 percent agreement among the experts. In the first round, the core areas of environmental health were established. In round two, key topics in each core area were identified from 177 potential topics that were initially generated by the investigators. The experts rated each topic using a six-point Likert scale. The authors also enabled the experts to list topics in addition to the 177. In round two, a 66 percent consensus criterion was used for the selection of each topic. One week was provided for this process to take place. Round three focused on having the experts identify knowledge, attitude, and behavior questions to be used in a consumer survey. To the authors' credit, because a total of 572 draft questions were initially developed by the authors and there was a concern about expert-related fatigue and drop-out, five separate instruments comprised of approximately 115 items each were developed so just one instrument could be provided per expert based on individual areas of expertise.

Overall, the results included the identification of 27 environmental core areas, which were further reduced to 11 core for consumer/public awareness. Within these 11 core areas, 25 topics were identified. Additionally, for the consumer-related survey that was developed, 443 knowledge, attitude, and behavior items were established. Throughout the Delphi process, the authors encouraged the experts to respond to the content derived from each previous round along with making recommendations for future investigations. The authors noted that there was a high degree of expert involvement throughout the assessment process: 88 percent responded to the original request in round 1, 83 percent in round 2, and 77 percent in round 3.

Online Resources

Visit go.jblearning.com/gilmore4 for links to these Web sites.

Community Advisory Committee of the Southern Health Board
An overview of methods for consumer and community participation in the planning of health services.

Delphi
Describes what a Delphi survey is and why it is used. Provides related links on the Delphi Technique.

Meeting the Needs of Women with Disabilities
Results of a Delphi survey of disabled women. Describes the characteristics of Delphi survey respondents.

Department of Agricultural and Food Economics
Describes an example Delphi survey in great detail, including objectives, techniques, methods, and design.

Focus Groups and Delphi Surveys
Discussion of focus groups and the Delphi surveys.

Scottish Network for Chronic Pain Research
Discusses the Delphi Technique in pain research.

Western Rural Development Center
Outlines community assessment techniques. This site describes participant observation, social network analysis, the Delphi survey, the nominal group process, advisory groups, community forums, and application of these techniques.

References

Butler, L., and Howell, R. (1996). *Coping with growth: Community needs assessment techniques.* Washington State University: Western Regional Extension.

Delbecq, A., Van de Ven, A., and Gustafson, D. (1986). *Group techniques for program planning: A guide to nominal group and Delphi processes.* Middleton, WI: Green Briar Press.

Gilmore, G. (1977). Needs assessment processes for community health education. *International Journal of Health Education, 20,* 164–173.

Green, L., and Kreuter, M. (2005). *Health promotion planning: An educational and ecological approach,* 4th ed. Boston: McGraw-Hill.

Kroth, M., and Peutz, J. (2011). Workplace issues in Extension: A Delphi study of Extension educators. *Journal of Extension, 49,* 1–10.

Linstone, H., and Turoff, M. (2002). *The Delphi method: Techniques and applications.* Newark, NJ: New Jersey Institute of Technology.

Moore, C. (1987). *Group techniques for idea building.* Newbury Park, CA: Sage Publications.

Ratnapradipa, D., Brown, S., and Wodika, A. (2011). Examining the breadth and depth of environmental health through a modified Dephi technique. *American Journal of Health Education, 42,* 50–57.

Turoff, M., and Hiltz, S. (1996). Computer-based Delphi processes. In Adler, M., and Ziglio, E. (Eds.), *Gazing into the Oracle: The Delphi method and its application to social policy and public health.* London: Kingsley Publishers.

Interviewing

Introduction

If you like conversation, interviewing can be an exhilarating experience and an effective way to assess needs. Talking with people about their health needs, using the best interviewing techniques, is often as satisfying as planning a program to meet those needs.

Interviews can also bring good results. Compared to surveys, which are a very common, and perhaps overused, strategy for assessing needs, interviews are a more novel approach. People may resist completing yet another questionnaire or refuse to participate in one more telephone survey. They may agree to an interview, however, because it is different. Most people like to talk about themselves. They feel flattered when selected to answer important questions and may be primed to give you good information.

At the same time, conducting interviews is not easy. The people you want to interview are often busy and difficult to contact to schedule an interview. When you do finally reach them, they may hesitate to interrupt their activities to participate. If they do participate, they may resist talking about their health.

Despite these difficulties, interviews are a good way to assess needs. If you have the time and other resources to conduct them, they can yield important information to use in planning educational programs.

Telephone and face-to-face surveys, discussed in Chapter 3, are a form of interviewing that follows a prescribed structure. This chapter focuses on some less structured interviewing approaches, which offer more flexibility and place more responsibility on the interviewer.

What do we mean by *interview*? A good interview is an exchange of information between two people: an interviewer and an interviewee. It may also include emotional expression and persuasion, similar to a good conversation (Gorden, 1998, p. 2). These characteristics are what make the interview process so fascinating. Not only do we obtain information from interviewees, but we learn about their attitudes and emotions as well.

Interviews can be either formal or informal. Informal interviewing is difficult to distinguish from ordinary conversation. The interviewer attempts to engage people in conversations, for example, about health-related issues. The conversation may occur in a very informal setting and usually is not arranged in advance. In some instances, the interviewee may not recognize this exchange of information as constituting an interview. Typically, the interviewer will know which questions to ask and will not refer to any notes or take any notes during the interview. As soon as possible thereafter, notes are written, typed, or dictated.

Although informal interviews can yield valuable insights, we will not consider them in this chapter. Because our focus is systematic needs assessment strategies, we will limit our discussion to formal interviews.

Oftentimes, we gain insights for our process through preliminary interviews with key informants (as described in Chapter 2). Key informant interviews are a very reasonable starting point in which formal and informal leaders and representatives of the population or group one is working with are interviewed and provided with open-ended questions. One example is provided based on the work of the author and a public health team with key informants located at the Pine Ridge Reservation in South Dakota (Gilmore, Kies, McIlquham, Nogle, Whitty, & Xie, 2010). Coupled with an outreach effort called *Global Partners* (Gundersen Lutheran Health System, 2010), as part of the Gundersen Lutheran Health System in La Crosse, Wisconsin, during July 2010, a public health team joined the ongoing efforts of a medical team that traveled to the Porcupine Clinic on the Reservation. This public health team of six individuals (Gilmore et al., 2010) first reviewed relevant secondary data (Red Cloud Indian School, 2010; Schrader-Dillon & Eagle Bull, 2009), and then conducted preliminary key informant interviews with key citizens, community leaders, and health professionals.

Seven open-ended questions were used during the process:

1. Tell me about you and your family's involvement with the Pine Ridge Reservation (e.g., how long have you lived here; number of generations on this land; type of employment)?
2. What are some of the unique qualities about living here?
3. Who assists you when you are in need of assistance?
4. Are there major problems that are affecting your health at this time?
5. Are there major problems that are affecting the health of your family and community members?
6. What could be done to make things better in living here?
7. What suggestions do you have to encourage people to practice healthier activities?

The results from these questions, which were asked of selected key informants across the reservation, were summarized into a report (Gilmore et al., 2010) that was provided to the health representatives on the reservation.

During the summary process, it is important to carefully review all responses and look for trends and patterns across the commentary that can be summarized by descriptors and phrases that accompany direct quotations. It is also important to go through a preliminary review of the collected information while on site, rather than waiting until the team returns home. This allows for better clarity about what transpired and also enables a preliminary report to be co-developed and shared with community members. During the Pine Ridge experience, as a planned event prior to the public health team's departure from the reservation, an open session was held with the health staff and interested community members to share and discuss some of the key findings and to provide an opportunity for clarifying questions and discussion. Other helpful examples of the key informant process and respectful connectivity with a population are provided from a community-based participatory research perspective (Cummins, Doyle, Kindness, Lefthand, Bear Don't Walk, Bends, Broadway, Camper, Fitch, Ford, Hammer, Morrison, Richards, Young, & Eggers, 2010; Israel, Eng, Schulz, & Parker, 2005).

Reviewing the Strategy

Formal interviews are clearly identified as interviews. An individual is asked to participate in the interview. The interviewer states the purpose of the interview, describes how the person has been selected to participate, and explains that responses will be treated confidentially. During the interview, the interviewer will refer to an interview guide, usually called an *interview schedule*, and use some method of recording information.

Formal interviews are classified as highly scheduled, moderately scheduled, or nonscheduled (Stewart & Cash, 2003, pp. 88–90). At one extreme, a *highly scheduled interview* follows a very specific list of questions and instructions. For each participant, the interviewer must proceed through these questions in exactly the same way. Background information and instructions to the participant are read verbatim from a script. Follow-up questions to clarify the meaning of responses and instructions on recording responses also are clearly specified. Highly scheduled interviews are conducted face-to-face or by telephone. They are practically identical to the face-to-face or telephone surveys discussed in Chapter 3 (Stewart & Cash, 2003, pp. 139, 158).

At the other extreme, a *nonscheduled interview* gives the interviewer much more freedom and responsibility. The goals of the interview are specified, but the interviewer must decide which questions to ask and in what order. The interviewer also decides how to summarize the information received.

A nonscheduled interview is not the same as the informal interview described earlier. Although the discussion may proceed in a relaxed, free-flowing, conversational manner, a nonscheduled interview is prearranged, has a stated purpose, and follows some type of overall structure. In these respects it differs from an informal interview.

A *moderately scheduled interview* falls between these two extremes. The interviewer follows a set of questions and suggested follow-up questions but is free to use them differently during the interviews. The wording of the questions can vary, as can the order in which they are asked. Additional follow-up questions are asked if the interviewer believes they would yield helpful information. He or she need not ask all questions of each participant if adequate answers to those questions have already been obtained. The interviewer receives some guidance about summarizing the information but must decide what to include and what to omit.

The word "schedule" can be confusing in this context. An interview schedule is a list of questions you plan to ask during the interview. It is easy to confuse this meaning of *schedule* (a noun) with the act of arranging a set time and place to conduct the interview (a verb). A *scheduled interview* means one that is conducted using a prepared list of questions, not one that is arranged in advance. A *nonscheduled interview* is one that does not use a prepared list of questions. This type of interviewing is different, however, from ordinary conversation that occurs spontaneously.

In this chapter, we will discuss only moderately scheduled and nonscheduled interviews conducted face-to-face. These interviews, which are sometimes called *qualitative interviews*, "sacrifice uniformity of questioning to achieve fuller development of information" (Weiss, 1994, p. 3). We will emphasize moderately scheduled interviews because they are more frequently used to assess health needs.

Advantages

Compared to highly scheduled interviews, moderately scheduled interviews have at least three advantages:

- *They offer more opportunities to discover information.* A scheduled interview restricts the questions asked, so the information obtained is necessarily restricted as well. A moderately scheduled interview gives the interviewer freedom to explore certain subjects more extensively with some participants than with others. The interviewer may pursue a particularly insightful response in great depth and discover important information that had not been anticipated.
- *They offer the opportunity to obtain more complete information.* The interviewer can ask as many follow-up questions as necessary to encourage participants to clarify and elaborate on their responses.
- *They are especially well suited for obtaining valuable information from busy people.* If necessary, the interviewer can focus on the questions that each participant can answer most completely. By discussing in depth the areas they know best, the participants may feel they are using their time to best advantage. If pressed for time, the interviewer can skip other questions.

Disadvantages

Moderately scheduled interviews do, however, have some disadvantages compared to scheduled interviews:

- *Interviewers need more in-depth understanding of the subject of the interviews.* Because the interviewers make more judgments during the interview about which questions to ask and which questions to omit, some knowledge of the subject is essential.
- *Interviewers need more extensive training.* Knowledge of the subject is not sufficient by itself. The interviewers also need a more complete understanding of the purpose of the interviews and more opportunities to conduct and critique practice interviews. They also need to practice recording and summarizing the information.
- *Data analysis is more difficult.* Information obtained from highly scheduled interviews primarily consists of quantitative data. By contrast, moderately scheduled interviews yield primarily narrative information. Analyzing the latter type of information requires making more judgments about organization and interpretation.
- *Moderately scheduled interviews are more costly.* Typically, more time is needed to complete a moderately scheduled interview and record the information. More time is also necessary to train interviewers and analyze data. Because the interviewers need a background in health education, they may also cost more to employ than a typical survey assistant.

These advantages and disadvantages also apply to nonscheduled interviews—the difference is simply one of degree. Because nonscheduled interviews give even more freedom to, and place even more responsibility on, the interviewer, they offer even more opportunities for discovery and in-depth information. In turn, they require interviewers with more knowledge of the subject and more extensive training. Data analysis becomes even more difficult, and the whole process is even more costly.

When deciding how extensively to structure the interviews for assessing health needs, consider the following questions:

- Do you want to measure what all of your participants know about certain healthy behaviors? Or do you want to discover what needs might exist? Generally, the more you want to discover needs, the less you should structure the interviews. For example, if you believe that poor diet and lack of exercise are major contributors to personal stress, you might use more structured interviews to determine what participants know about diet and exercise. If you are not predisposed to a diet-and-exercise focus, however, you might use less structured interviews and discover other contributors to stress, such as financial difficulties, family conflicts, and various work-related pressures.

- Do you have interviewers with a background in health? The less extensive their background, the more you should structure your interviews.
- How much time and money do you have for this project? The less you have, the more you should structure your interviews.

Motivational Interviewing

An important bridge between assessment and movement toward change transpires with motivational interviewing. The two prime movers in this approach to assessment and change, William Miller and Stephen Rollnick (2002), have stated:

> There is little that is truly original in motivational interviewing. We have built on the extraordinary contributions of Carl R. Rogers and his students, particularly Thomas Gordon, who developed the methods of client-centered psychotherapy over the past 50 years. Also influential in our thinking about motivational interviewing was the work of James Prochaska and Carlo DiClemente on the transtheoretical model of change, Milton Rokeach on human values, and Daryl Bem on self-perception theory (p. xvi).

Miller and Rollnick (2002) define motivational interviewing as "a client-centered, directive method for enhancing intrinsic motivation to change by exploring and resolving ambivalence" (p. 25). In describing the essence of the process, Miller and Rollnick (2002) emphasize that motivational interviewing is not simply the application of motivational interventions (e.g., cash incentives) attempting to mimic the techniques. Rather, the process involves being more collaborative and explorative in nature, evocative in drawing ideas and insights out of others, and autonomous where the responsibility for change rests with the individual (pp. 33–35). Miller and Rollnick (2002) also emphasize the foundation of four general principles: express empathy (acceptance); develop discrepancy (perceived discrepancy between one's present behavior and related goals or values); roll with resistance (reframe to create a new momentum toward change); and support self-efficacy (belief in the person's ability to change) (pp. 37–41). In terms of the applications of motivational interviewing to health care and public health, Resnicow, DiIorio, Soet, Borrelli, Ernst, Hecht, and Thevos (2002) cite the growing interest by professionals in these disciplines to use the process. They address the time constraints that are inherent in such professional settings and the "brief negotiation" (p. 253) process that has been developed. They point out that a challenge for public health and medical practitioners is having the available time for training in motivational interviewing, along with "adopting the more facilitative and collaborative spirit of motivational interviewing in place of the more prescriptive, practitioner-centered, and directive techniques that are traditionally employed in medical settings. This represents a formidable barrier to training PH and medical practitioners" (pp. 254–255).

Formidable, but not insurmountable. Resnicow and Thevos (2002) review the research efforts regarding the motivational interview process in primary and secondary prevention modalities that address diet and physical activity, smoking cessation, medication adherence, HIV prevention, cardiovascular and diabetes management, and international applications related to infection prevention. Several of these research studies led to "mixed" results, but there were a few that yielded significant findings, such as a study in Zambia where "a statistically significant sixteenfold increase in the use of water disinfectant was observed in the motivational interviewing area over the area receiving health education and social marketing alone" (p. 267). Overall, a motivational interviewing approach can contribute to health-related benefits, and the interested reader is referred to a sampling of key references for more in-depth discussion (e.g., Rollnick, Butler, Kinnersley, Gregory, & Mash, 2010; Miller & Rollnick, 2009, 2002; Rollnick, Miller, & Butler, 2008; Miller & Moyers, 2006) as well as references from the Internet (http://www.motivationalinterview.org).

Preparing for the Assessment

To prepare for interviews, follow the same basic steps discussed for surveys. Decide what you need to know, plan for Institutional Review Board (IRB) review and informed consent (Schiff, 2003), develop a budget, prepare your questions, test and modify these questions, develop a draft of an interview schedule or guide, conduct pilot interviews, develop data analysis procedures, and design the final schedule or guide. (See Chapter 3 for a more detailed discussion of these steps.)

How these steps are accomplished, however, is different for interviews. One difference relates to the development of questions. Although drafting, testing, and modifying questions is important, at least for moderately scheduled interviews, it is not as critical to develop the ultimate questions. Ultimately, the interviewers exercise some judgment over how questions are asked during the interview. They can clarify the meaning of questions if participants are confused.

A second difference relates to the development of an interview schedule or guide. Telephone and face-to-face surveys require a highly structured interview schedule. Moderately scheduled interviews, however, place more responsibility on the interviewer. They call for a list of questions to ask, along with suggested alternate wording and follow-up questions. With this kind of interview, the instructions need not be as specific nor the questions as precisely worded.

Nonscheduled interviews require even less structure. Typically, interviewer instructions include the goals of the interview and some guidelines to follow. The interviewers then proceed to ask the questions they believe will accomplish these goals. As the name implies, a nonscheduled interview does not even use a schedule, but what is more properly called a *guide*.

A third difference relates to the development of coding and data analysis procedures. You should have some idea of how you plan to organize and analyze the data before you conduct the interviews. Try to anticipate the responses you are likely to receive and organize them into categories and general themes as best you can. This structure represents your best guess of how you will organize and eventually communicate the interview results. It will have considerably less detail than the coding and data analysis procedures developed for telephone and face-to-face surveys.

The structure is also more tentative. You can anticipate how you want to use the data, but you must always wait to actually receive the data before committing to a particular structure. The data may suggest other categories and themes that you could not anticipate before conducting the interviews. The less structured your interviews are, the less you can plan your coding and data analysis procedures in advance.

Moderately scheduled and nonscheduled interviews follow the same basic preparation steps as surveys, but less effort is required for some of them. Do not think you are getting off easy, though. The time you save preparing for the interviews you will spend—and more besides—after the interview.

Details are provided elsewhere (e.g., Christopher, Burhansstipanov, & Knows His Gun-McCormick, 2005) regarding the development of assessment procedures and particularly an interviewer training manual that were in concordance with the population being assessed. In the instance of the work by Christopher and colleagues (2005), their assessment primarily focused on cervical cancer screening and the women of the Apsaalooke Reservation on the Northern Plains of the United States.

Conducting the Assessment

Many steps used for conducting telephone and face-to-face surveys also apply to moderately scheduled or nonscheduled interviews. You must select a sample of respondents to interview, recruit and train interviewers, and collect and record the data. How these steps are accomplished may vary considerably, depending on the interviews.

Select a Sample of Respondents

In some instances, the same probability sampling procedures used for surveys are appropriate for structured or nonstructured interviews. The less structured your interviews are, however, the more you may want to interview specific people. Remember that data analysis is a more extensive undertaking. Consider purposefully selecting a smaller number of key people, rather than drawing a systematic sample.

You may decide to interview "knowledgeable insiders," known as *key informants* (Weiss, 1994, p. 20), who have the best perspective on the health needs of a particular community or organization. These individuals are selected because they can offer a broader view, for example, of community issues or societal trends than you would obtain from a random sample (Queeney, 1995, pp. 136–138). In such cases, you do not claim to have selected a representative sample of a given population. Instead, you purposefully select as many as 10 to 15 individuals who can offer critical insights.

This approach of selecting a limited number of key informants is an example of a *nonprobability* or *purposive* sample, in which individuals are selected because they represent a range of diverse and important perspectives (Green & Lewis, 1986, p. 231). Make sure to include more people in your sample than you need to interview. Some individuals will decline to participate, and others will be virtually impossible to contact.

Select and Train the Interviewers

Because moderately scheduled and nonscheduled interviews place more responsibility on the interviewers, look for people who have both interviewing skills and a background in community health. Try to select individuals who are comfortable with and enjoy one-on-one, face-to-face situations. Look for people who are especially skilled in active and empathetic listening, people who can listen carefully to what interviewees are saying without preconceptions (Gorden, 1998, pp. 82–84). The more knowledge they have of the needs assessment project, the better. Knowledgeable interviewers have more credibility with interviewees and can make informed judgments about which follow-up questions to ask and which leads to follow.

Extensive interviewer training is necessary for moderately scheduled and nonscheduled interviews. As with telephone and face-to-face surveys, interviewers need to understand the purpose of the interviews, why the interviews are important, and how the information will be used. They need instructions on contacting participants, handling ambiguous responses, and recording data. Compared to those conducting surveys, though, the interviewers need more information about the assumptions and philosophy that ground the project. They also need more instructions about what kinds of follow-up questions to ask. Finally, they need more opportunities to conduct and then critique practice interviews.

Collect and Record the Data

From your sample, develop a priority list of people to interview. Then begin to arrange appointments to conduct the interviews, preferably by telephoning or e-mailing the individuals. State the purpose of the interviews, which organization is conducting them, why they are important, and how the information will be used. Explain how the individuals were selected to participate and describe procedures for keeping responses confidential. Then ask for an interview at a time and place convenient for the participant. Specify how long the interview will take.

Scheduling the interviews can take considerable time. If you are using the telephone, you will not reach everyone on the first try. Attempt to determine the best time to call back, and try again. Some people will not respond to an e-mail request for an interview. Resend your message after a few days, and then switch to the telephone to contact nonrespondents. Some people, particularly health professionals, are very busy and difficult to reach. Decide in advance how many "call backs" to make before skipping that person and contacting someone else.

If possible, conduct the interviews in places that have some association with your needs assessment. If interviewing health professionals about their needs for continuing education, offer to meet them in their offices or conference rooms. If interviewing consumers about their eating patterns, offer to interview them in their homes. These locations make participation in the interview convenient, but they also help the individuals focus on the subject of the interview. Be sure to arrive on time and conclude within the agreed-upon time.

When conducting interviews, take a few moments to set the stage. Although the participants have been contacted by phone to set up the interviews, they may have forgotten what was said or may not have listened very closely. Repeat the same information about the project to refresh their memories. Emphasize confidentiality. Have the interviewees sign a consent form that gives permission to use the information obtained (Seidman, 1998, pp. 56–58). If a telephone interview is being conducted, as with the telephone survey process in Chapter 3, respondents can respond verbally to consent-related questions, with notations made by the interviewer. A sample consent form is included at the end of this chapter.

The structure of an interview follows the same approach suggested for a survey in Chapter 3. Begin with questions that are relatively easy to answer. Ask potentially threatening or sensitive questions near the middle of the interview, and hold demographic questions until near the end.

Interviewers should not refer to their interview schedule or guide as often as they would for a telephone or face-to-face survey. As much as possible, they should memorize the basic sequence of questions. Seidman (1998, pp. 63–78) urges interviewers to concentrate on the interviewees and take advantage of promising leads.

Remember that nonverbal cues are important for interviews. Gorden describes seven nonverbal behaviors that affect the quality of the data: physical distance, body position, touch, eye contact, facial expression, tone of voice, and pace of the interview (Gorden, 1998, pp. 67–74). Give the participants enough space to communicate with a sense of freedom, and position yourself to talk with them one-on-one as equals. Face the participants, and use your posture to communicate a sense of relaxed anticipation. Use good eye contact, nod, and smile appropriately. An appropriate tone of voice is also important. Some participants may respond to a soft-spoken, low-key interviewer. Other participants may need more lively prodding to reveal good information.

Probing techniques are an essential part of interviewing. *Probing* involves the use of neutral prompts to persuade interviewees to answer questions fully and completely. It is necessary when interviewees offer no response at all or give answers that are incomplete, irrelevant, poorly organized, or unclear. Probes are intended to "elicit more details without changing the focus of the questioning" (Rubin & Rubin, 2005, p. 137). Examples of practical probing questions are provided by Angrosino (2007).

Probes are used to gain greater detail, elaboration, or clarification. Who, what, when, where, or how questions can encourage interviewees to provide more detailed information. Gentle, approving nods and neutral comments (e.g., "yes," "uh-huh") or questions (e.g., "anything else?," "then what?") are examples of elaboration probes; they are designed to keep the interviewees talking. Silence is also an effective elaboration probe. Resist the temptation to fill in gaps in the conversation. Instead, let the interviewees do the talking as long as they have relevant information to offer.

To clarify ambiguous, unclear, contradictory, or irrelevant answers, ask neutral questions (e.g., "What do you mean?," "Why do you say that?"). You can also restate the original question or summarize what has been said so far to encourage additional comments. Finally, appearing puzzled may result in clarification of a previous response. When probing, watch your emphasis on particular words, so as not to change the content or focus of a question.

Before concluding the interview, take a minute to review the schedule or guide to ensure that all pertinent questions have been asked. This review is especially important whenever questions have been asked in a different order from the schedule or guide, because it helps to prevent overlooking some questions. Finally, thank the interviewee for participating, and conclude the interview promptly.

Recording data poses special challenges for moderately scheduled or nonscheduled interviews. Unlike with surveys, writing every word in neat little boxes is not possible. Tape recording the interview is a possibility. A tape recording gives a complete record of the interview, which is important for some interviews. Some participants—particularly those with less education—may feel inhibited, however, by the presence of a tape recorder. More important, tape recordings require time and money to transcribe. Word-for-word transcriptions take from 2 to 6 hours for every hour of interview time (Gorden, 1987, p. 263).

Most needs assessments do not require the same precision in recording data as rigorous academic research. An alternative to word-for-word transcription is to summarize the interview. That is, one can transcribe critical statements in their entirety, but condense other statements. Repetitive and unimportant comments are skipped altogether. This summary will take significantly less time to transcribe, but it requires a knowledgeable transcriber who can judge what to include and what to omit.

For most needs assessments, effective note-taking during the interview is a good way to record data. This note-taking is more difficult than that performed for a survey. The questions are not as standardized, and the answers tend to be longer. The more structured the interview, the easier note-taking will be. When extensive note-taking is difficult during the interview, jot down key words or phrases. As soon as possible after the interview (preferably on the same day), expand these notes into a more detailed summary of the interview. Develop this summary on paper, at the computer, or on tape for later transcription.

Using the Results

What to do with the data is a major consideration when using moderately scheduled or nonscheduled interviews to assess needs. As noted earlier, talking with people about their needs can be exhilarating. After the interviews are over, however, you must make sense of the data stacked on your desk or stored in your computer.

With structured telephone or face-to-face surveys, this phase is more straightforward. The data collected from surveys are mostly quantitative, and procedures for analysis will have been developed during the preparation phase. Qualitative data typically are limited, both by the number of open-ended questions asked and by the scope of responses received.

In contrast, in moderately scheduled or nonscheduled interviews, the data are primarily qualitative. To some extent, you have tried to anticipate some responses and important categories during the preparation phase. Now you must determine whether these categories are still appropriate. Other categories may have become apparent during the interviews.

Use the questions asked during the interviews to suggest categories for data analysis. Remain open to other categories that emerge from the participants' responses. The more structured your interviews have been, the more appropriate your questions will remain for organizing the data.

The less structured your interviews, however, the more you will have to develop another way to organize the data. Look for themes that are suggested by one or more of the categories. This exercise may require reading the interview notes several times, developing a tentative structure, and refining that structure over a period of time. Less structured interviews require less time to develop questions before the interviews take place, but they require more time and effort to organize and analyze data after the interviews are complete.

With moderately scheduled or nonscheduled interviews, you may not have asked everyone the same questions. Thus, you cannot simply count how many participants expressed a certain need. Instead, you may have to present a narrative picture of the needs expressed. In this portrayal, use case examples from the best responses to illustrate the needs you are describing. The less structured your interviews, the more necessary this narrative picture. Seidman

(1998, pp. 101–105) suggests constructing profiles or vignettes to illustrate the needs of particular individuals.

The concepts of reliability and validity do not directly apply to qualitative data, but the same underlying principles apply (Seidman, 1998, pp. 16–20). Seek to establish the credibility of your data. Look for consistent responses within each interview as well as consistency across interviews. For example, if late in an interview a participant contradicts an earlier response, data from that interview are not as credible as data from an interview that is free of such contradictions. It also is important not to overgeneralize the information, where you generalize "beyond the groups and settings examined in your project" (Gibbs, 2007, p. 102). As an example, one should not let the example of one person, no matter how unique, unintentionally appear to be what many in the group are doing, unless that action has been verified.

Finally, consider how to present your findings to a planning committee or other interested groups. With a structured survey, you can rely heavily on a quantitative summary of the data and specific recommendations that follow. With moderately scheduled and nonscheduled interviews, however, more responsibility rests on you to present and interpret the findings in a way that is faithful to the data.

Reviewing an Example

A face-to-face semi-structured (moderately scheduled) questionnaire was used by Oladepo and colleagues (2008–2009) to assess the cervical cancer awareness, knowledge, perceived susceptibility, and screening practices of female students at the University of Ibadan in Nigeria. Pretesting of the draft questions took place in an adjacent region in Nigeria in order to address issues related to the comprehension and sequencing of questions. Eight interviewers were trained to ask the questions in a friendly manner in which they first introduced themselves to the respondents, followed by a statement of the purpose of the assessment, the confidentiality of the information to be provided, and the voluntary nature of participation. Following the interviews, the responses to the open-ended questions were coded and analyzed using descriptive statistics from the Statistical Package for Social Sciences (SPSS).

The findings indicated that 63.1 percent of the 350 respondents involved in the study had heard about cervical cancer, with 90 percent perceiving cervical cancer as a serious/very serious illness. Additionally, the "overall knowledge of cervical cancer causation, risk factors, symptoms, screening test, and prevention are low" (p. 301). Selected misconceptions prevailed regarding predisposing factors, with only 13.7 percent indicating abnormal bleeding as a symptom. Of additional concern to the authors, there was a low perception of personal susceptibility to cervical cancer, and only 2.6 percent of the respondents having had a cervical cancer screening test. The authors concluded that "integrated and interactive educational programs are urgently needed to increase knowledge, [and] stimulate positive attitudinal disposition to screening practices" (p. 302).

Online Resources

Visit go.jblearning.com/gilmore4 for links to these Web sites.

Community Advisory Committee of the Southern Health Board
An overview of methods for consumer and community participation in the planning of health services.

National Statistics Office
Republic of the Philippines notes of the National Demographic and Health Survey.

University of Surrey Social Research Update
Telephone methods for social surveys.

National Network for Child Care
An example of a student interview.

Health Bulletin
Role of the interviewer in data collection.

Canadian Community Health Survey
An example of a health survey methodology that includes various surveys and questionnaires.

Health Survey for England
Overview of a sample health survey done in England.

References

Angrosino, M. (2007). *Doing ethnographic and observational research*. Los Angeles: Sage Publications.

Christopher, S., Burhansstipanov, L., and Knows His Gun-McCormick, A. (2005). Using a CBPR approach to develop an interviewer training manual with members of the Apsaalooke Nation. In Israel, B., Eng, E., Schulz, A., and Parker, A. (Eds.), *Methods in community-based participatory research for health* (pp. 128–145). San Francisco: Jossey-Bass.

Cummins, C., Doyle, J., Kindness, L., Lefthand, M., Bear Don't Walk, U., Bends, A., Broadway, S., Camper, A., Fitch, R., Ford, T., Hammer, S., Morrison, A.,

Richards, C., Young, S., and Eggers, M. (2010). Community-based participatory research in Indian country. *Family and Community Health, 33,* 166–174.

Gibbs, G. (2007). *Analyzing qualitative data.* Los Angeles: Sage Publications.

Gilmore, G., Kies, B., McIlquham, B., Nogle, A., Whitty, J., and Xie, H. (2010). *Pine Ridge Reservation public health needs and capacity assessment, July 18–23, 2010: Process and summary.* La Crosse, WI: University of Wisconsin–La Crosse.

Gorden, R. (1998). *Basic interviewing skills.* Prospect Heights, IL: Waveland Press.

Gorden, R. (1987). *Interviewing: Strategy, techniques, and tactics.* Chicago: Dorsey Press.

Green, L., and Lewis, F. (1986). *Measurement and evaluation in health education and health promotion.* Palo Alto, CA: Mayfield Publishing.

Gundersen Lutheran Health System. (2010). *Global partners.* La Crosse, WI: Author.

Israel, B., Eng, E., Schulz, A., and Parker, E. (Eds.). (2005). *Methods in community-based participatory research for health.* San Francisco: Jossey-Bass.

Miller, R., Bedney, B., and Guenther-Grey, C. (2003). Assessing organizational capacity to deliver HIV prevention services collaboratively: Tales from the field. *Health Education and Behavior, 30,* 582–600.

Miller, W., and Moyers, T. (2006). Eight stages in learning motivational interviewing. *Journal of Teaching in the Addictions, 5,* 3–17.

Miller, W., and Rollnick, S. (2009). Ten things that motivational interviewing is not. *Behavioural and Cognitive Psychotherapy, 37,* 129–149.

Miller, W., and Rollnick, S. (2002). *Motivational interviewing: Preparing people for change.* New York: The Guilford Press.

Oladepo, O., Ricketts, O., and John-Akinola, Y. (2008–2009). Knowledge and utilization of cervical cancer screening services among Nigerian students. *International Quarterly of Community Health Education, 29,* 293–304.

Queeney, D. (1995). *Assessing needs in continuing education: An essential tool for quality improvement.* San Francisco: Jossey-Bass Publishers.

Red Cloud Indian School. (2010). *Pine Ridge Indian Reservation demographics.* Pine Ridge, SD: Author.

Resnicow, K., DiIorio, C., Soet, J., Borrelli, B., Ernst, D., Hecht, J., and Thevos, A. (2002). Motivational interviewing in medical and public health settings. In W. R. Miller and S. Rollnick, *Motivational interviewing: Preparing people for change* (pp. 251–269). New York: The Guilford Press.

Rollnick, S., Butler, C., Kinnersley, P., Gregory, J., and Mash, B. (2010). Motivational interviewing. *British Medical Journal, 340,* 1242–1245.

Rollnick, S., Miller, W., and Butler, C. (2008). *Motivational interviewing in health care: Helping patients change behavior.* New York: The Guilford Press.

Rubin, H., and Rubin, I. (2005). *Qualitative interviewing: The art of hearing data,* 2nd ed. Thousand Oaks, CA: Sage Publications.

Schiff, L. (2003). *Informed consent: Information, production, and ideology.* Lanham, MD: Scarecrow Press, Inc.

Schrader-Dillon, L., and Eagle Bull, A. (2009). *2009 health report*. Pine Ridge, SD: Oglala Sioux Tribe Health Administration.

Seidman, I. (1998). *Interviewing as qualitative research: A guide for researchers in education and the social sciences*, 2nd ed. New York: Teachers College Press.

Stewart, C., and Cash, W. (2003). *Interviewing: Principles and practices*, 10th ed. Boston: McGraw-Hill.

Weiss, R. (1994). *Learning from strangers: The art and method of qualitative interview studies*. New York: Free Press.

Informed Consent Area-Wide Telephone Worksite Survey

**Note: This informed consent form will be read verbally via telephone. Respondents will be required to state "I agree" or "I disagree" after each statement. The subjects' responses will be recorded by the telephone surveyor. Agreement with all five statements is required prior to the collection of any data.

1. I have been informed that the purpose of this study is to conduct an area-wide telephone survey, providing up-to-date statistics on smoke-free worksites in order to ensure the health and safety of employees and other community members.

I agree ——————   I disagree ——————

2. I have been informed that the survey will take approximately 15 minutes to complete.

I agree ——————   I disagree ——————

3. I have been informed that I am free to withdraw from the study at any time without penalty.

I agree ——————   I disagree ——————

4. I have been informed that the data will be held separately from the identification of the source. The County Health Department will retain names, addresses, and phone numbers of business participants in order to develop a list of smoke-free worksites, what smoke-free policies they have in place, when the policy was put in place, the status of current cessation support programs available to employees, and the level of interest in support services by the county. The survey results will not identify business finances nor health insurance information.

I agree ——————   I disagree ——————

5. I have been informed that the results of this survey may be published in scholarly journals without the mention of specific business names involved. The names of businesses that are smoke-free may be published in various media outlets as a way to positively recognize their contribution to the health enhancement of others.

I agree ——————   I disagree ——————

Recorder:

Name ———————————————— Date ————————————————

Signature ——————————————————————————————————

Source: Based on a consent form developed by Jill Hubbard, MPH candidate, and thesis committee, University of Wisconsin–La Crosse. Used with permission.

Assessments with Groups

A variety of methods are available to conduct needs and capacity assessments with assembled groups. In the next five chapters, the following types of assessments will be discussed: the nominal group process, focus groups, community forums, participant observation, and photovoice. These strategies often are coupled with other assessment approaches in an effort to gain a more in-depth understanding of the reported needs and available resources. Additionally, two important contexts for group needs assessments through technology and large-scale community-based formats will be addressed.

6

Group Participation Process: Nominal Group

Introduction

The nominal group process was developed in 1968 by Andre Delbecq and Andrew Van de Ven (Delbecq, Van de Ven, & Gustafson, 1986) for assessments in business settings. It was based on the involvement of a few target audience representatives in a highly structured process to qualify and quantify specific needs. Since its development, the process has been used by a variety of professionals, including those in health care, human service agencies, voluntary organizations, university extensions, and educational settings (Moon, 1999; Queeney, 1995; Butler & Howell, 1993; Delbecq et al., 1986; Gilmore, 1977).

The nominal group process is a consensus method (Bowling, 2006) that utilizes groups of five to seven people who have some knowledge of the issues being examined. Group members are asked to write responses to a question without discussing it amongst themselves. Each participant then shares one of his or her responses in a round-robin fashion until every response from each individual has been recorded. The responses are clarified through discussion. Next, the participants select and rank a stated number of items that they think are the most important. The process may stop at this point or a discussion of the preliminary vote may be followed by a final vote. The assessment produces quantified estimates of consensus by using both quantitative and qualitative processes (Bowling, 2006).

Reviewing the Strategy

Although not a great deal of reading is required of the participants, possession of a clear and concise writing ability by the representatives greatly aids the process. Group involvement and understanding of health issues are important requirements of the representatives as well. The nominal group process provides both quantitative data, in the sense of voted-upon priorities, and qualitative data, in terms of a descriptive discussion of the problem (Delbecq et al., 1986). The qualitative data flow from the discussion is characteristic of most of the nominal group process. As part of this flow, members often provide critical incidents or personal anecdotes. The combined qualitative and quantitative data encourage professional reaction to client needs.

One difficulty that planners face when using the nominal group process is finding people who are willing to commit more than an hour of their time to the process. You may want to elicit participation by invitation—either of specific people or in an open situation in which people can reply with a commitment to participate. You can also seek cooperation from groups already in existence. MacPhail (2001) has reported that the process works well with school-aged youth, primarily because every participant has an opportunity to be involved in the process, accuracy is reflected in the ideas of the participants, and the process is clearly established.

Advantages
The nominal group process offers a number of advantages:

- *Direct involvement of target groups.* Those who may be most affected by a particular problem can be actively involved in its identification and scope.
- *Planned interactivity.* All participants have an equal opportunity to share their ideas and be actively involved.
- *Diverse opinions.* Because of the disciplined process, minority opinions and conflicting ideas are tolerated. The process attempts to avoid the evaluation of the ideas until the very end, when voting takes place. The process avoids arguments over semantics and wording through a clarification step.
- *Full participation.* Because everyone is given an opportunity first to write down their ideas and then to discuss them, all are encouraged to participate. This higher degree of participation also tends to reduce the potential for control or use of hidden agendas by one or two participants.
- *Creative atmosphere.* The nature of this group process, especially because it encourages the writing down of ideas and discussion, generates a creative tension that stimulates more ideas.
- *Recognition of common ground.* Participants can discover areas of "common ground" among those who are present in the process, thereby enhancing the *esprit de corps* (Hair & Walsh-Bowers, 1992).

Disadvantages
The disadvantages of the nominal group process are as follows:

- *Time commitment.* Because of the amount of time required, scheduling problems may arise and it may be difficult to find participants who are willing to commit more than an hour of their time.

- *Competing issues.* The group responses may deviate from the intended direction of the written questions, and participants may end up focusing on an issue different from the original.
- *Participant bias.* Biases can enter into this process because it encourages sharing personal opinions, beliefs, and experiences.
- *Segmented planning involvement.* Often the people who identify the need have no further involvement in the continuing program planning process.

Preparing for the Assessment

Four to 8 weeks before conducting the nominal group process, the following preliminary work should be completed.

Identify Potential Groups for Participation

Ask yourself which specific populations comprise your target audience during a particular programmatic phase or time period (e.g., health education for primary prevention through immunizations). Next, consider what sample size of the target audience would reflect that group's needs. Identify specific people who can make up that sample and hence should be invited to a nominal group meeting.

Enlist and Train Facilitators

Attempt to have a facilitator for each grouping of five to seven people. Explain to the facilitators the purpose of the nominal group process and the specific steps they will follow. Also, have them assist you in the development of the question to be posed to the representatives.

To fully prepare facilitators for the various details related to the process, we recommend taking them through a trial run as participants. Compose a question and then move the facilitators through the entire process. Following this experience, allow time for specific questions about the process. Emphasize the need for preplanning, particularly in regard to arrangement of facilities and materials.

Develop the Question

This question must be clear and simply stated. Delbecq et al. (1986) have emphasized that the question should be generated after considering (1) the objective of the meeting, (2) an example of the type of items sought, (3) the development of alternative questions, and (4) the pilot testing of alternative questions with a sample group. A planning committee can be very helpful during this part of the process. One example of a question is, "What do you consider to be the major health problems you are facing at this time?" Minkler and Hancock (2008) in discussing the community dialogues approach of the National Coalition for Healthier Cities and Communities/National Civic League, identify other questions that can be used that have a more positive focus, including "What do you believe are the two or three most important characteristics of a healthy community?" and "What makes you most proud of our community?" (p. 160). One of these questions can be placed at the top of a sheet of paper and copied to hand out to the participants.

Arrange for the Facilities and Necessary Materials

Consider where to hold a meeting of your representatives. You may find that it is best to hold several meetings at different locations for the convenience of the target audience. This approach has been used in multicounty assessments by the author, for example. The following materials will be needed: one marking board, a flipchart (or other large writing surface for each small group), index cards (10 to 18 cards per person), handouts stating the group questions, pencils, and an information sheet to collect demographic data. You will need a large meeting room with enough space to accommodate smaller groups of five to seven people. The room should be equipped with tables or desks and should be comfortable. If it is necessary to use the large room for several smaller groups, try to keep the groups as separate as possible so the work of one group does not influence or hinder other groups.

Conducting the Assessment

Complete the following steps to conduct the assessment.

Convene as a Large Group

Explain the purpose of the meeting and the process that will be used. Establish a comfortable environment.

Arrange Participants into Groups and Assign a Facilitator to Each Group

Assign five to seven members per group. Those selected as participants should be representative of, and knowledgeable about, the community in question. The facilitator should introduce him- or herself and emphasize the need for full participation. It is important to keep in mind that the nominal group process is designed to encourage everyone to participate openly without being impeded or overwhelmed by the titles of others in the group. (It is helpful for the participants to introduce themselves without stating their positions of employment.)

Pose a Single Question and Have the Participants Write Down Their Responses

It is best if the group's question can appear in writing on a marking board or flipchart and on handout sheets. Overall, handouts are the easiest for the participants to use because they keep the question in front of the group members and provide space to write responses. Handouts also tend to keep the participants focused on the task, rather than gazing about the room. An alternative approach is to just write the question on a marking board, flipchart, or overhead projector transparency.

Although the actual amount of time necessary to write the responses will vary depending on the particular question, an approximate amount of time would be 15 minutes. It is important that the group proceed in absolute silence. Such an approach enables each member to reflect carefully upon his or her own ideas, to be motivated by the observance of others who are working diligently by writing down their responses, and to be involved in a competition-free atmosphere where premature decisions do not have to be made.

Elicit Individual Responses in a Round-Robin Fashion

One participant begins by giving a single response, the next gives a single response, and this process continues until each participant has contributed a single response. As the responses are stated, the group leader writes them on the marking board or flipchart, numbering each item. The same process is repeated until all contributions have been recorded. This procedure enables each group member to fully participate. During this time, no discussion is permitted regarding the form, format, or meaning of a participant's response.

Clarify the Meaning of the Responses

Take time to be certain each response is clearly understood. Allow participants time to discuss what they meant by a particular response, the logic behind it, and its relative importance. However, this is not the time for argumentation and lobbying. The group leader must direct the proceedings so that only clarification takes place. Combine items with the same meaning.

Conduct and Discuss a Preliminary Vote

From the original list of responses, participants are directed to select and rank a stated number of items that they consider the most important. This ranking is accomplished by writing each of the statements on a separate index card and then rank ordering them. Make sure to distribute to each participant the appropriate number of index cards in accordance with the number of statements to be ranked. Delbecq et al. (1986) point out that group members can prioritize only five to nine items with some degree of reliability. Participants are asked to list one statement per index card. This is done by citing the statement number in the upper-left portion of the card, with a brief notation of key words from the statement in the center of the card. When all participants have accomplished this task for the statements they have selected, they should be encouraged to focus on the cards for ranking purposes. This will assist in decreasing any interference with their concentration during this important phase. Participants rank the cards by placing the rank number in the lower-right portion of the card and circling or underlining it. It is easiest to have individuals use a reverse rank order process. For example, if five items are being ranked, have participants list the highest-ranked item as 5 (i.e., the weighted value of the first ranked item). This will assist the facilitator as he or she lists the values on the marking board or flipchart during the feedback phase (see below). Otherwise, the facilitator must translate the actual rank values into weighted values prior to writing them on the board.

On the marking board (or flipchart), the group leader then records the rankings assigned to the statement selected by each participant (or has each participant come to the board to record his or her rankings). The facilitator totals the votes after all participants have contributed their rankings. The item with the largest numerical total represents the top-priority issue.

Discuss the various explanations related to the voting patterns. It may be valuable to discuss the high vote getters and the low vote getters. It also may be useful to redefine the meaning of selected items to be certain that all participants are clear on their meaning. Should any overriding concerns about the end result arise, it would be of value to provide the participants with another opportunity to vote.

Conduct a Final Vote

For this step, two procedures can be used: (1) as in the preliminary vote, select a stated number of the most important items and then reverse rank order them; or (2) select a stated number of the most important items and then rate them. To rate them, if seven major items are selected, each item could be rated on a scale from 0 (not important) to 10 (very important). This procedure provides insight regarding the magnitude of differences between the major items.

Calculate the Total Vote

Remembering that several groups of representatives may be participating in this process, it is important to calculate a grand total vote. First, the items from all groups are arranged into similar categorical areas (as closely as possible), and then the numbers from the rank ordering or rating exercises are added together in each categorical area. For example, if three items from group 1, two items from group 2, and four items from group 3 relate to health problems with rodent infestation, the total value (from ranking or rating) is calculated for all nine items. The resulting value is then listed for the categorical need area of "health problems related to rodent infestation." As the total votes are calculated for each categorical area, it will be realized that they can be placed in descending order. The categorical area with the largest number is considered to be of the highest priority.

Compile and Prioritize the Data

Once the data are compiled for each group, the next task is to combine similar need areas and the ratings (see **Table 6-1** and **Table 6-2**). Similar specific needs from each group are assimilated into a combined need statement. Also, the

TABLE 6-1
Nominal Group Process: Organizing and Combining the Data

Plot Group Results (for given geographical area)					
Group I		*Group II*		*Group II*	
Specific Need	*Rating*	*Specific Need*	*Rating*	*Specific Need*	*Rating*
A	40	A	2	A	28
B	33	B	15	B	7
C	0	C	17	C	19
D	50	D	28	D	44
E	2	E	48	E	12
F	19	F	41	F	22
G	21	G	3	G	37
H	33	H	0	H	18
I	5	I	29		
J	16	J	35		
		K	21		
		L	38		
		M	9		

Note: These are *specific* need priorities.

Combine *Similar Specific* Needs and Their Ratings

Example: Item D (Group I) + Item F (Group II) = Item H (Group III) =

Specific Need	*Rating*
Combined need statement	109

TABLE 6-2
Nominal Group Process: Establishing General Need Areas

Final Ranking	Final Rating
First general need area	221
a. Combined need statement	109
b. Specific need statement	44
c. Specific need statement	35
d. Specific need statement	33
Second general need area (follow same procedure)	

Note: May have to use "miscellaneous" and "unclassifiable" categories as general need areas.

individual ratings for each specific need are combined (see the second step in Table 6-1). Finally, general need areas are established and aligned with a grouped rating value for each area (combined and general need areas). The quantitative analysis relates to the final rating values.

Needs assessed through the nominal group process are carefully reviewed by the planning committee. Although the qualitative and quantitative data presented in Table 6-2 appear to be absolute, one should not be guided solely by this tabular arrangement. Consider the commentary of your planning committee regarding additional needs that may not have been directly stated, but rather were implied. Consider potential reformulations of the general and combined need areas, as well as potential resources and barriers in addressing each one of the identified needs. Then have the planning committee establish the final priority listing.

Using the Results

One particular advantage resulting from the nominal group data compilation is that you have a quantified summary of the group discussion. This summary can be used in your planning process as one source of information. However, make certain to remind your planning committee that it is not to be construed as the end result of an explicit research process but rather as the summary of a group interaction process. Inform them that the numbers are not absolutes. Whether you choose to address those needs with the highest-priority listing will depend on multiple factors, such as lead time, available resources, target audience readiness, and opportunities for success. For example, you initially may wish to address a lower-priority need because of the availability of resources and the high chances for success. Where and when you start can be a planning committee decision.

Reviewing an Example

Place (2007), a faculty member in the Department of Agricultural Education and Communication at the University of Florida, uses the nominal group process (NGP) in assessing the ideas of new extension agents regarding the effective involvement of advisory committee members. In addition to offering a review of the NGP steps to take, Place (2007) specifies some of the benefits of the process, including everyone having an equal opportunity to participate; greater opportunity for more ideas to be offered; and greater buy-in by the members to the process and the outcomes. The NGP has been beneficial because of the active involvement from each individual that is stimulated by the process. In addition, because the focus is on the generation of ideas by the new agents for actively involving advisory committee members, capacity is being reviewed and enhanced. Six cohort groups of new agents have gone through the process resulting in three major categories with aligned subcategories. They have included (1) Advisory Committee Management with a focus on recruiting, orientation and training, building rapport and relationships, and recognition and rewards; (2) Meeting Management with a focus on comfortable settings, and the prompt, effective use of time; (3) Committee Involvement in Extension Programming with a focus on identifying grassroots needs, and actual committee member involvement (e.g., in needs analysis, marketing, program facilitation). By going through the process, the agents learn about the NGP along with sharing ideas about the value of developing and working with advisory committees, a valuable part of the capacity dimension of Extension services.

Online Resources

Visit go.jblearning.com/gilmore4 for links to these Web sites.

Community Advisory Committee of the Southern Health Board
An overview of methods for consumer and community participation in the planning of health services.

Michigan State University Extension
Outlines the nominal group process and presents the advantages of using the process.

Center for Rural Studies, University of Vermont
Gives an overview of the nominal group process, the role of the facilitator, pros and cons of the process, and when to use the process.

Western Rural Development Center
Outlines community assessment techniques. This site discusses participant observation, social network analysis, the Delphi Technique, the nominal group process, advisory groups, community forums, and application of these techniques.

Nominal Group Technique
Provides an explanation of the nominal group process and lists resources for further reading on the process.

Iowa State University Extension
Describes the nominal group process and outlines the steps of the technique.

References

Bowling, A. (2006). *Research methods in health and health services*. New York: Open University Press.

Butler, L., and Howell, R. (1993). *Coping with growth: Community needs assessment techniques*. Washington State University, Pullman: Western Regional Extension.

Delbecq, A., Van de Ven, A., and Gustafson, D. (1986). *Group techniques for program planning: A guide to nominal group and Delphi processes*. Middletown, WI: Green Briar Press.

Gilmore, G. (1977). Needs assessment processes for community health education. *International Journal of Health Education, 20,* 164–173.

Hair, H., and Walsh-Bowers, R. (1992). Promoting the development of assessment. *Journal of Community Psychology, 20,* 289–303.

MacPhail, A. (2001). Nominal group technique: A useful method for working with young people. *British Educational Research Journal, 27,* 161–170.

Minkler, M., and Hancock, T. (2008). Community-driven asset identification and issue selection. In M. Minkler and N. Wallerstein (Eds.), *Community-based participatory research for health: From process to outcomes,* 2nd ed. (pp. 153–169). San Francisco: Jossey-Bass.

Moon, R. (1999). Finding diamonds in the trenches with the nominal group process. *Family Practice Management, 6,* 49–50.

Place, N. (2007). Using nominal group techniques for helping new extension agents understand how to effectively involve advisory committee members. *Journal of Extension, 45,* 1–3.

Queeney, D. (1995). *Assessing needs in continuing education: An essential tool for quality improvement*. San Francisco: Jossey-Bass Publishers.

Group Participation Process: Focus Group

Introduction

Focus group assessments are exploratory forms of qualitative research that can be used as a single method or as a part of a multiple methods approach (Barbour, 2007). One purpose of these types of needs and capacity assessments is to engage in brainstorming and generate ideas (Edmunds, 1999). The focus group process has its roots in the group depth interview that was developed as a form of group therapy (Boyd, Westfall, & Starch, 1981). In the 1950s, this technique was borrowed from psychiatry and developed as a marketing research technique (Gage, 1980). It is in this area that the focus group gained prominence, and it remains one of the most widely used marketing research techniques. Its use has expanded into other areas, including education, government, and social change and diversity arenas (Wycoff-Horn, Fetro, Drolet, & Russell, 2002; Edmunds, 1999; Schinke, Orlandi, Schilling, & Parms, 1992).

The focus group is typically an exploratory process that is used for generating hypotheses, uncovering attitudes and opinions, and acquiring and testing new ideas. It utilizes groups of 6 to 12 people that are fairly homogeneous in nature. The groups gather in a relaxed, informal setting to participate in an unstructured interview. A moderator has the task of focusing the group on the discussion topic and skillfully guiding the discussion in a way that stimulates interaction and encourages the sharing of feelings, attitudes, and ideas from all group members. With the participants' permission, the discussion usually is tape recorded and/or videotaped (Lacey, Manfredi, Balch, Warnecki, Allen, & Edwards, 1993). If facilities are available, the focus group process can be viewed by administrative staff through a one-way mirror or via closed-circuit television. The focus group process aligns with the Social Diagnosis phase of the PRECEDE-PROCEED model (Green & Kreuter, 1999).

Reviewing the Strategy

Advantages

The following are the advantages of using focus groups:

- *Low cost.* The focus group is a relatively inexpensive method of using an exploratory approach to assess needs.
- *Convenience.* Focus groups are easy to arrange and can be completed in a short amount of time (usually 1.5 hours). Because of the relative ease of implementation, a larger number of groups may be involved in this process than in other needs assessment strategies.
- *Creative atmosphere.* The lack of rigid structure in the process encourages spontaneity and stimulates a wide range of ideas, emotions, attitudes, perceptions, and thoughts. A comment from one person may solicit ideas, feelings, or opinions from other people in the group. These comments are accepted as valuable information (Edmunds, 1999). The atmosphere is most important when sensitive issues are being addressed, such as the assessment of one's beliefs, attitudes, and perceptions about euthanasia (Wycoff-Horn et al., 2002).
- *Ease of clarification.* The focus group structure enables the moderator to obtain clarification, if needed.
- *Flexibility.* Unlike with the nominal group process, there is greater tolerance to deviate from the intended direction and to explore related ideas and concerns. Deviations are analyzed as carefully as other responses. However, it is the moderator's job to direct the group back to the topic if the discussion becomes irrelevant.

Disadvantages

The following are some of the disadvantages of focus groups:

- *Qualitative information.* The data are exclusively qualitative, making coding, tabulating, and analyzing more difficult.
- *Limited representativeness.* Sample sizes are quite small, and the randomization of the sample may be limited. Results are not easy to generalize (Schechter, Vanchieri, & Crofton, 1990).
- *Dependence on moderator skill.* The results depend on the skill of the moderator. An inexperienced moderator or a moderator who has preconceived ideas can produce misleading results. Additionally, depending on how the meeting is conducted, some participants may not have an equal chance of participating. Some individuals may dominate the interaction, not allowing the more reserved individuals an opportunity to participate.

- *Preliminary insights.* Because of the preliminary nature of the findings, as well as the focus on brainstorming rather than seeking consensus, the information obtained from focus groups usually does not stand alone. It is recommended that additional assessments that can add insight to the focus group findings be conducted before making any final decisions. A survey and/or nominal group process can serve this purpose very well.
- *Participant involvement.* Recruitment of participants may be difficult, especially when trying to identify homogeneous groups in a short amount of time.

Preparing for the Assessment

Some market researchers are able to assemble a focus group within a few days. However, a little planning 1 to 2 months prior to the focus group discussion will help to keep the entire project on target.

Develop an Interview Guide

The interview guide outlines the scope of the need area that you will be assessing. Its purpose is to assist the moderator in introducing the topic or topics and focusing on these areas as needed throughout the discussion.

Enlist a Well-Trained, Experienced Moderator

The moderator is a crucial part of the focus group process. He or she must have good interpersonal communication skills and be able to quickly establish rapport and gain the confidence of the participants. Ideally, the moderator should fit in with the group. For example, if one is working mostly with women, the moderator should be a woman. This type of alignment is not always possible, especially when diverse groups are used. The same moderator should work with all groups. Familiarize the moderator with the goals and objectives of the needs assessment, as well as the mission, philosophy, and operations of your organization (if the moderator is from outside your organization). Make sure that you and the moderator become acquainted before beginning the focus group process.

Determine the Number and Composition of the Groups

A good rule of thumb is to continue conducting focus groups until no new ideas are generated. A saturation point generally occurs after three or four groups. You may want to conduct more focus groups, depending on the kind of information you are seeking, the diversity of your groups, and time and cost allowances. If you want information from people of different backgrounds, you should identify those subgroups and conduct three to four focus groups for each subgroup. Do not rely on only one focus group (Lacey et al., 1993).

The makeup of the groups should be as homogeneous as possible. This consistency reduces variations in responses based on social, intellectual, lifestyle, or demographic differences. People from similar backgrounds are more likely to relate better to one another, and this composition will enhance the focus group discussion.

Select Participants

Establish categories for participants based on criteria that will produce the most homogeneous groups. These categories may include gender, age, income, education, or other demographic factors that may affect how people respond to the need area. For example, you may want to separate mothers who work outside the home from those who do not when assessing needs for health care services for children. The perceptions of these two groups may differ significantly and interfere with participants' abilities to relate to one another. Putting them together in one focus group may hinder the discussion.

Participants may be recruited from ads, lists, or other means, using the quotas to screen the most appropriate candidates. They should have adequate background or experience so that they can contribute to the discussion. The participants should not know one another prior to the meeting because their familiarity may influence group interaction. However, this recommendation is not always possible to achieve in small communities. In these situations, at least try to avoid placing close friends in the same group. The participants should not have taken part in a similar group interview for at least 6 months. Sometimes participants are paid for their involvement. Payment can be achieved in a variety of ways, such as monetary recognition of $5 to $10 or social recognition of the participant's involvement in a worthy cause.

Arrange the Facilities

Where the focus group is held has important implications for the success of the process. The setting should be very relaxed and informal. Sometimes it is appropriate to meet in the home of one of the participants. Avoid meeting around a large conference table, which is usually too large and formal to create a comfortable environment. The site of the focus group also may be influenced by what type of recording will be done. Use of a one-way mirror or closed-circuit television will require specific types of facilities, whereas tape recording or videotaping allows for more flexibility in choosing the meeting site. The most critical factors are that the room be comfortable to allow for open communications and that it be easily accessible to the participants.

Conducting the Assessment

The following list presents a summary of the key considerations for conducting a focus group (it can be helpful as an overview to use in training others to assist in facilitation):

- The moderator should fit in well with the group. This person focuses the group on the discussion topic and guides the discussion so that interaction is stimulated and there is a sharing of ideas, feelings, and attitudes from all participants.

- Attempt to convene groups in which participants have similar backgrounds (within the group).
- Each group should consist of approximately 6 to 12 people.
- Have the groups gather in a relaxed, informal setting, and enable them to have time to "visit" briefly before getting started.
- At the start of the meeting, the moderator and participants should introduce themselves, and participants can be encouraged to make very brief comments related to the discussion topic.
- The moderator provides a brief introduction to the purpose of the meeting (e.g., to get participants' ideas about health-related issues and services related to families in a certain county) and offers discussion guidelines:
  1. Speak so that everyone can hear.
  2. Speak one at a time.
  3. Be open and honest in expressing what you think and feel.
- Ask the group members if they mind your use of a tape recorder so that you do not miss any important comments (you want to spend your time guiding the discussion, not writing too much).
- The moderator poses the questions and guides the discussion. The group members are free to interact with one another while making their responses. Remember, we are trying to get ideas, not achieve complete consensus.
- As a rule of thumb, continue the discussion on each question until no new ideas are being generated.
- Bring the discussion to a close by asking participants to summarize the key issues raised. You also can go around and have each participant offer one final comment.
- As soon as possible, prepare a summary of key ideas offered for each question.

Conducting the assessment involves the following steps.

Allow Time for Participants to Gather and Talk Among Themselves

This "fraternization" period gives the participants an opportunity to get to know one another and to become more comfortable with the surroundings. The moderator should introduce him- or herself and then ask the participants to introduce themselves. Participants also can be asked to share with the group something about themselves that relates to the topic. For example, if the need area concerns children and you are meeting with young parents, you may want to ask them to tell the group something about their children.

Introduce the Process and Topic

The moderator should provide a brief description of the process and offer some guidelines for the discussion: speak so that everyone can hear, speak one at a time, and be open and honest in expressing what you think and feel. The moderator can then make some general comments about the purpose of the meeting, being careful not to imply any expectations. Next, the moderator makes a statement or asks a question that will open the discussion.

Guide the Discussion Carefully

Once the moderator initiates the discussion, group members are free to interact with one another in pursuing the topic. The moderator should take a less dominant role in the group, becoming involved only to ask questions that will keep the discussion moving, to introduce a new dimension to the topic, or to refocus the group if it has completely lost track of the topic. The moderator must carefully direct the discussion in a way that both maintains optimal freedom of the group interaction and elicits information that is relevant to the need area. For the moderator to focus on the group interaction, taping is strongly recommended. Trying to record notes about the event while it is happening will result in missed data. However, if only audio taping is available, the moderator may want to make some notations on behaviors throughout the interview.

Observe the Process

If the process is being directly observed by other staff members through a one-way mirror or closed-circuit television, they should keep in mind several points. First, realize that what is being watched is work in progress. Second, listen actively and selectively, rather than for what you want to hear. Third, watch for nonverbal cues. Fourth, trust the moderator. If the process is not going well, however, let the moderator know. Seek participant permission for any recording.

Bring the Discussion to a Close

When all the areas outlined in the guide have been addressed, the discussion can be brought to an end. The moderator should ask the participants to offer a summary of what was discussed and what was resolved.

Make Follow-Up Calls

After several days, a follow-up call can be made to all participants to thank them for their involvement. At that time, you may ask for any additional information and ideas they may have generated since the focus group meeting took place.

Using the Results

Following each focus group, the moderator should meet with you to clarify what occurred in the session. A transcript should be created from the audio or videotape and then synthesized, analyzed, and interpreted. The information will usually be more significant if the people in the focus group become quickly involved without much prodding from the moderator, if the participants speak in the first person instead of the third person, and if they indicate some past experiences with this need area. Consider these points as you develop the report. The report should be written to include implications, interpretations, hypotheses, theories of how things are or could be, and recommendations. It should be integrated with quantitative and other qualitative data before making any decisions related to program planning. An example of this type of follow-up has been provided by Schinke et al. (1992), who conducted focus group assessments with Hispanic and African American adolescents in New York City. Following a series of seven focus group sessions held over a 2-month period, six expert panels of professionals were convened to corroborate the most reasonable educational recommendations for the prevention of HIV infection.

Additionally, in another example, Berry and colleagues (2010) attempted to understand the public's perception of physical activity guidelines and the formats that were most appealing. Information was collected from 22 participants who comprised five focus groups. The authors found that there was little awareness of *Canada's Physical Activity Guide* (CPAG); the *Guide* could be produced in a more appropriate and appealing manner (e.g., it is hard for adults to take the messages seriously with the use of cartoons); the provision of success stories (especially with celebrities) along with realistic examples would be quite motivating; and there is value in using Internet-based media to promote the *Guide* and physical activity, particularly with younger participants. The authors felt that other health promotion specialists could draw helpful planning suggestions from the participant insights derived from their assessments.

Overall, Barbour (2007) has offered the following recommendations for the analysis of the collected information and observations:

- Be careful not to take excerpts out of context.
- Pay attention to what is happening (in terms of group dynamics and the end product/point).
- Although the group is the main unit of analysis, you should also pay attention to individual voices.
- Remain open to other explanations for identified patterns.
- Sometimes unexpected similarities between groups can be just as illuminating as differences.

- The key to identifying patterns in your data is to use some form of counting.
- Silences can be equally illuminating.
- Reflexively use your own reactions to excerpts from focus group discussions (p. 143).

Reviewing an Example

The author conducted a series of focus group sessions in Vernon County, Wisconsin, while serving as the planning and evaluation consultant as part of a Family Preservation and Support (FPS) grant. To assess family health-related needs and resources across the three target groups of youths, adults, and older adults, members of the FPS Steering Committee were trained to serve as focus group facilitators. The basic principles for the process were outlined on a handout, which the facilitators used as a reference during the focus group sessions. A series of questions designed to elicit family health-related issues, as well as possibilities for individual and organizational resources that could be tapped (i.e., capacity building), were developed for each one of the three types of groups. An example of a health-related question for youths was as follows: "Generally, how has your family contributed to your current health and well-being?" An example of a capacity-building question for youths was as follows: "What kinds of contributions could you make to improve the quality of living in Vernon County?"

The process for each group throughout the county was dynamic. Individuals did not mind the use of a tape recorder because it was announced that people would not be identified and that the tape recording enabled the leader to participate fully in facilitating the discussion. Indeed, some participants commented that the use of some type of recording device during group discussions and interviews is quite commonplace.

The preliminary results indicated a wide range of family health issues and commentary on how society has changed today (e.g., it is harder for people to volunteer their time as they once did, given the need for many in the family to work outside of the home). Additionally, suggestions were offered for individual and organizational contributions that could be made (e.g., setting up a "banking" process to record volunteer time contributions and responding in kind when the volunteers have special needs).

Online Resources

Visit go.jblearning.com/gilmore4 for links to these Web sites.

Focus Groups and Delphi Surveys
Describes focus group methods and Delphi surveys.

Centers for Disease Control and Prevention

The CDC's Evaluation of HIV Prevention Programs using Qualitative Methods, which includes the Teacher's Focus Group Guide.

National Network for Child Care, Parents

An example focus group questionnaire for parents.

National Network for Child Care, Assessment

An example of a follow-up assessment of a focus group.

U.S. Department of Health and Human Services

Ways to manage focus groups effectively for maximum impact.

References

Barbour, R. (2007). *Doing focus groups*. Los Angeles: Sage Publications.

Berry, T., Witcher, C., Holt, N., and Plotnikoff, R. (2010). A qualitative examination of perceptions of physical activity guidelines and preferences for format. *Health Promotion Practice, 11,* 908–916.

Boyd, H., Westfall, R., and Starch, S. (1981). *Marketing research text and case studies*. Homewood, IL: Richard D. Irwin.

Edmunds, H. (1999). *The focus group research handbook*. Chicago: NTC Business Books and the American Marketing Association.

Gage, T. (1980). Theories differ on use of focus group. *Advertising Age, 51,* 519–522.

Green, L., and Kreuter, M. (1999). *Health promotion planning: An educational and ecological approach*. Mountain View, CA: Mayfield Publishing.

Lacey, L., Manfredi, C., Balch, G., Warnecki, R., Allen, K., and Edwards, C. (1993). Social support in smoking cessation among black women in Chicago public housing. *Public Health Reports, 108,* 387–394.

Schechter, C., Vanchieri, C., and Crofton, C. (1990). Evaluating women's attitudes and perceptions in developing mammography promotion messages. *Public Health Reports, 105,* 253–257.

Schinke, S., Orlandi, M., Schilling, R., and Parms, C. (1992). Feasibility of interactive videodisc technology to teach minority youth about preventing HIV infection. *Public Health Reports, 107,* 323–330.

Wycoff-Horn, M., Fetro, J., Drolet, J., and Russell, R. (2002). Beliefs, attitudes, and perceptions of selected undergraduate students about euthanasia. *The Health Educator: Journal of Eta Sigma Gamma, 34,* 11–16.

Community-Based Needs and Capacity Assessment Processes

Introduction

Two very specific and popular group needs and capacity assessment strategies, nominal groups and focus groups, were discussed in Chapters 6 and 7, respectively. These assessments are typically used with groups that are formulated by the person(s) coordinating the assessment efforts. Complementing these assessments are community-based capacity assessments, which are conducted in natural community settings. The original work by Kretzmann and McKnight (1993), as described in Chapter 2, has been expanded through in-depth descriptions of how to plan for and conduct capacity assessments (Kretzmann, McKnight, & Sheehan, 1997; Kretzmann, McKnight, & Puntenney, 1998; Dewar, 1997). Note that because of the clear distinction drawn by Kretzmann, McKnight, and Sheehan (1997) between needs and capacity assessments, these community-based approaches are specifically capacity assessments. Because they usually take place in distinct areas or community settings, these types of capacity assessments can be considered *neighborhood capacity assessments.* There also are excellent examples of regional capacity development for health promotion occurring within countries. As but one example, Van den Broucke, Jooste, Tlali, Moodley, Van Zyl, Nyamwaya, and Tang (2010, pp. 7–8) have addressed capacity development in South Africa through three main goals: (1) integrating health promotion into the health policy plans at the national, provincial, and district levels; (2) strengthening the health promotion capacity in two select Provinces in South Africa; and (3) supporting the development of tools for the monitoring and evaluation of health promotion. As a part of this effort, four areas of health promotion capacity enhancement were evaluated by the authors: network partnerships (e.g., having a sustainable network to support health promotion programs), knowledge transfer (e.g., developing and implementing health promotion programs addressing assessed community needs), problem solving (e.g., networking and working together to solve problems), and infrastructure (e.g., developing financial capital and social capital). Overall, capacity assessments provide an excellent opportunity for

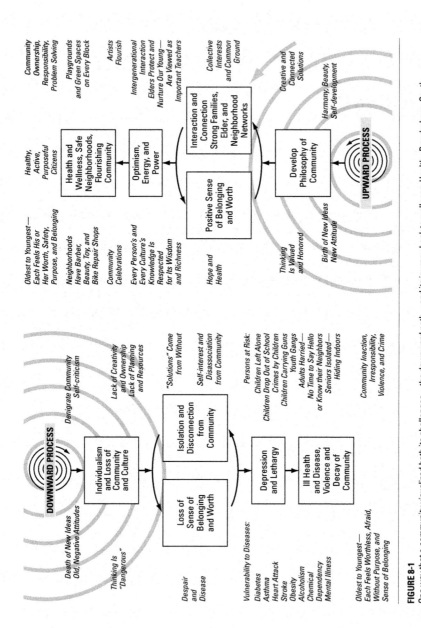

FIGURE 8-1

One way that a community visualized both its challenges—the downward path—and its journey back to wellness. Healthy Powderhorn, South Minneapolis.

Source: From Dewar, T., Kretzmann, J., and McKnight, J. (1997). *A Guide to Evaluating Asset-Based Community Development: Lessons, Challenges, and Opportunities.* Chicago: ACTA Publications. ABCD Institute. Used with permission.

128

determining basic talents and resources that are inherent in the population (see **Figure 8-1**). They also represent a positive and productive way to meet and greet others in a neighborhood.

Whether a singular part of capacity assessment strategies or a part of community-based participatory research (CBPR) in which there is an intentional and increased likelihood that community members are invested in the process, mutual benefits can accrue with this partnership approach (Faridi, Grunbaum, Gray, Franks, & Simoes, 2007; Israel, Eng, Schulz, & Parker, 2005). Capacity building and asset development can ensue where community and research partnerships are in place (Downey, Castellanos, Yadrick, Threadgill, Kennedy, Strickland, Prewitt, & Bogle, 2010). In the example reported by Downey and her colleagues (2010), community members from a tri-state region in the Lower Mississippi Delta were trained as co-researchers in a nutrition and physical activity research project. Notable outcomes included increased exercise activity and weight loss. Community resources (assets) can be infused into the sustainability of such efforts, providing a clear example of how assessment and intervention can be connected for health enhancement.

Complementing these types of survey and group discussion approaches for ascertaining individual talents and resources are several other community-based methods. The *community forum* (also referred to as a *public hearing*) is intended to address a focused issue in a community and to assess actual and perceived resources through a rather formal process. Additionally, *participant observation* affords the person(s) carrying out the assessment with a nonreactive group process. This method offers one the ability to think creatively in planning and conducting the community-based assessment processes so that reality is more fully reflected in the resulting information and insights.

COMMUNITY CAPACITY ASSESSMENT

Reviewing the Strategy

Capacity assessments have their origins in Ivan Illich's Center for Intercultural Documentation in Cuernavaca, Mexico, in which educators participated in seminars to brainstorm creative educational models (Kretzmann et al., 1998). Drawing from this collective thinking and sharing approach, Denis Detzel brought back to Northwestern University the idea of developing a local capacity listing and referral service. This process, which soon became known as the *Learning Exchange*, had as one of its key goals the development of an "economical and efficient vehicle to collect, organize, and make accessible information about educational and recreational resources and opportunities in metropolitan Chicago" (Kretzmann et al., p. 3). A complementary goal addressed the encouragement of individuals "to assume the responsibility to teach, learn, and share their interests with others" (p. 3). Overall, the process of information gathering, storage, and retrieval stimulated an exchange of skills and talents and fostered relationship building. Of note, the assessment process can range from simple to complex. An example of a simpler version of a community capacity survey is included in Appendix E. In addition, a community mapping process can be used. An example of the process is provided in **Figure 8-2**, as presented in Rowitz (2006), drawing data from the seminal work of Kretzmann and McKnight (1993). Key community resources can be identified using such a mapping approach (also see http://ctb.ku.edu/en/tablecontents/sub_section_main_1043.aspx).

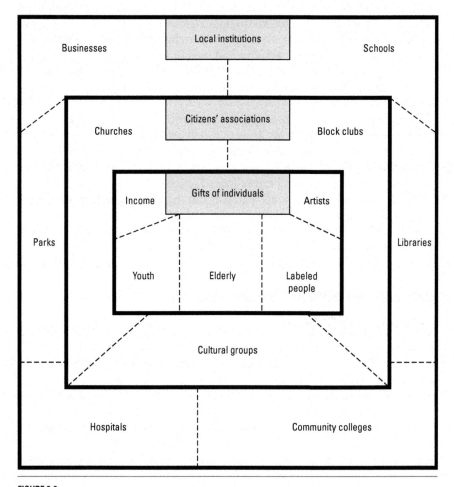

FIGURE 8-2
Community assets map.
Source: From Rowitz, L. (2006). *Public health for the 21st century: The prepared leader.* Sudbury, MA: Jones & Bartlett Learning. Used with permission.

Advantages

Community capacity assessment offers the following advantages:

- *Easy to develop and implement.* As long as the purpose of the assessment is clearly stipulated and followed by the planners, the capacity assessment procedures can incorporate a variety of information-gathering methods (e.g., brief survey, interviews, group discussions).
- *Provides opportunities for active involvement of residents.* Individuals who reside in the neighborhood feel more engaged in the process and the value of the information derived. Additionally, because residents often are involved in conducting the assessments, they have an *added benefit of "meeting and greeting" others.*
- *Process can be repeated at various times.* Because the assessment is considered to be for the benefit of the neighborhood, residents are often more inclined to allow and facilitate multiple requests for information. For the multiple assessment contacts to continue, it is important for the residents to receive ongoing updates regarding how the information is being used to better their circumstances.

Disadvantages

Community capacity assessment has the following disadvantages:

- *Possible surface assessment, affording more breadth than depth.* Although it is possible to develop a capacity assessment process of any degree of complexity, because of the usual intent to engage residents in the process (see the discussion regarding participatory community-based research in Chapter 2), the assessments tend to be simpler in format. Although this consideration does not detract from the value of the process, commitment over time on the part of those involved will be necessary to encourage continuing engagement in future aspects of the assessment.
- *Initially, residents may be skeptical and want anonymity.* Today, more than ever, community members are being inundated with requests for their time, resources, and identity. The emergence of multiple means of contacting people (e.g., electronic, postal, face-to-face), has led to well-founded concerns about being taken advantage of and being the target of identity theft. Such concerns may lead individuals to be reticent about becoming involved initially. One means of addressing this concern is to make certain that key community leaders (formal and informal) are involved in the early and continuing phases of the project and to ensure that the community is updated on the effort from its early stages throughout its implementation.

Preparing for the Assessment

Clear steps must be built into the planning phases. At the outset, it is essential to identify a core group of volunteers. Kretzmann and colleagues (1998) point out that paid staff can always be added during the later planning phases, but initially identifying a core group of dedicated volunteers who have most of the following skills will be most advantageous: record-keeping, advertising, fundraising, writing, and graphic design. This part of the preparation process also achieves a degree of buy-in.

The next steps include the development of a plan. The plan should have clearly stated goals (future directions) with aligned objectives (e.g., developing an appropriate contact system). Each objective is then addressed by specific strategies and time lines for achievement. Even though the assessment process is itself a type of formative evaluation process, it will be necessary to develop an evaluation system for the overall assessment effort. The evaluative commentary from volunteers and residents will be helpful in detecting the degree and type of accomplishment of the objectives.

Kretzmann, McKnight, and Puntenney (1998) carefully describe approaches for developing information systems that will be used in an ongoing manner in the community. Overall, they view the information-gathering process as an ongoing venture, rather than as a single effort conducted at one point in time. They delineate several types of files that can be developed as a part of the information system: a master card file with basic background, skill/talent, and contact information for those who are retained in the system; teacher/learner cards for individuals to signify their particular desired role in the process; interest cards on which individuals can indicate their interests in joining others for various activities; and feedback cards, which can be used to provide input regarding activities undertaken and a brief evaluation of one's involvement. For purposes of brief assessment, inventories such as the one in Appendix E can be used.

Bartholomew, Parcel, Kok, and Gottlieb (2001) complement the capacity assessment steps by delineating an intervention-mapping approach for health promotion. This process has five key steps:

1. Creation of matrices of proximal program objectives based on the determinants of behavior and environmental conditions
2. Selection of theory-based intervention methods and practical strategies
3. Translation of methods into organized programs
4. Integration of adoption and implementation plans
5. Generation of an evaluation plan (p. 9)

Conducting the Assessment

At the outset, it is important to have a stated purpose for the assessment. Keep the purpose simple and understandable for those involved in the capacity assessment process. Also, refer to the purpose frequently as a guide while developing the process. Kretzmann, McKnight, and Sheehan (1997) caution against collecting too much information, or information without a purpose: "Too much information, especially if it is not clearly related to community-building goals, often becomes cumbersome and awkward to use"; additionally, people can "get so focused on the collection of data about individual capacities that they forget their vision for how assets will be tapped and gifts and resources shared" (p. 65). Clearly, it is important to consider how the information will be used.

Early in the assessment process with a population, a community assets map can be developed which "adds information about the given assets and ways that different individuals and groups can better work together" (Rowitz, 2006, p. 408). Figure 8-2, which was presented earlier, provides an example of such a map in which community resources are identified.

Ayala, Maty, Cravey, and Webb (2005) provide several examples of community-based mapping experiences based on their CBPR involvement with community groups in North Carolina. One particular project involved the Hispanos Unidos effort in which representatives from Latino families wanted to improve the well-being of Latino families in North Carolina. The principal community partner was a woman from Costa Rica; the group was composed of eight men and women whose children participated in a youth soccer league. The first stage of the process involved the development of focus group discussion guide by the university researcher, with pilot testing via the Hispanos Unidos group. Results from the focus group processes guided the structure and content of the mapping activity. The eventual focus was gaining greater insight into:

> . . . where certain behaviors take place and in understanding how youths and their parents see their respective environments (for example, do youths perceive fast-food restaurants as bad or good, and how does this compare with how their parents see them). Mapping was identified as a method for determining where people go in their normal everyday lives so that a program can be designed to fit their current activity patterns (p. 203).

The group also decided that it would be important to include in-depth parent–child interviews for context. Of note, the group asked to be involved in some of the data analysis procedures, rather than having the university researcher prepare a preliminary report to be presented and discussed at a community forum. Eventually, the overall plan that emerged was to have the families review the findings and then become involved in the program development/action steps.

Wherever possible, involve community representatives in conducting the assessment. These individuals are known by the community, and thus they should be better able to access a cross-section of the population.

In terms of the methods for collecting capacity information, Kretzmann, McKnight, and Sheehan detail the following key questions (1997, pp. 66–67):

- What is the most effective way to collect information from our residents, given the resources at our disposal?
- How many of our community residents do we want to interview?
- How will our interviewers be educated and trained in the capacity inventory approach and process?
- What will happen to the capacity information once it has been collected? Who will be responsible for analyzing and maintaining it and making sure it is available to be used toward meeting the organization's goals?

Using the Results

Once the data are collected, it is important to become immersed in them. Kretzmann, McKnight, and Sheehan (1997) point out that during this phase a computer can be of great help "but it cannot understand individuals and capacities" (p. 71). Thus, it is imperative that the compiled information be reviewed by a planning or advisory committee so the various skills, gifts, talents, and interests of the assessed neighborhoods and communities can be categorized and aligned with the planned community-building efforts. Businesses also can be assessed regarding their capacities, and these resources can be aligned with the assessed individuals' gifts and talents (Kretzmann & McKnight, 1997). Overall, all of the assessed capacity information can be input into a data system for retrieval on an as-needed basis.

COMMUNITY FORUM

Reviewing the Strategy

The *community forum*, or *public hearing*, assessment approach is an attempt to identify the needs and capacities of communities and neighborhoods through public meetings. Although the main effort is to inform the public, these meetings also can seek the needs and capacity-related insights of those in attendance, usually at minimal cost (Butler & Howell, 1993). Witkin (1984, p. 130) notes that a variety of formats can be used in the community forum:

- Hearings in which people can speak as long as they desire, an approach typically employed during more formal and official hearings
- Meetings in which each speaker has a set amount of speaking time

- Meetings that use a group survey, asking participants to rank or rate statements or respond to questions
- A small group approach whereby participants are divided into small groups for discussion and eventual feedback to the total group

Typically, the community forum approach is used to identify general areas of need and capacity, which are subsequently refined through additional strategies. It also can be a gathering opportunity for the presentation of findings from other needs and capacity assessment procedures so additional input can be provided along with considerations for next steps. An example of this approach was provided by Haque and Eng (2011), as they developed a community forum in order to display and discuss the results of their photovoice process used with an urban neighborhood in Toronto, Canada (see the discussion on photovoice later in this chapter).

A community forum is a public meeting that invites participation from anyone in the community wishing to offer his or her perspective on a particular issue. It seeks to involve a broad cross-section of the community in an effort to review various points of view. In some cases, a community forum is conducted by a unit of local government as a public hearing, following the statutes governing that unit. At other times, a community forum is conducted less formally.

Advantages
Community forums offer the following advantages:

- *Relatively straightforward to conduct.* People are invited to come to a community facility to express their views on an issue, one at a time. You record what they say. Compared to a nominal group process, for example, a community forum is much simpler to run and requires fewer staff members with less extensive training.
- *Relatively inexpensive.* The only costs are for publicity, staff time to attend the forum, staff time to record and analyze the information gathered from the forum, and possibly rental fees for the facility used.
- *Access to a broad cross-section of the community.* Because the forum is publicly advertised, it offers the opportunity to hear the views of all segments of the community.
- *People can participate on their own terms.* They can come to the forum and simply state what is on their minds. They do not have to master a certain technique or follow a structured set of questions.
- *Identify people who are interested.* A community forum can help identify people from the community who are most interested in addressing the determined needs. The people who take the time to participate in a forum are likely to be those who feel most strongly about the issues and want to see them addressed. They are people who may later be involved in planning ways to meet the identified needs, thus enhancing the overall community capacity.

Disadvantages

Community forums have the following disadvantages:

- *Often difficult to achieve good attendance.* Although a community forum usually has the potential to attract a cross-section of the community, in reality it rarely does. As a result, the people who do participate will offer only a partial view of the needs that exist.
- *Participants in the community forum may tend to represent special interests.* They have the most to gain or lose, so they usually are most highly motivated to come. People with less of an investment in the issue may have valuable insights to offer, but because they are not as highly motivated, they may not take the time to attend. Therefore, although the participants in a community forum may be good candidates for helping to meet the identified needs later on, they also may represent special interests that can skew the planning process.
- *The forum could degenerate into a gripe session.* Because the format allows people to say what is on their minds, they may avoid focusing on particular needs to be addressed. Although other strategies for needs and capacity assessment can be more difficult for the participants to relate to, they do introduce some structure that can prevent the process from devolving into an unending series of complaints.
- *Data analysis can be time consuming.* Because the information gathered from a community forum may not follow any particular pattern, it will be necessary to develop a structure after the forum and determine the best way of summarizing and presenting the findings.

The best way to consider the role of a community forum in the needs assessment process is as a test of needs that have been identified through some other process. Previously identified needs can be presented to the public through the forum to determine whether the public confirms them as needs. It is a way of legitimizing needs that have already been suggested as well as allowing new needs to surface.

Preparing for the Assessment

Preparing for the assessment involves the following steps.

Develop One or More Questions the Forum Will Address

It is better to use questions rather than present a general topic so that it is easier for the participants to focus their comments. The question orientation also makes it easier for them to respond and may increase their motivation to participate.

Determine How Many Forums to Schedule

You should keep several criteria in mind when determining how many forums to conduct. If you want to obtain the broadest possible participation, you may need to schedule several forums at different times and in different places. If you want to draw people from a wide geographical area, then you will want to schedule them so as to minimize travel distances. Keep in mind the type of people you want to attend. An evening forum usually will be necessary to attract working people, but its timing may discourage elderly people from attending; they may need an opportunity to attend a forum during the day. A final criterion is the amount of time and money you have to complete your needs and capacity assessment. Although a community forum is relatively inexpensive, each forum does involve certain costs.

Schedule the Forum(s) in an Accessible Place

Often a well-known public facility located in a convenient location (e.g., a public library, city hall, local school, community center) works well. Even hospitals and colleges can be used if they are known for their community service work. When scheduling the facility, consider the availability of parking at the time the forum will be held.

Publicize the Forum Widely

Take advantage of as much free publicity as possible from the mass media. Send press releases to local daily and weekly newspapers, radio stations, and television stations. Follow up these news releases by contacting news reporters. Try to arrange an appointment to discuss the importance of the upcoming forum and encourage the release of an article in advance of the forum. Try to arrange to be interviewed by radio and television reporters, and participate in call-in talk shows or local community features, if possible.

Do not rely solely on the mass media, however, to publicize the forum. Consider mailing flyers to organizations interested in the issues to be addressed, and ask these organizations to publicize the forum to their members (perhaps by placing an announcement in their newsletters). Place notices in widely used public sites, such as public libraries, banks, restaurants, and supermarkets. If your budget permits, you may want to mail letters or flyers directly to individuals or groups you especially want to attract to the forum.

In the publicity materials for the forum, make sure to specify what participants will be asked to do. Clearly identify the question or questions they should address. Give them the opportunity to speak at the forum and/or to submit written commentary if desired.

Make the Necessary On-Site Arrangements

Make sure enough chairs are available. Typically, the staff would be seated at a table slightly removed from the participants, with paper and pens to take notes as desired. If the room is large, microphones should be provided both for the participants and for the staff members who may wish to ask questions. A staff member should register the participants as they arrive and receive any written materials they wish to submit. Be sure the room is well marked both outside and inside the building. If the budget permits, providing light refreshments can contribute to a congenial gathering.

Conducting the Assessment

Conducting the assessment involves the following steps.

Start the Forum on Time

The person conducting the forum should welcome the participants, thank them for coming, introduce him- or herself and the other staff members, briefly state the purpose of the forum, and explain how the event will be conducted.

Keep the Forum Moving

Invite the participants to participate in the order in which they registered upon arrival, unless you have in mind some other plan for the order of presenting comments. Encourage the participants to keep their remarks within the allotted time, typically 5 or 10 minutes. After the participant comments, allow each staff member present to ask the participant any questions for clarification or follow-up. Usually, you will not want to have your staff or members of the audience engage in a discussion of what was said. The purpose of a forum is to allow everyone an opportunity to speak in an orderly fashion, with opportunities for clarification by staff members.

Conclude the Forum When Appropriate

It is difficult to predict what will happen during a community forum. If only a few people show up, there will be more opportunity to ask questions of the participants. If a large crowd attends, it may be best to restrict the follow-up questions to keep the forum from dragging on too long. Thank the people for their participation and assure them that their commentary will be used in planning to address the needs identified. You also may want to remind them that some may be called upon in the future for program development involvement.

Using the Results

As noted earlier, it is difficult to structure the data analysis until after the forum is complete. Analyzing the data from a community forum can be similar to analyzing the data from key informant interviews, as explained in Chapter 5. Read through the information to see what categories emerge and then summarize the data under each of those categories. Again, a community forum may be best used to confirm needs determined by other needs assessment strategies. Compare the needs that surfaced from the forum with these other needs before making final decisions about which ones should be addressed.

PARTICIPANT OBSERVATION

Reviewing the Strategy

Health professionals sometimes place themselves in group situations for varying amounts of time in an effort to gain a sense of group health needs and available resources. Examples include attending a community group's series of meetings as a known representative of a health agency without serving in any official capacity and attending such meetings as a concerned citizen with one's professional responsibilities undeclared. In both cases, the health professional attempts to accumulate visual and auditory cues, which eventually may lead to clear patterns of an expressed need and opportunities for group contributions. No matter how well integrated into the group this person becomes, however, an inherent bias may be interjected into the group discussions and interactions due to his or her presence (Webb, Campbell, Schwartz, & Sechrest, 1966, p. 113).

Advantages

Participant observation offers the following advantages:

- *Direct observation of interactions.* Participant observation enables one to observe the unique interaction of group members directly, rather than serving necessarily as an outside observer.
- *Minimal interference.* Typically, outside interference (e.g., activities of other groups) is minimal as one views the selected group members working together in their natural environment.
- *Observe trends over time.* Observation at a series of group meetings is possible. This flexibility provides several opportunities to examine trends over time and, if necessary, have them clarified and corroborated by certain group members.
- *Multiple means to access information.* The information-gathering procedures are flexible. You do not get "locked in" on a single process during the event.

Disadvantages

Participant observation has the following disadvantages:

- *Group influence by observer.* The observer may potentially exert (knowingly and unknowingly) some influence on the discussion patterns and decisions and be inclined to pick up on only certain types of information (Webb & Weick, 1983).
- *Time consuming.* Participant observation is a time-consuming activity. In addition to the time spent sitting through an entire meeting, you

have to allow travel time to and from the meetings and time (very soon after the meeting) to commit your observations to writing.
- *Need for multiple meetings.* Attendance at more than one meeting of the group is usually necessary. Unlike a nominal group process or a community forum, both of which are very structured group meetings designed to yield very specific information on one occasion, participant observation is much more unpredictable and open-ended. Although one meeting can yield much information about health-related needs and potential resources, the next two or three meetings may provide little information. Due to the time and staff resources that must be committed to such a venture, you should determine whether the benefits will be worth the cost.

Preparing for the Assessment

Preparing for the assessment involves the following steps.

Determine Specifically What You Are Looking For

If you want to try to answer very specific questions about health-related needs from observing a group, be very focused in your observations. Pay particular attention to those group interactions that help to answer those questions. More often, however, you may not have such a sharply focused list of questions. In that case, you will want to pay attention to a wider range of group interactions. Also, determine the scope of your participant observation activities. Determine how many groups are to be observed, how many meetings of each group to attend, and how active you want your observers to be during these group meetings.

Select Your Observers

The participant observer may be you, or you may need additional observers if you plan to observe more than one group. More significantly, you may decide in some situations that you are not the best person to observe the group. Many of the group members may know you, and you may believe this relationship will unduly bias the group interaction. In those situations, it may be best for the observer to be someone the group members do not know. Also, your professional status may hinder the group's willingness to contribute. If so, it may be advisable to recruit people who can more easily blend in with the group members. Just as good teaching is often considered an art, so is good participant observation. Some people are more naturally gifted in this area than others. Thus, in the observer selection process, consider whether individuals have the appropriate personality to become good observers and how much experience they have had working with groups.

Train the Observers

Explain the purpose of the observation to your observers and tell them what to look for. Discuss good group observation techniques (see "Conducting the Assessment"). Develop handouts describing how to use these techniques in more detail, and arrange opportunities to discuss these observations. Also, discuss how to record observations, and provide opportunities to practice and critique.

Gain Access to the Group

Obtain permission to attend group meetings. Explain as much as you can about your purpose in observing the group without undermining what you are trying to accomplish. You want to be honest about your intentions; do not deceive participants about your activities. Tell them what organization is conducting the assessment and how the data will be used. Assure the group members that the data will be kept confidential. In some cases, it may be best to have the group members sign a statement of permission to participate in your process.

Conducting the Assessment

Conducting the assessment involves the following steps.

Be as Inconspicuous as Possible

However, try to position yourself so that you can observe the group members. Facial gestures are an important part of any group observation. If your role is strictly to observe, you may be able to sit off to the side. If you are going to participate in a limited way, however, you will need to be more a part of the group.

Limit the Recording of Data During the Meeting

One of the best ways to record data is to take limited notes during the meeting by using a small notepad to jot down key phrases and impressions you want to remember. Keep the note-taking as inconspicuous as possible. If the group members see you writing down every word they say, they may not feel as free to share what they really have in mind.

Develop Extensive Descriptions After the Meeting Ends

Use the notes taken during the meeting as a guide, and begin writing the descriptions of the meeting as soon as possible. If you have been able to focus your observation on some key issues, describe what happened that is relevant to these issues. If your observation is not as focused, then you will have to describe the meeting in greater detail. These field notes can be dictated for later transcription. (Remember that this dictation will increase the cost of your observations, because someone will have to transcribe it later.) If possible, develop these field notes right after the meeting. Even with no notes available, you will be surprised how much you recall from the meeting and how extensive your eventual field notes will be.

Critique Your Observations Between Group Meetings

The day after the meeting, take time to reread your field notes and reflect on what you have observed. Ask yourself what you are learning and whether you are observing the right things. This self-critique will help you be more focused for the next meeting.

If you started participant observation without a truly specific focus, you should find that you can become more focused with each meeting observed. If more than one person is observing groups, it may be helpful to have them periodically meet to share notes. What one person is observing may be confirmed by another observer's experience. Also, this collaboration may assist the other observer to have a better idea of what to look for at the next group meeting.

Using the Results

Analysis of the data from participant observations is similar to the analytical method used for interviews. If you have specific questions in mind that you want answered from the assessment, organize your findings around these major questions. If you do not have specific questions in mind, look for categories and then group the categories into themes. This latter approach is a more inductive process.

Trends emanating from the participant observation process can be aligned with the prioritized needs evolving from other needs assessment strategies. This additional information is incorporated into the decision-making process so that the next steps can be established. The decision-making process can be as straightforward as initiating planning committee discussions regarding what the prioritized needs are and then reviewing the pros and cons of the objectives and methods to address the needs.

Reviewing an Example

Dewar (1997) described the Healthy Powderhorn Story, which took place in south Minneapolis. One of the major efforts of this community-organizing initiative was to "uncover the resources and talents already existing in the community" (p. 15). An asset-based approach was taken to focus on community building. The community had identified several challenges that needed to be addressed:

- How to mobilize the community and its assets around health action and cultural practices;
- How to deinstitutionalize community residents and their organizations in their approach to both individual and collective health;
- How to develop and run an effective community intermediary that is connected to, and truly respectful of, the values and aspirations of community residents; . . .
- How to document the impact, and report on progress toward goals in ways that would be credible, community sensitive, and doable. (pp. 17–18)

Assessments of talents and resources emerged from discussions conducted at community meetings (over a 26-month period, 249 neighborhood meetings were held with structured listening opportunities serving as capacity assessments). Emerging from the suggestions were Community Health Action Teams (CHATs), which facilitated walking clubs, Native American spirituality classes, and the like.

PHOTOVOICE

Reviewing the Strategy

Photovoice is a unique assessment process that uses a community-based participatory research approach. The process was developed during the 1990s by Caroline Wang and Mary Ann Burris (1997). Wang and Burris (1997) have defined *photovoice* as "a process by which people can identify, represent, and enhance their community through a specific photographic technique," having the three main goals: "(1) to enable people to record and reflect their community's strengths and concerns, (2) to promote critical dialogue and knowledge about important issues through large and small group discussion of photographs, and (3) to reach policymakers" (p. 369). Overall, the process is intended to detect needs and assets in a given community setting.

The basic process involves cameras (often disposable ones) being distributed to representatives of a given community so that they can depict something of meaning to them. In an extensive photovoice literature review, Catalani and Minkler (2010) described the purpose, process, training, participation, and outcomes for 37 published articles. They concluded that "the quality of participation appeared to increase with project duration" (Catalani & Minkler, 2010, p. 439).

Wang and Redwood-Jones (2001) addressed the important consideration of ethics with regards to the photovoice process. In particular, they discussed issues grounded in *image ethics*, which relates to people's moral rights as they appear in visual media. Drawing on work by Gross, Katz, and Ruby (1988), Wang and Redwood-Jones (2001) describe four "ethical implications for photovoice" (p. 564). The first ethical implication is the intrusion into one's private space. They point out that this matter can be partially addressed through consent forms. The second ethical implication involves the "disclosure of embarrassing facts about individuals" (p. 565). They note that this can be addressed by receiving written permission as well as avoiding the use of potentially embarrassing photos in public. The third ethical implication is "being placed in a false light by images," whereby "the interpretation of the events pictured conflicts with the subject's thoughts or feelings" (p. 566). Careful facilitation of the interpretive discussion with the inclusion of other corroborating findings can be particularly helpful in assuring greater accuracy.

Finally, "protection against the use of a person's likeness for commercial benefit" goes to a core photovoice understanding that "participants own the negatives they produce" (p. 566). Here, written consent for the publication of the photographs and even the use of an honorarium for the photographer are recommended, as appropriate. For a more in-depth treatment of this important consideration, practitioners contemplating the use of the photovoice assessment process are strongly encouraged to carefully review the Wang and Redwood-Jones (2001) publication.

Advantages
Photovoice offers the following advantages (Wang & Burris, 1997):

- *Community perceptions.* Photovoice enables practitioners to assess what the community members think is important.
- *Visual images.* The process uses visual images as the major mode of communicating perceived needs and assets.
- *Simplicity.* Anyone in the community who can use a camera is able to participate without relying on reading and writing.
- *Array of findings.* "People with cameras can record settings—as well as moments and ideas—that may not be available to health professionals and health researchers" (p. 372).
- *Continuing participant involvement.* It is possible to maintain community involvement as the assessment phase moves into program implementation.
- *Dual purpose.* Photovoice assesses the needs and assets in the community.

Disadvantages
Photovoice does have the following disadvantages, as noted by Wang and Burris (1997):

- *Limited documentation.* There are limitations as to what the participants can document due to potential risks related to various sources of power in the community.
- *Individual judgment for photo selections.* "Personal judgment may intervene at many different levels of representation: who used the camera, what the user photographed, what the user chose not to photograph, who selected which photograph to discuss, and who recorded whose and what thoughts about whose and which photographs" (p. 374).
- *Potential inequality inducement.* "The participatory process attempts to address material and status inequalities, yet the extent to which it may perpetuate those inequalities deserves scrutiny" [e.g., "the process entrusts cameras to the hands of ordinary people, but in whose hands does money, support, and editorial control remain?"] (p. 374).
- *Analysis complexities.* Analyzing and summarizing the information and insights can be complex and difficult.

Preparing for the Assessment
The steps for preparing for the photovoice assessment are as follows.

Plan for Necessary Logistics, Including the Needed Equipment
Part of the preparation may include writing a small grant to support the cameras that will be used, in addition to other logistics expenses. Digital cameras offer the advantage of participants being able to see the photos as they are captured and being able to connect the cameras to a computer and LCD projector for use during the sharing sessions.

At the end of Wang and Burris' (1997) project in Yunnan, China, they noted that the cameras were not given as gifts, but were made available to community members for purchase at a discounted price. This imparted a sense of value for the equipment on the part of the community members, and the cameras could also be used for future program evaluation.

Clearly Identify the Community Parameters/Confines
Determine how much of the given community can be realistically addressed given the available time and personnel. It is important not to try to do too much during the first assessment (particularly if it part of an ongoing effort).

In a recent outreach effort this author was involved with in a village in northern Nicaragua, a combined public health and medical care team from the United States had to delimit a realistic segment of the population for key informant interviews. Potential photovoice assessments were then projected for follow-up assessments in that same locale. Delimiting the sample population in advance facilitated the proper preparation of assessment procedures and materials and informed the type of training required in advance for the team members.

Conduct Training Sessions in Advance

For the sake of time while on site for a given assessment project, as well as resource development for the required assessment-related materials and logistics needs, training sessions for the members of the team must occur well in advance of the on-site experience. In preparation for such sessions, make sure to clarify the purpose of the experience and the goals for a given visit (as established in advance with community representatives). Make sure to write them down (usually accomplished by a steering committee) and distribute the information to the team members for the sake of a clearer understanding and consistency (this step oftentimes is neglected, with subsequent impact on the smooth operation of the assessment). As a part of the training session, make certain to address the purpose, goals, and process to be used. It is helpful to have the members go over their responsibilities and to provide opportunities for members to raise questions and offer suggestions.

Identify Facilitators and Participants and Establish Training Sessions

Because photovoice is a participatory type of needs assessment, it must be conducted in concert with the population. As Wang and Burris (1997) have emphasized in relation to their work with women in Yunnan, China, the participatory nature of this assessment needs to be conveyed to the target community. Specifically, the challenge "is to offer guidelines that might expand, rather than limit, the perceived range of a community's assets and to avoid language that pathologizes its members" (p. 378). To address this challenge, Wang and Burris (1997) asked the women to photograph "the spirit of village women's everyday lives" (p. 378). Training sessions also can address the care and protection of the equipment that will be used, encouraging, rather than unintentionally stifling, the participants' creativity and making sure that they are aware of the broader implications that the photographs and their meanings could have on others.

Overall, Catalani and Minkler's (2010) photovoice literature review determined that 62 percent of the 37 reviewed studies had some type of basic training experience for the participants. Of note, 12 of the studies included training on photography techniques, as well as on ethics and safety.

Conducting the Assessment

There can be some latitude in the overall process one employs for photo-voice. Lopez, Eng, Robinson, and Wang (2005) have discussed a process they followed as part of a community-based participatory research project with African American breast cancer survivors from three rural counties in North Carolina:

- Participate in a training session
- Conduct photo-assignments
- Participate in photo-discussion sessions
- Assess the trustworthiness of the findings (particularly from the analysis of the discussion transcripts)
- Plan a forum to present the findings and foster collaboration with influential individuals who can advocate for change (pp. 328–329)

The researchers wanted to have the women "communicate the social and cultural meaning of living in silence with breast cancer" (p. 330). Of note, prior to launching a full-scale effort, the researchers used a pilot study to make certain the approach would be well received and provide the necessary assessment information and insights from the participants.

As has been shown through the literature review by Catalani and Minkler (2010), the photovoice assessment process can be quite varied depending on the project goals, the types of populations involved, and the degree of investigator–participant interaction. They found that the duration of the photovoice process ranged from 2 weeks to several years, with a median of 3 months. Variability was also found in the investigators' meetings with the participants. At the low end, investigators met twice with the participants: once to provide an introduction to the project and a second time to collect the photos and to obtain information through interviews or discussions. Forty-three percent of the studies reviewed were considered to be at a medium level of participation by the investigators, much along the lines of the seminal work by Wang and Burris (1997). Catalani and Minkler (2010) described this medium level as having a duration of "4 months, during which time facilitators and participants met more than twice to clarify photo assignments, discuss pictures, and engage in action. Action commonly took the form of organizing a public photo exhibit" (p. 440).

The photovoice process also can be connected to frameworks such as the logic model (refer to Chapter 2 for a more detailed discussion of this model). Strack, Lovelace, Jordan, and Holmes (2010) connected the photo-voice process with the logic model in the *Picture Me Tobacco Free* project. Incorporation of the logic model offered a number of benefits: the logic model was able to indicate system change; it helped investigators and participants stay "on the same page"; it facilitated the development of new tactics and outcomes as the project continued; and it assisted in determining whether change actually resulted from project activity.

The photovoice process can be coupled with other needs assessment procedures, as demonstrated by Valera, Gallin, Schuk, and Davis (2009). Valera and colleagues used photovoice and focus groups to assess nine low-income women from the SisterLink community action program in New York City. During the focus group process, the women were asked to discuss concerns that affected their families. As a result of their prioritization of the issues that emerged, they decided to focus on access to fresh fruits and vegetables for further exploration. The photovoice process was used for this aspect of the assessment.

The analysis of the information and insights conveyed by the photos that are taken can be quite diverse, but the three-stage process originally recommended by Wang and Burris (1997) still represents an important starting point:

1. Participants *choose* those photographs that "most accurately reflect the community's needs and assets" (p. 380).
2. Participants *contextualize* the chosen photographs, "telling stories about what the photographs mean" (p. 380).
3. Participants *codify* the photographs, "identifying those issues, themes, or theories that emerge" (p. 380).

Wang and Burris (1997) use the acronym VOICE—Voicing Our Individual and Collective Experience—for the group discussion process used in this approach, because the photographs "alone, considered outside the context of women's own voices and stories, would contradict the essence of photovoice" (p. 381).

Building on that foundation, an approach to dialogue termed SHOWED can help participants identify and take next steps for change and improvement. This process is based on a series of questions (Wallerstein & Bernstein, 1988):

- What do you see in this photograph?
- What is happening in this photograph?
- How does this relate to our lives?
- Why do these issues exist?
- How can we become empowered by our new social understanding?
- What can we do to address these issues?

Using the Results

The results from photovoice can lead to numerous responses in thought and action. In particular, as offered by Freire (1970, 1973), visual images can stimulate a group to further analyze their own situations and circumstances, increasing the potential for change. Such a result can contribute to the empowerment of individuals. Themes emerging from the analyses can guide the development of participant-driven action plans for next steps. In addition, the results from photovoice can add to and corroborate the findings from other assessment formats. As has been pointed out by Haque and Eng (2011) based on their work in an urban neighborhood in downtown Toronto, a photovoice project can engage and eventually empower residents by influencing local policy for the improvement of local health services. Their findings included both positive and negative health impactors that were categorized as:

- Physical issues such as overcrowding, housing conditions, open space, public facilities
- Environmental issues such as noise, pollution, and garbage
- Social issues such as meeting spaces, isolation, neighbourliness
- Economic issues such as employment, recognition of foreign qualifications, and health services accessibility (p. 17)

As they have stated, the photovoice process "can be effectively used to enter research-resistant communities, engage disadvantaged populations, and establish trust in a community" (Haque & Eng, 2011, p. 18).

Reviewing an Example

In terms of gender, Catalani and Minkler's (2010) review of photovoice research determined that the majority (78%) of the reviewed photovoice studies involved female participants. Insightful photovoice studies involving males have taken place, such as the research by Ornelas, Amell, Tran, Royster, Armstrong-Brown, and Eng (2009) involving African American men and their perceptions of racism, male gender socialization, and social capital. The photovoice process was incorporated as a part of the Men As Navigators (MAN) for Health project in which 12 African American men living in urban and rural settings took photographs. Following introductory meetings that provided background information on photovoice, ethical issues with taking photographs, and an opportunity to develop rapport, the navigators brainstormed what their photo assignments would be in relation to their role as lay health advisors. After the photos were taken, follow-up meetings were held for the navigators to select photos that they wanted to share with the group, with the group then selecting one to two photos for group discussion.

Based on audio recordings and meeting notes, codes were established and then grouped into broader concepts. Further qualitative analysis took place using Atlas.ti computer software (Scientific Software Development, 2003). The preliminary results in terms of rural and urban photos and themes were shared and discussed at community forums. The three areas of focus were: race and racism, roles and responsibilities of being an African American man, and social networks and social capital. The investigators summarized a strength of the study as:

> . . . its analysis of data collected through the CBPR [community-based participatory research] approach, which engaged African American men as co-investigators. The CBPR methodology of photovoice enhanced the quality and validity of research by drawing on rural and urban African American men's expertise to generate an understanding of issues that they, themselves, deem important, as well as to move toward identifying action steps. (Ornelas et al., 2009, p. 563)

Online Resources

Visit go.jblearning.com/gilmore4 for links to these Web sites.

Community Advisory Committee of the Southern Health Board
An overview of methods for consumer and community participation in the planning of health services.

The Community Tool Kit
This site offers guidance on the essential skills necessary to build a healthy community.

Western Rural Development Center
This Web site describes community assessment techniques, including participant observation, social network analysis, the Delphi Technique, the nominal group process, advisory groups, community forums, and application of these techniques.

Latino Needs Assessment Child Care Program
An example of a needs assessment.

U.S. Public Health Service
A report on community forums for youth violence and public health.

The Nature and Society Forum
A nonprofit community-based organization that promotes the health and well-being of individuals and the natural environment.

Women's Health Forum
Commissioned papers providing links to sessions and workshops.

References

Ayala, G., Maty, S., Cravey, A., and Webb, L. (2005). Mapping social and environmental influences on health. In Israel, B., Eng, E., Schulz, A., and Parker, E. (Eds.), *Methods in community-based participatory research for health* (pp. 188–209). San Francisco: Jossey-Bass.

Bartholomew, L., Parcel, G., Kok, G., and Gottlieb, N. (2001). *Intervention mapping: Designing theory and evidenced-based health promotion programs.* Mountain View, CA: Mayfield Publishing.

Butler, L., and Howell, R. (1993). *Coping with growth: Community needs assessment techniques.* Pullman, WA: Washington State University, Western Regional Extension Service.

Catalani, C., and Minkler, M. (2010). Photovoice: A review of the literature in health and public health. *Health Education & Behavior, 37,* 424–451.

Dewar, T. (1997). *A guide to evaluating asset-based community development: Lessons, challenges, and opportunities.* Chicago: ACTA Publications.

Downey, L., Castellanos, D., Yadrick, K., Threadgill, P., Kennedy, B., Strickland, E., Prewitt, E., and Bogle, M. (2010). Capacity building for health through community-based participatory nutrition intervention research in rural communities. *Family and Community Health, 33,* 175–185.

Faridi, Z., Grunbaum, J., Gray, B., Franks, A., and Simoes, E. (2007). *Community-based participatory research: Necessary next steps. Preventing chronic disease: Public health research, practice, and policy.* Atlanta: Centers for Disease Control and Prevention.

Freire, P. (1970). *Pedagogy of the oppressed.* New York: Seabury Press.

Freire, P. (1973). *Education for critical consciousness.* New York: Seabury Press.

Gross, L., Katz, J., and Ruby, J. (Eds.). (1988). *Image ethics.* New York: Oxford University Press.

Haque, N., and Eng, B. (2011). Tackling inequity through a photovoice project on the social determinants of health. *Global Health Promotion, 18,* 16–19.

Israel, B., Eng, E., Schulz, A., and Parker, E. (Eds.). (2005). *Methods in community-based participatory research for health.* San Francisco: Jossey-Bass.

Kretzmann, J., and McKnight, J. (1997). *A guide to mapping local business assets and mobilizing local business capacities.* Chicago: ACTA Publications.

Kretzmann, J., and McKnight, J. (1993). *Building communities from the inside out.* Chicago: ACTA Publications.

Kretzmann, J., McKnight, J., and Puntenney, D. (1998). *A guide to creating a neighborhood information exchange: Building communities by connecting local skills and knowledge.* Chicago: ACTA Publications.

Kretzmann, J., McKnight, J., and Sheehan, G. (1997). *A guide to capacity inventories: Mobilizing the community skills of local residents.* Chicago: ACTA Publications.

Lopez, E., Eng, E., Robinson, N., and Wang, C. (2005). Photovoice as a community-based participatory research method: A case study with African American breast cancer survivors in rural eastern North Carolina. In B. Israel, E. Eng, A. Schulz, and E. Parker (Eds.), *Methods in community-based participatory research for health* (pp. 326–348). San Francisco: Jossey-Bass.

Ornelas, I., Amell, J., Tran, A., Royster, M., Armstrong-Brown, J., and Eng, E. (2009). Understanding African American men's perceptions of racism, male gender socialization, and social capital through photovoice. *Qualitative Health Research, 19,* 552–565.

Rowitz, L. (2006). *Public health for the 21st century: The prepared leader.* Sudbury, MA: Jones and Bartlett Publishers.

Scientific Software Development. Atlas.ti [computer software]. (2003). Berlin, Germany: Author.

Strack, R., Lovelace, K., Jordan, T., and Holmes, A. (2010). Framing photovoice using a social-ecological logic model as a guide. *Health Promotion Practice, 11,* 629–636.

Valera, P., Gallin, J., Schuk, D., and Davis, N. (2009). "Trying to eat healthy." A photovoice study about women's access to healthy food in New York City. *Affilia: Journal of Women and Social Work, 24,* 300–314.

Van den Broucke, S., Jooste, H., Tlali, M., Moodley, V., Van Zyl, G., Nyamwaya, D., and Tang, K-C. (2010). Strengthening the capacity for health promotion in South Africa through international collaboration. *Global Health Promotion, Supp (2),* 6–16.

Wallerstein, N., and Bernstein, E. (1988). Empowerment education: Freire's ideas adapted to health education. *Health Education Quarterly, 15,* 379–394.

Wang, C., and Burris, M. (1997). Photovoice: Concept, methodology, and use for participatory needs assessment. *Health Education and Behavior, 24,* 369–387.

Wang, C., and Redwood-Jones, Y. (2001). Photovoice ethics: Perspectives from Flint photovoice. *Health Education & Behavior, 28,* 560–572.

Webb, E., Campbell, D., Schwartz, R., and Sechrest, L. (1966). *Unobtrusive measures: Nonreactive research in the social sciences.* Chicago: Rand McNally and Company.

Webb, E., and Weick, K. (1983). Unobtrusive measures in organizational theory. In Van Maanen, J. (Ed.), *Qualitative methodology* (pp. 209–224). Beverly Hills, CA: Sage Publications.

Witkin, B. (1984). *Assessing needs in educational and social programs.* San Francisco: Jossey-Bass.

Technology-Supported Assessments

Introduction

Rapid technological change dominates our lives today. Advances in technology have led to many changes in health care and health promotion. Advances in communication technologies offer seemingly endless opportunities to change the ways we conduct business, use community services, and communicate with friends. The emergence of the Internet has revolutionized many aspects of society, to include providing unique information sources regarding the health status of populations. As one example, Black and Peacock (2011) have demonstrated the value of exploring the health-related insights aligned with a *strong Black woman* script by reviewing the popular media sources of African American women, particularly magazines and blogs (i.e., Web logs). Based on their secondary data analysis in the areas of role management, coping strategies, and self-care, the authors concluded that "we are charged with listening to these voices to create gender-specific and culturally responsive health and wellness initiatives tailored to the needs of African American women generally, and supportive of reenvisioned notions of strong Black womanhood specifically" (p. 148).

This global expansion in technology has created opportunities to assess needs and capacities in new ways, especially with regards to working with people located some distance from one another. Examples include audio conferences, computer conferences, and videoconferences. Equipment for these strategies is typically located in educational institutions, county courthouses, public libraries, medical facilities, and corporations. Some conferences require facilities with special equipment, whereas others can use desktop computing equipment available at individual workstations. Also, the surge in social media connections (referred to as the *participative Internet*) provides avenues for interfacing with people of all ages across the country and globally (Chou, Hunt, Beckjord, Moser, & Hesse, 2009). Additionally, for health education, Kittleson (2009) has described the role of technology and its multiple purposes. In their national study regarding adults in the United

States, Chou and colleagues (2009) found that the only significant predicator regarding site involvement in blogging and social networking was younger age. In a study reported by Rice (2010), the positive role of social networks and social networking technology related to condom use by homeless young people aged 16–26 years was demonstrated. Of note, respondents in this study who had a street-based peer who was a condom user (52%) were less likely to have unprotected sex. Additionally, approximately "22% of respondents had a condom-using, home-based peer with whom they communicated only via social networking technology" (p. 588). Overall, it is important to note that social media practices can vary from country to country (Ontario Health Promotion eBulletin, 2010). In order to bring some structure to the rapidly changing communication realm of social media, the Centers for Disease Control and Prevention (CDC) has developed guidelines and best practices (2010) for the use of social media tools that can be useful when using these tools in health and public health research.

Reviewing the Strategy

Audio Conferencing

Audio conferencing is perhaps the most basic use of technology to assess needs. Essentially, it connects people by telephone. Sometimes a dedicated line is available to connect the participants, but more commonly the audio conference uses standard telephone lines. Newer telephones often have a conference call feature that enables the conference moderator to connect the participants directly. Alternatively, each participant might dial a central telephone bridge number and use a special code to connect to the conference.

A speaker phone with a mute button is highly recommended if at all possible to free the participants' hands for writing and shuffling papers and to ensure optimal audio quality. A speaker phone also enables participants to shift their posture and move around from time to time. With this arrangement, a productive audio conference can continue as long as an hour. After an hour, the conference may become difficult to sustain. If additional time is needed, schedule another conference call at a later time.

Audio conferencing can suffer from inappropriate acoustical conditions and the relative lack of control over the order in which participants speak. It requires discipline on the part of the participants to pay close attention to whom is speaking and to what is being said. An effective moderator is essential to help maintain control of the conference and to ensure that everyone has a chance to participate.

A variation of audio conferencing makes use of online computers. This type of computer-enhanced audio conferencing is sometimes called *audiographics*.

Participants use a two-way audio conference connection and a "real-time" computer connection via a modem. The computer connection enables the conference moderator to send diagrams, charts, or other schematics. Computer graphics and prescanned images are "called up" on the screen when needed during the conference. Using special "writing pads" and pens, participants can respond to questions directly on the computer screen. What one person writes on the pad, everyone else sees simultaneously on the computer screen. Usually this audiographics system also involves the use of a slow-speed video camera for transmitting still images to each computer screen.

Advantages

Audio conferencing offers the following advantages:

- *Very accessible*. Virtually everyone has a telephone. A conference call can bring together people who are widely scattered geographically.
- *Comparatively inexpensive*. A local conference call has no direct costs. Although long-distance charges can mount for conference calls connecting several individuals, they are still less than the costs for other technologies.
- *A relatively quick process*. A typical conference call is shorter than a face-to-face meeting and does not require participants to travel.
- *Encourages busy people to participate*. People who do not have time to travel out of town to attend an extended face-to-face meeting might agree to participate in a hour-long conference call.

Disadvantages

Audio conferences have the following disadvantages:

- *Limited interaction*. An audio conference call offers verbal communication without the benefit of facial expression and other nonverbal cues.
- *Requires people who are comfortable with verbal expression*. Participants are isolated from others on the line and do not have the opportunity to observe expressions or receive encouragement from other people.

COMPUTER CONFERENCING

The Internet has enabled people to connect through their personal computers to other people in various parts of the country and all over the world. Major advances in computer technology continue to expand the possibilities for information sharing at a rapid pace.

As more and more people have personal computers and Internet access both at work and at home, opportunities to assess needs using their computers become available. The key to a computer conference is having each participant connect to the Internet, either using a direct connection through work or via a home subscription service. Today, many computers are equipped to offer audio and video connectivity, such as with video calling plans like Skype.

Both synchronous and asynchronous computer conferences are possible. The simpler and more common approach is the asynchronous conference, which calls for participants to send and respond to messages during a pre-scribed period of time when everyone is not online simultaneously. This period may theoretically be as short as an hour but is more likely as long as a week or even a month. During this period, participants agree to respond to questions, either directly by e-mail or through a listserv subscription.

In contrast, a synchronous computer conference requires all participants to be online with their computers at a prearranged time. Typically, a subscription service is used to set up a chat room or instant messaging. Participants receive directions for logging onto their computers and gaining access to the discussion. They then proceed to converse with one another in written form using specified commands and directions. The dialogue that appears on the screen resembles a script for a dramatic production.

A variation on synchronous computer conferencing is the *Web conference* (also know as a Webinar), which combines computer conferencing with audio conferencing. Participants connect to the audio conference and then individually connect their computers to a preassigned Web address. PowerPoint slides or other visuals can be uploaded to a conference server and then discussed during the conference. The visual material also can include various interactive tools. People can participate anywhere they have access to the Internet and a phone.

Advantages
Computer conferencing offers the following advantages:

- *Becoming more accessible.* Personal computers are now standard equipment in the workplace, and virtually all professionals have access to them. An increasing number of people have computers and access to the Internet in their homes.
- *Comparatively inexpensive.* Once people have access to a personal computer, they will need an Internet connection at home or at their workplace. Assuming this basic equipment is available, most people will not incur any direct costs to participate in a computer conference. Although some people may incur long-distance telephone charges to connect to the Internet at home, most subscribers pay a flat monthly fee for unlimited Internet use.
- *Relatively quick process.* The length of a synchronous computer conference is approximately the same as the length of an audio

conference. An asynchronous computer conference could span a period of several weeks, but the actual time necessary for participants to read and respond to their messages is probably no more than 20 minutes at any one time.

- *Encourages busy people to participate.* As with audio conferencing, people who are reluctant to participate in a face-to-face meeting might welcome the opportunity to join a computer conference.
- *Novel approach.* Some people grow weary of having to attend one more meeting or participate in yet another conference call. For them, a computer conference offers the opportunity to do something different, and their curiosity may overcome their initial resistance.
- *Participants not influenced by socioeconomic status differences.* Because they cannot observe or talk with one another, participants do not pick up visual or verbal cues to socioeconomic status, unlike in face-to-face communications.

Disadvantages

Computer conferencing has the following disadvantages:

- *Limited interaction.* Computer conferencing involves responding in written form to other written information, unless it is combined with audio conferencing or videoconferencing in some way.
- *Requires people who enjoy written interaction.* Participants are isolated from one another and, unless combined with audio conferencing or videoconferencing, cannot benefit from voice or facial interaction. As a result, computer conferencing is most useful for people who are comfortable using computers and enjoy written communication.
- *Difficult to reach certain populations.* The proliferation of personal computers and the growing number of people with access to the Internet are making involvement of professionals in computer conferences quite realistic. For reaching a cross-section of the general public, however, and especially lower-income, younger, or older populations, a computer conference is not as feasible.
- *Multi-tasking.* During simulcasts, some participants may feel the need to engage in multiple responsibilities at the same time, unknowingly disrupting the proceedings as well as becoming a more "detached participant."

VIDEOCONFERENCING

Satellite technology has been used to offer credit courses and professional seminars for more than two decades. Unfortunately, this technology offers only one-way video and one-way audio communication from the instructors or speakers to the participants. To ask questions or offer comments, participants must initiate a telephone call on a separate line, typically to a toll-free number, or send an e-mail or facsimile message. This form of video-conferencing is very expensive, requiring uplinking satellite equipment and a studio facility at the origination site and downlinking satellite equipment at each receive site.

Telephone lines for videoconferencing represent another format for two-way interactive video and audio communication that is made possible through fiber-optic cables. Fiber-optic networks have been developed in most states, connecting schools, institutions of higher education, hospitals, government agencies, and other community organizations. These fiber-optic networks offer very high-quality, full-motion videoconferencing at a far lower cost than current satellite technology. If participants have access to network sites, a fiber-optic videoconference is an exciting way to conduct a needs assessment exercise. Developing such a network does require an extensive financial investment, however, to establish dedicated telephone lines between a limited number of fixed sites. Internet work connections are possible, allowing for communication with additional sites separated by greater distances, but they require additional coordination and financial investment.

Another use of telephone lines for conferencing relies on compressed video technology. Unlike with fiber-optic networks, compressed video is not limited to established fixed sites. Instead of using dedicated telephone lines, anyone with the appropriate equipment and technical expertise can use regular tele-phone lines to connect to a compressed videoconference. Participants can dial another site directly or use a video bridge to connect several sites. The bridge simply manages all incoming and outgoing calls.

Establishing a compressed video system requires considerably less financial investment than creating a dedicated fiber-optic network, but users typically incur long-distance toll charges for two to six telephone lines whenever the system is used. Additionally, conducting a compressed videoconference over the Internet has become possible, saving the long-distance telephone costs. Using telephone lines is still the preferred method at this time, however, because the connection is more stable than one established via the Internet.

Although compressed video is less costly and more agile than fiber optics, the quality is not as good. The major disadvantage is that at lower transmis-sion rates the video image can appear "jerky." Audio communication also is slightly delayed. Transmission of still images and graphics is usually of good quality. Users can choose the transmission rate they prefer, but all connecting sites must receive and transmit at the same rate. A higher transmission rate results in higher-quality video and audio communication, but the additional telephone lines needed mean higher long-distance charges. Compressed video conferencing has improved significantly in recent years, resulting in consider-ably less audio and video delay, and should develop further during this decade. It represents a promising approach to needs assessment, because participants potentially can use regular telephone lines or the Internet to connect anywhere in the world.

Even more promising is another form of videoconferencing called *desktop conferencing*. Using the Internet, video images are transmitted and received through a regular personal computer monitor or through a small video monitor mounted on top of the computer monitor. Desktop videoconferencing is a form of compressed video conferencing, albeit one typically carried out at the slowest transmission speed. Picture quality is at best fair, but it at least provides live two-way video interaction. Due to the widespread use of personal computers, desktop conferencing is potentially much more accessible for needs assessment exercises than compressed video systems or fiber-optic networks. Improvements in compressed video technology in the years ahead should improve the quality of desktop conferencing as well.

Overall, an array of videoconferencing formats can facilitate needs and capacity assessments that can inform distance education activity to include planning, delivery, and evaluation (Gilmore, Olsen, & Taub, 2010). Awareness of learner needs (e.g., public health practitioners, teachers, students) to include the type of academic recognition, along with capacity issues, such as available technology; one's Internet experience; cost factors; and the timeframe/timing of the educational events can lead to a more reasonable opportunity for success in distance education (Gilmore et al., 2010). **Figure 9-1** depicts this more systematic approach.

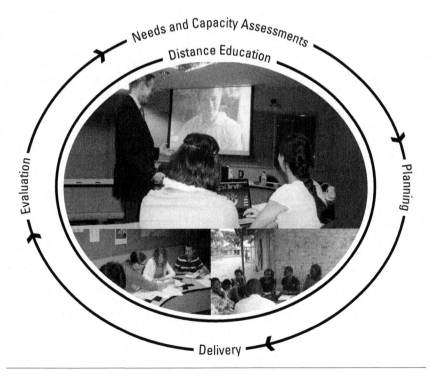

FIGURE 9-1
Process of distance education involving assessment, planning, delivery, and evaluation.

Advantages

Videoconferencing offers the following advantages:

- *More extensive interaction.* A videoconference enables both verbal and nonverbal communication and provides opportunities to transmit graphics, video, and other forms of multimedia.
- *Typically a shorter process than a face-to-face meeting.* "Dial-up" long-distance charges for compressed videoconferences, tightly scheduled transmission and reception facilities, and "technology fatigue" from using a more structured mode of communication all limit the length of a videoconference.
- *Attractive to busy people.* Even if travel to a special facility is necessary, the time and expense are usually less than that required for an extended face-to-face meeting.

Disadvantages

Videoconferencing has the following disadvantages:

- *Less accessible.* People can participate in a conference call in the office, at home, or at other locations, but a videoconference often requires a specially equipped facility. Many people currently do not have access to these facilities.
- *Significantly more expensive.* Developing a fiber-optic network requires a major capital investment. Once established, long-distance communication is available at no cost to network members, but the network may charge user fees to recover overhead costs. Compressed video equipment is less costly, but the long-distance charges for multiple telephone lines add up. Participants typically need technical support when using videoconferencing equipment, which also adds to the cost.
- *Requires more advance planning.* A videoconference usually requires reserving a specially equipped room and scheduling time on a network or securing the use of a video bridge.
- *More limited nonverbal communication than in a face-to-face meeting.* Picture quality for compressed videoconferencing varies considerably, depending on the transmission speed. The video and audio delay makes facial expressions more difficult to decipher. Fiber-optic videoconferences have better picture quality, but subtle forms of nonverbal communication are less obvious.
- *Occasional awkward verbal communication with compressed video and desktop conferencing.* Participants can see a speaker at another location but experience a slight delay hearing what is said. When viewing someone responding to a question, they may wonder at first if the respondent heard the question.

Despite the apparent disadvantages of videoconferencing, take heart. The advantage of two-way video communication is very significant for communication at a distance. The improvements in this technology that will occur in the years ahead and its expansion into ever more schools, hospitals, government agencies, businesses, and nonprofit organizations should result in its widespread use for needs assessment activities. As one example, many laptop computers already come equipped with inset Web cameras ready for immediate use.

Preparing for the Assessment

As with any needs and capacity assessment strategy, several general steps are necessary to prepare for the assessment of these technology-supported assessments. For example, you need to select the participants and develop the issues on which to focus. Also, as with other assessments, consider the type of database format (e.g., an Excel spreadsheet, use of FileMaker) that will be used prior to the collection of data. Additional specific steps are necessary to prepare for audio conferences, computer conferences, and videoconferences.

Schedule the Conference for the Convenience of Most Participants

If you are using a dedicated audio or video network, or even an audio or video bridge, you must consider the time available on those systems. Dialing each participant directly offers the most flexible scheduling.

A computer conference requires arranging for computer time and specifying the timeframe during which people must respond to your information. Stivers, Bently, and Meccouri (1995) list some of the more frequently used public health-related discussion lists and online discussion groups available. Kittleson (2009) addresses the quality issue with distance education technology, citing its convenience and value to the participants.

Select One or Two Major Questions to Consider

Because several people will participate in the conference, you cannot ask as many questions as during a telephone survey. You will need to allow time for everyone to respond to your questions and time for the participants to respond to one another, if desired. The people who participate in these conferences are often busy, so you want to use the time you have to best advantage.

Prepare Graphics, Videos, and Other Multimedia Materials

These enhancements add variety and quality to a videoconference and counter the tendency to rely on "talking heads."

Send the Participants Information Before the Conference

Remind participants when the conference will take place, who it includes, and what you hope to accomplish. If possible, list the questions you plan to ask, so that they can think about how to respond. Request that all participants dedicate themselves to the experience and keep multi-tasking to a minimum during the proceedings.

Schedule Training and Technical Support

Participants in a videoconference need instructions, demonstrations, and practice in using the equipment, preferably before the conference actually begins. Otherwise, valuable time will be wasted. In the worst case, untrained and inexperienced participants could undermine the entire videoconference. If possible, arrange for technical support personnel to be present or close by during the conference to handle any technical problems that arise.

Conducting the Assessment

The following steps describe how to conduct these technology-supported assessments.

Use the First Few Minutes for Warm Up

Start the conference on time, but do not plunge into the first question right away. Instead, introduce yourself and restate the purpose of the conference. Conduct a roll call to ensure that everyone who is to be involved is on the line. This roll call also gives each person the opportunity to become comfortable with the equipment and to make sure it is operating satisfactorily.

Ask Your Questions in a Structured Fashion

One option is to ask a question and then to proceed to call on each person by name for a response. A structured approach is important for audio conferencing because you cannot observe facial cues to determine who is ready to respond. Interjecting comments during an audio conference is also more difficult than during a face-to-face meeting. Less spontaneous people may have trouble making their comments if they are not asked directly. By comparison, the discussion will likely flow more easily during a videoconference.

After everyone has had an opportunity to respond, pause and ask whether anyone has any other comments to add before moving to the next question. If possible, try to summarize what the group has said before discussing the next question.

Less structure is necessary for a small group, especially if the members are relatively comfortable with one another. In such situations, it is possible to throw the question out to the group and let the participants respond. Before moving to another question, though, be sure to ask those who have not responded if they have any comments.

Record the Information

If at all possible, try to have someone other than the conference moderator present during an audio conference to take extensive notes. That leaves the moderator free to concentrate on conducting the conference. Tape recording is another possibility for an audio conference or videoconference when the issues are not sensitive, provided that the group is clearly informed of its use. Recording information is less of a challenge for computer conferencing because the written dialogue is easily stored or printed. Participants must be informed that the session will be taped.

Using the Results

As soon after the conference as possible, summarize the information gathered. Because the conference has been conducted in a structured manner, this summary should be easy to organize. If possible, send the summary to the participants. Ask them to review it for accuracy and to send you any corrections. Then share the information with your planning committee.

Without question, the rapid expansion in technology we are experiencing is creating exciting possibilities for examining health-related needs. Additional possibilities are on the horizon. Of some concern, however, is whether these advances will primarily benefit certain individuals (e.g., younger aged, those of a higher socioeconomic level) at the expense of others. Such a development would require judicious use of technology to assess needs of certain populations, so as to avoid bias in the results.

Reviewing an Example

Using technology to explore the media sources of particular populations provides an opportunity to tap into unique health-related insights. In the study by Black and Peacock (2011), the authors focused on the daily responsibilities and stressors related to the maintenance of health and wellness among African American women as depicted in the media and blogs. The methodology involved being guided by a *strong Black women (SBW)* script which included the attributes of "self-reliance, self-sacrifice, and self-silence" (p. 144). These attributes were considered best assessed through the women's daily life-management experiences of role management, coping, and self-care (considered a priori codes) as presented in magazine articles and blogs. Coupled with these sources, the authors also intertwined research studies from women's studies, family science, and health sciences. Selected findings included media and blog-related articles that focused on trying to do it all and "pleasing the masses" with the consequential health impacts (p. 147); coping strategies that "also manifested as maladaptive health behaviors" (p. 147); and a blogger's sentiment that was "expressed by many women in popular media sources about the health consequences of sacrificing self-care: 'Being strong can kill you.'" (p. 147). Overall, the authors concluded that the voices of these women not only have to be heard, but distinctly addressed.

Online Resources

Visit go.jblearning.com/gilmore4 for links to these Web sites.

Agency for Health Care Research and Quality

A Web-assisted audio conference on surge capacity assessments and regionalization issues.

National Information Center on Health Services Research and Health Care Technology

Outlines the 10 basic steps to health care research assessments.

National Institutes of Health, Collaboration Project

This forum allows people to use collaborative technologies to solve management challenges.

TRECC

Information on videoconferencing.

Videoconferencing

Information on videoconferencing, telemedicine, and audiovisual equipment.

National Network for Child Care, Videoconference

An example of a videoconference evaluation.

References

Black, A., and Peacock, N. (2011). Pleasing the masses: Messages for daily life management in African American women's popular media sources. *American Journal of Public Health, 101,* 144–150.

Centers for Disease Control and Prevention (CDC). (2010). Social media guidelines and best practices. Available at: http://www.cdc.gov/SocialMedia/Tools/guidelines.

Chou, W., Hunt, Y., Beckjord, E., Moser, R., and Hesse, B. (2009). Social media use in the United States: Implications for health communications. *Journal of Medical Internet Research, 11,* 4. Available at: http://www.jmir.org/2009/4/e48.

Gilmore, G., Olsen, L., and Taub, A. (2010). Going the distance for health enhancement: Capacity building using distance education. Presented at the 20th International Union for Health Promotion and Education-IUHPE World Conference on Health Promotion, July 13, 2010, Geneva, Switzerland.

Kittleson, M. (2009). The future of technology in health education: Challenging the traditional delivery dogma. *American Journal of Health Education, 40,* 310–316.

Ontario Health Promotion eBulletin. (2010). Social media overview. Available at: http://www.ohpe.ca/node/11601.

Rice, E. (2010). The positive role of social networks and social networking technology in the condom-using behaviors of homeless young people. *Public Health Reports, 125,* 588–595.

Stivers, C., Bently, M., and Meccouri, L. (1995). Internet: The contemporary health educator's most versatile tool. *Journal of Health Education, 26,* 196–199.

Large-Scale Community Assessment Strategies

Introduction

Over the last few decades, several needs and capacity assessment procedures have emerged that have been applied to communities and regions as part of a larger health planning framework. These large-scale community assessment strategies typically are highly planned, resource-intensive, and long-term in nature. A number of those described here are based on collaborative efforts involving both the public and the private sectors. They strive for a variety of approaches to assessment that will yield insights into diverse populations within a specified geographic area.

The following community needs and capacity assessment strategies are current examples of large-scale approaches. The assessment components are part of a larger planning framework. They have been developed through the collaborative efforts of several agencies and organizations and have been implemented in community settings for a number of years. The major advantages of these approaches are that they (1) provide a comprehensive review of the needs and strengths of the population, (2) tie into a planning framework that includes the development and implementation of action plans, and (3) encourage partnerships and collaborative efforts among organizations and community members. The major disadvantages are that they (1) are very time intensive, (2) are highly resource intensive, and (3) require continual monitoring and maintenance to keep the process moving and individuals motivated to participate in the various committee procedures. A few key large-scale frameworks and their salient characteristics are described in the following sections.

Reviewing the Strategy

ASSESSMENT PROTOCOL FOR EXCELLENCE IN PUBLIC HEALTH (APEX-PH)

With the financial support of the National Association of County Health Officials and the Centers for Disease Control and Prevention (CDC), six professional and official organizations joined together to develop an assessment process intended for use by local health departments entitled the Assessment Protocol for Excellence in Public Health (APEX-PH) (National Association of County and City Health Official [NACCHO], n.d.; Centers for Disease Control and Prevention [CDC], 2003). This approach was developed in a response to several national reports that emphasized the need for a focus on prevention and health promotion (e.g., *Healthy People 2010, Healthy People 2020*) as well as the important role played by local health departments in conducting needs assessments, policy development, and assurance activities (Institute of Medicine, 2003). Today, greater focus is placed on using the MAPP approach, which is described in a subsequent section in this chapter on page 171.

The process consists of three parts. In the first phase, an organizational capacity assessment addresses how an agency can review and improve its performance. An eight-step process is recommended that seeks to analyze an organization's strengths and weaknesses and then to rank-order problems according to three criteria: magnitude of the problem, seriousness of the consequences of the problem, and feasibility of correcting the problem. Afterward, a plan can be developed to strengthen the organization's status. Worksheets are provided to assist in the organizational assessment.

The second phase involves the community assessment process, in which the organization works with the community, particularly through a community health committee, to identify, prioritize, and analyze community health problems. Worksheets are provided to assist in identifying health problems through a review of secondary information—particularly demographic, morbidity, and mortality data. In addition, the community health committee is encouraged to serve as a sounding board by reacting to the proposed community health problems suggested by the organization's staff. The selection of a prioritization process in which community health problems are ranked is open to the discretion of the organization's staff and the committee. The nominal group process with its systematic ranking is one recommended approach.

Also included in the second phase is an analysis component, which delves into why a particular health problem exists by reviewing its risk factors (scientifically established determinants that relate directly to the level of a health problem—for example, low birth weight as an influence on infant mortality), direct contributing factors (scientifically established determinants that directly affect the level of a risk factor—for example, teen pregnancy as an influence on low birth weight), and indirect contributing factors (community-specific determinants that directly affect the level of direct contributing factors—for example, low self-esteem as an influence on teen pregnancy). Based on this information as well as a review of actual and potential resources, the committee can develop a specific community health plan for implementation.

The third phase addresses activities that will support the implementation of the plan of action. These include policy development procedures, assurances of continuing support for the community health committee, ongoing data surveillance, public health service provision, monitoring of progress, and formal evaluation of the effectiveness in meeting the stated goals and objectives in the plan.

PLANNED APPROACH TO COMMUNITY HEALTH (PATCH)

The origins of the Planned Approach To Community Health (PATCH) date back to the early 1980s when the then-titled Center for Health Promotion and Education in the CDC attempted to guide the proposal development and support efforts of the Health Education–Risk Reduction (HERR) categorical grants program. Even as this federal categorical grant process evolved into a more state-managed prevention block-grant approach with the addition of seven other categorical grant programs, the overriding principle remained encouraging the development of an organized, planned approach to community-based interventions by local, state, and federal health organizations (Kreuter, 1992). The two original goals that directed the PATCH efforts were (1) to "create a practical mechanism through which effective community health education action could be targeted to address local level health priorities," and (2) to "offer a practical, skill-based program of technical assistance wherein health education leaders in state health agencies would work with their local health counterparts to establish community health education programs" (Kreuter, 1992, p. 136).

The PATCH approach incorporated a community intervention strategy within the context of the PRECEDE model described in Chapter 2. While PATCH is no longer active, the lessons learned from the process continue to provide valuable insights. Green and Kreuter (2005) point out that "existing programs and activities in a community can also be a source of even richer information than prior interventions conducted elsewhere because they are indigenous to the community or setting and they were designed with the same population and more similar circumstances than most prior interventions" (p. 203).

With national leadership from the CDC, PATCH worked with national partners from voluntary agencies, Cooperative Extension, and the National Education Association. More than 42 states, the District of Columbia, the Virgin Islands, and international sites such as Queensland, Australia (Swannell, Steele, Harvey, Bruggemann, Town, Emery, & Schmid, 1992), participated in the PATCH network, including both civilian and military populations. The framework for activity involved vertical (national to local level) and horizontal (across the various partnership agencies and organizations) communications and support (see **Figure 10-1**).

The driving force behind the approach was the encouragement of local ownership. Particularly during the needs assessment phase, which encompassed an average of 1 year of data collection and analysis, a sense of empowerment emerged as involved individuals and groups come to realize that they were a part of the decision-making process. **Figure 10-2** depicts the usual steps in the PATCH process that preceded the determination of health promotion needs and community diagnosis methods, followed up with the identification of priorities for work plan development. Five elements in PATCH were considered essential:

1. Community members participate in the process.
2. Data guide the development of programs.
3. Participants develop a comprehensive health promotion strategy.
4. Evaluation emphasizes feedback and program improvement.
5. The community capacity for health promotion is increased.

This approach was exemplified by the effort undertaken by the National Coalition of Hispanic Health and Human Service Organizations, which selected the PATCH approach to address a growing concern about the leading causes of death among Hispanics in El Paso, Texas (Ugarte, Duarte, & Wilson, 1992). The approach taken was considered to be unique because the assessment strategies needed to be modified to reflect the bilingual, bicultural, and unique health needs of that population and resulted in the development of the Hispanic Health Needs Assessment (HHNA) process. It incorporated a community profile, review of morbidity and mortality rates, a behavioral risk factor survey, and community opinion surveys for local leaders and residents. It was felt that the comprehensive assessment approach was an important first step in being able to initiate health promotion programs in Hispanic communities. Many of the principles and practices emerging from PATCH can provide guidance to assessment efforts taking place today.

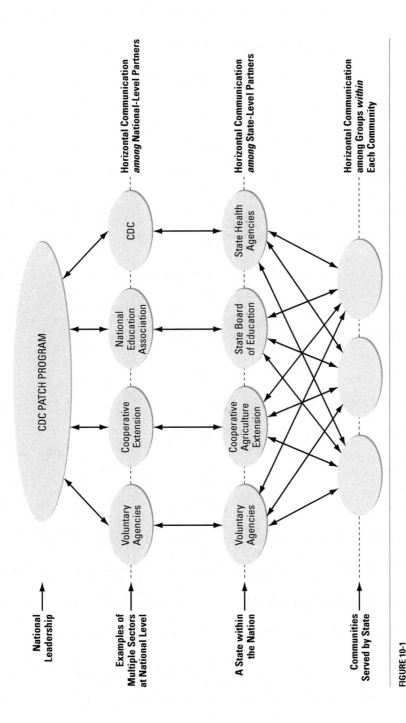

FIGURE 10-1

PATCH. Mobilizing vertical and horizontal communication and support among the national, regional, and community levels.

Source: Kreuter, M. (1992). PATCH: Its origin, basic concepts, and links to contemporary public health policy. *Journal of Health Education, 23,* 135–139. Reprinted with the permission of the American Association for Health Education.

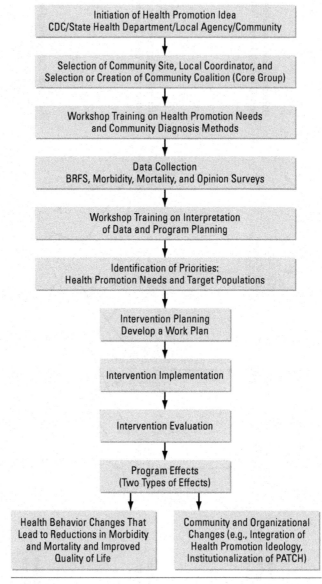

FIGURE 10-2
The presumptive PATCH model.

Source: Steckler, A., Orville, K., Eng, E., and Dawson, L. (1992). Summary of a formative evaluation of PATCH. *Journal of Health Education, 23,* 174–178. Reprinted with the permission of the American Association for Health Education.

MOBILIZING FOR ACTION THROUGH PLANNING AND PARTNERSHIPS (MAPP)

An emerging large-scale process with key needs and capacity assessment phases is the community-wide strategic planning tool known as Mobilizing for Action through Planning and Partnerships (MAPP); it is offered through the National Association of County and City Health Officials (NACCHO) in cooperation with the CDC (http://www.naccho.org/toolbox/index.cfm?v=3). The process begins with communities bringing various partners together for organizational and shared visioning purposes. These steps are followed by the community's involvement in four key needs and capacity assessments:

- Community themes and strengths, which identifies community assets, interests, and perceptions about quality of life
- Local public health system assessment, which measures the capacity and performance of the local public health system along with other community organizations
- Community health status assessment, which assesses health status, quality of life, and risk factor data
- Forces of change assessment, which identifies forces affecting the community or the local public health system

Following the various assessment phases, an illustrated community roadmap is developed so that all stakeholders can envision a healthier community as a destination. Overall, "MAPP is not an agency-focused assessment process; rather, it is an interactive process that can improve the efficiency, effectiveness, and ultimately the performance of local public health systems" (National Association of County and City Health Officials [NACCHO], 2011). Currently, demonstration sites throughout the United States are preparing for and implementing the MAPP process so that review and revision can take place.

COMPASS COMMUNITY ASSESSMENT

United Way of America has developed a community-based needs and capacity assessment process that enables representatives from community agencies to become engaged in comprehensive planning, implementation, and evaluation procedures. Initially, six communities in the United States (including La Crosse, Wisconsin) were selected to pilot the assessment process. The approach draws upon key community resource materials developed earlier by United Way (United Way of America, 1996; 1997). As one example, the Great Rivers United Way (with headquarters in Onalaska, Wisconsin) entered into its fourth multicounty COMPASS assessment during 2011. The format was based to a large degree on the *2008 Community Compass Now* assessment, the third community-based assessment conducted (the full report is available online at http://gruw.org/documents/Final%20Full%20Report%205-12-08.pdf). The goal of the 2007–2008 assessment was to "further develop the COMPASS process and standardize the approach to enable comparison of the outcomes from this third COMPASS and future COMPASS projects," (Great Rivers United Way, 2008, p. iii). Eight phases were used in this process: Form a community partnership; inventory key community assets; collect, map, and analyze data; create a community vision; identify critical community issues and desired outcomes; detail a community action plan; take action; and measure outcomes (Great Rivers United Way, 2008, p. iv). The results were reported as *Community Strengths* (related to community services, health care, education, natural environment, and safety), *Regional Issues Identified*, and *Recommendations*. Additionally, some local public health agencies have found it of value to use the collaborative COMPASS approach as a part of their required community-wide needs and capacity assessment processes.

COMBINED HEALTH SYSTEMS: EMERGENCY RESPONSE

During times of community challenge, various health-related organizations can come together to conduct needs and capacity assessments. One such example arose following Hurricane Katrina, which occurred along the Gulf Coast on August 29, 2005. This was a Category 5 storm, and numerous residents were evacuated to regional cities. To assess the health status of 124 evacuees who were placed in shelters in Houston, Texas, an assessment process involving a survey and interview was developed by the Houston Department of Health and Human Services, Harris County Health Department, and the School of Public Health at the University of Texas Health Science Center. In the report detailed by Coker, Hanks, Eggleston, Risser, Tee, Chronister, et al. (2006), the assessment process used a brief survey designed to determine the medical, social, and psychological needs of the evacuees (e.g., level of posttraumatic stress disorder [PTSD]), along with encouraging those who were willing to discuss their experiences during and after the hurricane, using an interview process.

Notable findings included 41 percent who were afraid they would die, 16 percent who saw someone close to them injured or dead, 17 percent who saw violence, and 6 percent who directly experienced physical violence. Moderate PTSD and severe PTSD were experienced by 38.6 percent and 23.9 percent, respectively. In their summary commentary, the authors stated that the "stability of an individual's physical and mental health may become more vulnerable when that person is displaced from their community and social networks. . . . All of our team who interviewed Katrina evacuees learned from their experiences and their courage; in this process, we were reminded of the interconnectedness of life. What happens to our neighbors in New Orleans directly influences our lives in Houston, Texas" (Coker et al., 2006, pp. 92–94).

Preparing for the Assessment

All of these large-scale community assessment formats require carefully established time lines with several months of lead time built in. Additionally, if grant-related funding will be sought, one must plan 1 to 2 years in advance of the assessment implementation phase to prepare the appropriate proposals.

Although the time lines certainly will vary depending on the size of the population base, the degree of difficulty in accessing and working with partners and the target audience, and the availability of resources, the approach offered by *Healthworks* in Erie, Pennsylvania, does offer a helpful preliminary planning framework.

Six to 9 months before kick-off:

1. Select a coordinator and support staff.
2. Develop a draft implementation plan.
3. Select a target community.
4. Define your target audience.
5. Marshall your resources.

Three to 6 months before kick-off:

6. Select your survey instruments and screening methods.
7. Gain support from community leaders.
8. Form a steering committee.
9. Solicit donations of incentive prizes.
10. Schedule town meetings and feedback sessions (p. 5).

It is important to add to this list that the early review of secondary data regarding, at a minimum, the demographics, morbidity, and mortality information for a community will yield valuable insights. The worksheets provided for the APEX-PH process can facilitate this phase in terms of its logical data collection format and its ability to provide for data reporting to committee members.

Those wishing to learn more about the PATCH approach, given its extensive national, state, and local partnership configuration, can visit http://wonder .cdc.gov/wonder/prevguid/p0000064/p0000064.asp.

Conducting the Assessment

In addition to having an established time line with aligned responsibilities, it will be essential to have mutually agreed-upon means of communication with all partners during the assessment implementation phase. Written time line/responsibility information, secondary data summaries, meeting summaries, and the sharing and discussion of preliminary primary data findings will need to be built into the assessment process. This effort will ensure that all of the partners are kept as up-to-date as possible while the assessment progresses and will enable revisions in the process to occur as needed. Data updates should be scheduled as routinely as the steering committee deems appropriate.

Due to the multiple assessment procedures that usually are incorporated into large-scale community-based approaches, it is recommended that assessment purpose statements be established to guide the methods selected. One example would be "to characterize the living standards of this population," which could be addressed through a review of that population's demographic data.

Using the Results

The large-scale community assessment formats occur within the context of a larger planning framework. For that reason, the collected needs information can be fed directly into the action planning phase of the respective framework. Typically, this entails the prioritization of the assessed needs using established criteria (see Chapter 2), leading to the development of overarching goals and action-related objectives for health enhancement. Note that while the data sources are valuable in gaining insights into the needs of the population, the discussion that ensues from steering, planning, and/or advisory committees reviewing such information represents a rich resource of ideas, concerns, and issues that should not be taken lightly. These inputs can be particularly welcome contributions as one attempts to derive trends and patterns from the multiple data sources. Over time, you should learn to trust the instincts and insights of a longstanding, representative committee that is being properly facilitated.

Reviewing an Example

A rural health promotion project was established in Vernon County, Wisconsin, to demonstrate that health care providers could work in partnership with community organizations to identify health needs and then mutually address those needs (Gilmore, Traastad, & Johnson, 2003; Favor, Robinson, & Gilmore, 1994). Representatives from these organizations were members of the Community Health Intervention Partnership (CHIP) Council, which served as the oversight and planning body. It was suggested that seven clustered, but not mutually exclusive, target groups be addressed in the effort: Amish, youth, elderly, farming families, unemployed, socioeconomically disadvantaged, and general public.

The planning framework deemed most appropriate for the county-wide effort was the APEX-PH approach, with certain modifications in the organizational assessment phase. Because all of the organizations represented on the CHIP Council had interacted with one another previously, a general sense of trust was already engendered, as was an understanding of available resources. Following the collection and review of public and private sources of secondary data, a survey was developed, pilot tested, and implemented in the county. The survey assessed general well-being, risk factor and protective factor involvement, social networking opportunities, environmental factors, and personal, family, and community health promotional issues within a sample population ranging in age from 13 to 103 years. Additional insights into the top-priority health issues were revealed through a nominal group meeting of selected citizens from throughout the county who represented the seven target populations. Based on a continuing review of these primary and secondary data sources, the CHIP Council was able to identify three top-priority areas for immediate attention to be addressed through the development and implementation of action plans, as coordinated by respective subcommittees: (1) enhancement of primary prevention and health promotion activities, (2) strengthening of the family unit, and (3) improvement of access to services and information.

The overall effort was deemed a success due to the continuing nature of the CHIP Council as the 3-year foundation funding concluded, the enduring partnerships that were established across the county, the sense of trust and resource sharing that prevailed, and the successful accomplishment of many of the outcomes specified in the action plans. During the 1999–2002 period, the needs and capacity assessment process was repeated using a revised survey format, followed by action plan development for the county during 2003. An additional example of regional assessment is provided in Gilmore, Schwan, and McLaughlin (2007) regarding emergency preparedness.

Online Resources

Visit go.jblearning.com/gilmore4 for links to these Web sites.

Assessment Protocol for Excellence in Public Health (APEX)
Overview of APEX-PH process with contact information.

COMPASS Community Assessment
Description of the United Way community-based regional assessment process.

Study Circles Research Center
Documentation and assessment of the community-wide study circles and best practices links.

Higher Education Center for Alcohol and Other Drug Prevention
Statewide initiative assessment, strategic planning, and evaluation.

Centers for Disease Control and Prevention
CDC Assessment Protocol for Excellence in Public Health (APEX) publication and links.

APEX
A PowerPoint presentation on APEX presented by NACCHO and the CDC in alignment with the three core public health functions.

PATCH
CDC PATCH document presented and described, to include a guide for the local coordinator.

References

Centers for Disease Control and Prevention (CDC), Division of Public Health Surveillance and Informatics. (2003). Assessment protocol for excellence in public health (APEX-PH). Atlanta, GA: Author. Available at: http://wonder.cdc.gov/wonder/prevguid/p0000089/p0000089.asp.

Coker, A., Hanks, J., Eggleston, K., Risser, J., Tee, G., Chronister, K., Troisi, C., Arafat, R., and Franzini, L. (2006). Social and mental needs assessment of Katrina evacuees. *Disaster Management and Response, 4,* 88–94.

Erie County Department of Health. (1992). *Healthworks: Guide for conducting a community-based health risk appraisal program.* Erie, PA: Author.

Favor, S., Robinson, J., and Gilmore, G. (1994). *Report of the Vernon County Community Health Intervention Project.* Westby, WI: Coulee CAP.

Gilmore, G., Schwan, W., and McLaughlin, M. (2007). An assessment of emergency preparedness in western Wisconsin. *Wisconsin Medical Journal, 106,* 71–77.

Gilmore, G., Traastad, K., and Johnson, E. (2003). Vernon County, Wisconsin, Health Needs Assessment Report: 1999–2002. University of Wisconsin–Extension.

Great Rivers United Way. (2008). 2008 Community COMPASS NOW: A snapshot of LIFE in the Great Rivers Region. Onalaska, WI: Author.

Green, L., and Kreuter, M. (2005). *Health program planning: An educational and ecological approach.* Boston: McGraw-Hill.

Green, L., and Kreuter, M. (1992). CDC's planned approach to community health as an application of PRECEDE and an inspiration for PROCEED. *Journal of Health Education, 23,* 140–144.

Institute of Medicine. (2003). *The future of the public's health in the 21st century.* Washington, DC: National Academies Press.

Kreuter, M. (1992). PATCH: Its origins, basic concepts, and links to contemporary public health policy. *Journal of Health Education, 23,* 135–139.

National Association of County and City Health Official (NACCHO). (2011). Mobilizing for Action through Planning and Partnerships (MAPP). Available at: http://www.naccho.org/topics/infrastructure/MAPP/index.cfm.

National Association of County and City Health Official (NACCHO). (n.d.). APEX-PH resources. Available at: http://www.naccho.org/topics/infrastructure/APEXPH/index.cfm.

Steckler, A., Orville, K., Eng, E., and Dawson, L. (1992). Summary of a formative evaluation of PATCH. *Journal of Health Education, 23,* 174–178.

Swannell, R., Steele, J., Harvey, P., Bruggemann, J., Town, S., Emery, E., and Schmid, T. (1992). PATCH in Australia: Elements of a successful implementation. *Journal of Health Education, 23,* 171–173.

Ugarte, C., Duarte, P., and Wilson, K. (1992). PATCH as a model for development of an Hispanic health needs assessment: The El Paso experience. *Journal of Health Education, 23,* 153–156.

United Way of America. (1997). *ACCESS97: User's guide.* Alexandria, VA: Author.

United Way of America. (1996). *Measuring program outcomes: A practical approach.* Alexandria, VA: Author.

Self-Directed Assessments

Self-directed assessments are personal review procedures. A majority of these approaches address primary prevention issues, such as the assessment of risk factors and protective factors in one's lifestyle pattern, and the secondary prevention process of the early detection of disease symptoms. Some of these strategies combine the two aspects of prevention so that risk factors and symptoms can be detected and addressed. Still others expand into an assessment of positive (protective) factors in one's lifestyle, thereby becoming more wellness oriented (e.g., assessing positive exercise, diet, and relaxation patterns). Although some of the assessment procedures, such as breast self-examination, require initial instruction, others do not (e.g., taking a self-scored General Health Status Inventory). Some of the assessment inventories are self-scored, whereas others are analyzed by computers. In Chapters 11 and 12, a variety of approaches for health and wellness assessment will be reviewed.

CHAPTER 1

Self-Directed Assessment Inventories

Introduction

Individual concern for heightened levels of wellness and willingness to take personal responsibility for certain lifestyle changes have been the recent focus of health promotion in our society. Although the degree of individual commitment and follow-through varies greatly, it is clear that a rather potent health consciousness has arisen in many societies.

Several key efforts have been designed to kindle national concern about health and overall well-being. Notable among these is *Healthy People 2020*, which provides national objectives for health promotion and disease prevention (U.S. Department of Health and Human Services [USDHHS], 2010). It clarifies the risks to good health, including those lifestyle aspects over which an individual has a good deal of control—for example, smoking, alcohol misuse and abuse, poor diet, lack of regular exercise, and stress. Although the initiative largely focuses on risk factors and disease and injury outcome reduction, guided by a "determinants of health" (Commission on Social Determinants of Health, 2008) approach, the framework also targets certain protective factors, such as eating a balanced diet, engaging in physical activity, and establishing healthy schools and worksites. The report calls for more attention to be paid to multiple levels of responsibility involving individuals, families, health professionals, health institutions, schools, business and labor, communities, and government. Particular attention is centered on the individual's role in making day-to-day decisions. The public needs to be reminded about the value of health screenings as a complement to primary prevention strategies (i.e., preventive efforts taken before a particular disease develops). Figure 2-7 in Chapter 2 provides an overview of *Healthy People 2020* in terms of its vision, mission, goals, and foundation points. It is of value to note the overarching goal to "promote quality of life, healthy development, and healthy behaviors across all life stages" (USDHHS, 2010).

Ten great public health achievements in the United States between 2001 and 2010 have been noted by the Centers for Disease Control and Prevention (CDC). These include the lifestyle-related factors of tobacco control, motor vehicle safety, cardiovascular disease prevention, and cancer prevention. The report refers to the judicious use of the legal system (e.g., taxation, regulatory action) in modern public health practice (Centers for Disease Control and Prevention [CDC], 2011, p. 621).

This chapter examines health promotion assessment inventories that can be used with individuals, to be potentially followed up with intervention, planned change, or strategies and their reinforcement (Powers & Dodd, 2003; Squire, Gilmore, Duquette, & Riley, 2001; Gilmore, Dosch, & Hood, 1985; Gilmore, 1979). Some of the available formats provide a brief assessment of several health promotional dimensions, known as general health status inventories (GHSIs). The basic intent of these formats is to quickly sensitize an individual to risk factors and certain protective factors, typically through self-scoring and interpretation. More in-depth risk factor assessments are available through health risk appraisals (HRAs), which are usually longer and scored by computer. Both formats tend to concentrate almost exclusively on risk factors or disease/death/disability inducers. In a third type of format, provided by wellness inventories (WIs), risk factors and protective factors, or health-related inducers, are assessed (Squire et al., 2001; Gilmore et al., 1985).

The groundings for these types of assessments are described in a brief historical sketch by Hall and Zwemer (1979). They cite the landmark efforts by Dr. Lewis Robbins, who, while serving as Chief of the U.S. Public Health Service Cancer Control Program, fostered the development of a preventive approach that would identify and appraise disease precursors, eventually leading to risk reduction efforts. In 1959, 25 HRAs were completed at the Department of Preventive Medicine at Temple University School of Medicine, incorporating the probability tables (chances of dying) that had been developed by Harvey Geller, then a statistician with the Cancer Control Program. By 1962, the term *prospective medicine* had been coined.

These events eventually led to a series of key events:

- The publication of *How to Practice Prospective Medicine* in 1970 by Robbins and Hall
- Early use of prospective medicine in Canada, starting in 1971
- The incorporation of the Society of Prospective Medicine in 1974
- A collaborative agreement between the U.S. Centers for Disease Control and Prevention (CDC) and Health and Welfare Canada for further health risk appraisal research and development in 1978
- The first CDC Health Risk Appraisal Users Conference to stimulate the use of the process and to share information in 1983
- The introduction of a reformulated version of the adult HRA in 1987

Reviewing and Selecting a Strategy

General Health Status Inventories

One simple process for health promotional assessment involves self-scored general health appraisals. These usually brief, self-reported, hand-scored inventories address a few health promotion categories, such as cigarette smoking, alcohol and drug use, diet and fitness, stress management, and safety. Using very few questions or statements in each category, this process attempts to develop preliminary sensitization to selected risk factors and protective factors. It is helpful in initially directing the attention of an individual or group toward prevention and health promotion issues, to be followed with an educational message and possibly certain health promotional activities. If the individual or group is to be involved in additional sessions, more advanced assessment procedures, such as those described later in this chapter, could be employed.

Examples of GHSIs include *Healthstyle,* originally developed by the U.S. Department of Health and Human Services (see Appendix A); the "Nutrition and Activity Quiz" by the American Cancer Society, which briefly assesses one's dietary and activity patterns; and a host of lifestyle assessments (see http://www.cancer.org/healthy/toolsandcalculators/quizzes/app/nutrition-activity-quiz) for various audiences (e.g., see Powers & Dodd, 2003).

Computer-Analyzed Health Risk Appraisals

A more in-depth analysis of health risks is provided by computer-analyzed health risk appraisals. This appraisal format typically relies on participant self-reported information related to demographics; use of tobacco, alcohol, and other drugs; use of seatbelts; involvement in physical activity; use of disease-screening activities (e.g., a Pap smear); hazardous practices (such as hitchhiking); and a brief health history.

The original health risk appraisals, offered through the CDC, were based on an actuarial model incorporating national mortality statistics related to age, gender, and race (white or nonwhite). The printout from this format provided individualized information about one's chances of dying within the next 10 years from each of 12 ranked causes of death per 100,000 population. A summary of these data yielded an appraised health age (an estimate of how healthy one is in comparison to others of the same race, age, and gender) and an achievable age (an estimate of how healthy one could be if recommended lifestyle changes are made). For example, if a 45-year-old Caucasian man is informed that his appraised health age is 49 years, the risk factors in his lifestyle align him with the death statistics of Caucasian men aged four years older. If he was willing to alter some of those risk factors, it could result in an achieved health age of 45 years. The printout provides information about recommended lifestyle changes based on the risk factors as well as an expanded review of each possible cause of death and related risk categories.

Whereas early versions of the HRA used the paper-and-pencil method for recording an individual's health risk information, electronic technology has advanced the process into the twenty-first century. Gorsky (2010) has addressed the changes that have taken place over time in going from a paper-based HRA to Internet and palm-based formats (see Appendix B). His review concludes that each format can have a place, depending on the audiences and settings to be accessed. Health promotion assessment instruments and HRAs are described in Appendix D.

Wellness Inventories

Another grouping of health assessments includes wellness inventories. These formats are typically self-reported, computer-scored inventories that address a broad spectrum of health-related factors and their effects on morbidity, mortality, and health enhancement. Here the health-related factors can be either risk factors (leading to negative impacts in a person's life) or protective factors (leading to positive impacts). A number of the available formats are described by Beery, Schoenbach, and Wagner (1986). As with HRAs, these types of assessments need to be reviewed for reliability (consistency) and validity (accuracy).

One example of a WI is the La Crosse Wellness Inventory (LWI), which is part of the La Crosse Wellness Project (see Appendix C). The inventory was developed as a wellness assessment format to be included in the overall process of assessment, intervention, and reinforcement. Initiated through the efforts of a community planning committee in 1976, the LWI—along with its follow-up, intervention, and reinforcement procedures—has been researched in university and community settings. Its primary content validity was established through a national jury process. Its overall reliability (internal consistency) was calculated at 0.87 (Gilmore, Dosch, & Hood, 1983, 1985). Additional types of WIs and information for ordering them are listed in Appendix E.

The development of WIs usually follows a four-step process: (1) formulating questions based on literature reviews, (2) refining the questions, (3) validating the questions through comparisons with standards, and (4) calculating reliability coefficients. Richardson (1986) notes that this process is more appropriate when epidemiologic data are not available for diverse lifestyle factors such as frustration, adaptive stress, and depression. With WIs, the goal is to assess areas of health-related strengths and weaknesses. It is not to determine the length of one's life based on health practices.

Preparing for the Assessment

A few major issues must be considered when preparing to use self-directed assessment inventories. First, these inventories are not self-reliant. They can be but one part of a total program experience; they are just one type of assessment. Other program aspects, such as intervention and reinforcement, will need attention as well (McKenzie, Neiger, & Thackeray, 2009; Hyer & Melby, 1985).

Second, individualized explanation, interpretation, and behavioral counseling regarding the inventory results are beneficial. It is not recommended to involve participants in GHSIs without follow-up discussion or to send HRA and WI results through the postal mail and e-mail. Depending on the program's focus, time should be allocated for a clarification of the meaning of the results, particularly for the HRA and WI, including discussions about individualized steps or strategies for health-related changes.

Third, multiple program sessions appear to enhance the impact on participants, in contrast to singular events (Gilmore et al., 1985; Hyer & Melby, 1985). Repeated sessions allow time not only for the necessary inventory analyses, but also for more in-depth individualized discussion regarding the meaning of the results and possible next steps.

Fourth, these assessment inventories are not solely aligned with one professional group. Although they have their groundings in epidemiological research and physician-to-patient counseling, they have been routinely incorporated into programming by health departments, business and industry (Abby, 1986), insurance companies, voluntary agencies, and other private agencies (Hyer & Melby, 1985).

Fifth, HRAs can be used to create community risk assessments (as distinguished from individualized appraisal) through the calculation of the population attributable risk proportion (PARP), as presented in Appendix G. This approach allows for the review of the impact on a population of risk factor combinations over time.

Finally, HRAs are targeted primarily for mainstream, employed, literate adults, even though other target groups serve as major reservoirs of preventable risks (Moriarty, 1986; Rowley, Mills, Kellum, & Avery, 1986). As a consequence, caution should be exercised in considering the use of these assessments with underrepresented populations. The assessments can be incorporated quite easily into employee health promotion programs. One example would be with the American Cancer Society's "Active for Life" Program, which is a 10-week program encouraging people to be more active on a regular basis (American Cancer Society [ACS], 2011). Individual assessments can be used to enable participants to set their own goals based on how currently active they are in relation to how active they want to be in the future. The assessments can be repeated at various intervals to record one's progress.

Various characteristics of the three inventory formats are detailed in **Table 11-1**. Usually, the HRA and WI formats will be more in-depth than the GHSI. Keep in mind that the basic purpose of the GHSI is to identify the risk factors over which individuals have some control, as well as those unchangeable risk factors (e.g., heredity) that could encourage modified behaviors. The usual GHSI and HRA inventory formats focus on a negative reinforcement approach of avoiding hazards. The WI formats basically focus on positive and negative reinforcers so that undesirable behaviors can be reduced and desirable behaviors can be enhanced (Powers & Dodd, 2003; Gilmore et al., 1985; Hyer & Melby, 1985; Richardson, 1986).

TABLE 11-1
Characteristics of Three Assessment Inventory Formats

	GHSI	HRA	WI
Assessment Purpose	General health awareness	Risk of dying in next ten years	Health strengths and weaknesses
Type of Reinforcement	Negative	Negative	Negative and positive
Scoring Process	Self-scored	Computer-scored and self-scored	Computer-scored and self-scored
Administration Process	One-time basis	Repeatable	Repeatable

Considerations for the implementation of the three inventory formats are cited in **Table 11-2.** One very important step prior to administering the HRA and WI formats is to make certain that enough advisors are trained for the explanation, interpretation, and counseling sessions. Typically, each advisor can work with as many as 10 participants.

TABLE 11-2
Implementation Considerations for Three Assessment Inventory Formats

	GHSI	HRA	WI
Preliminary Steps	Identify target audience and secure site	Identify target audience, train advisors, and secure site	Identify target audience, train advisors, and secure site
Materials	Inventory and writing implements	Inventory, answer sheets, writing implements, and computer	Inventory, answer sheets, writing implements, and computer
Administration Time	10 minutes	20–35 minutes	20–45 minutes
Interpretation Time	15 minutes	30 minutes–1 hour	30 minutes–2 hours

Plan and conduct an advisor training session that includes the following steps:

1. Advisors-to-be should take the inventory prior to your training session so that the printouts will be available on the date of the training.
2. During the training session, include participant and trainer introductions as well as a review of the training agenda (usually two trainers can work with up to 15 advisors-to-be).
3. Present a brief history of the inventory format (15 minutes).
4. Return and discuss the inventory results just as if the advisors-to-be were program participants during the next 45 minutes to 1 hour.
5. Encourage questions for 15 to 30 minutes.
6. Discuss the process you would like the advisors to follow with the program participants during the next hour.
7. If there is enough time, demonstrate the computer program that was used to analyze the inventory responses and produce a printout.

Conducting the Assessment

After making the various logistical arrangements for the program, you will need to have the program participants take the HRA or WI in advance of the program date if it is a singular event (the GHSI can be taken on site) or at the first session of a multiple-session program. In contacting program participants in advance, send a letter with the inventory and answer sheet attachments that communicates the following message: This assessment is a very special feature of the program that will take approximately 25 minutes to complete; the results will be presented at the first program session and will be confidential; the assessment is a process for understanding the impact of one's health habits, and not a diagnostic process; from this a personal health promotion strategy can be developed; the inventory should be completed as accurately as possible because more complete responses will yield a clearer picture of the impact of one's health habits; and the answer sheet and the inventory should be returned by a specific date in an enclosed self-addressed, stamped envelope.

Many of these same ideas can be presented at the first session of a multiple-session program. It is particularly important to emphasize that the purpose of the assessment is to understand the impact of one's health habits, that accuracy of responses is important, and that the results are confidential. Participants can be informed that a follow-up session has been planned so their results can be returned, general principles discussed, specific questions answered, and preliminary plans for health enhancement made.

Using the Results

Because the GHSI is self-scored, program participants will be able to quickly sense whether certain risk factor areas need attention. It is very important to clarify the meaning of the score totals (usually this information is printed on the inventory) and to emphasize that this assessment primarily is designed to provide a short, general introduction to the personal meaning of risk factors and lifestyle improvement. Participants should be informed that more in-depth assessments (e.g., HRA, WI) are available, but even these are not intended for diagnostic purposes. Participants also should have the opportunity to discuss their results individually or in small group sessions with trained advisors. Usually, one risk factor area can be isolated and discussed, and simple steps for health enhancement can be identified.

The HRA and WI formats necessitate a greater degree of participant and advisor involvement during the feedback session for individuals. One approach to conducting this session is to start off by introducing the meaning of risk factors (those that enhance negative health-related outcomes) and protective factors (those that enhance positive health outcomes, such as consumption of a diet with appropriate fiber content). This step can be followed by a history of the assessment process and then a return of the individual printouts.

The printout for the *Healthier People* HRA in Appendix B provides a person's present risk age, based on how one completed the HRA in comparison with a target risk age. The present risk age reflects appraised risk factors that, when reduced or eliminated, usually yield a lower target risk age. It should be made clear to the participants that the HRA is not a diagnostic tool and thus is not meant to replace health-related examinations. Participants then can be led through the more specific information on the printout, which aligns risk rates (number of deaths in the next 10 years per 1000 population) with common causes of death for one's gender and age, as well as specific risk factors for reduction. This part of the printout enables participants to see the potential effects of their risk reduction efforts (in terms of having a higher potential of reducing the risk related to the listed common causes of death). Additionally, participants can review their desirable weight range, a summary of their present habits that are considered good (for a measure of positive reinforcement), a summary of specific and general risk reduction recommendations, and gender- and age-specific routine preventive services. Thus, the three major areas for printout-related discussions with the participants involve (1) making a distinction between present risk age and target risk age, (2) clarifying the alignment of specific risk factors with gender- and age-related common causes of death, and (3) addressing specific next steps that can be taken for risk reduction.

Following these kinds of clarifications, participants can be encouraged to develop a personal health plan, which focuses on changes they are able to make. One approach is to have participants write down a risk factor or protective factor to address, ways they will address it (i.e., how to decrease or eliminate the risk factor, or how to maintain or increase a protective factor in their lives), the point at which they will address it, a person who will motivate them to stay on task, and any special considerations (e.g., avoiding situations where the risk factor is encouraged). Examples of changes would be most helpful at this stage. These examples could come from the advisors or from the participants themselves. Also, this may be a good point in the program to offer educational experiences dealing with general risk-reduction issues.

The WI format printouts are quite variable. However, it can be said that general feedback sessions benefit from a clarification of the purpose of the assessment process (particularly noting that they are not diagnostic in nature), an individual or small-group interpretation of the results that personalizes them, and recommendations for steps to take for health enhancement. One WI format also includes a listing of local resources that can be tapped by the participant, a follow-up wellness development process (WDP) for the determination of specific next steps to take, and established reinforcement strategies (McKenzie, Neiger, & Thackeray, 2009; Gilmore et al., 1985). In accomplishing this, the participant works with the individualized data from the printout by using a workbook and through advisor interaction.

Results from HRA and WI formats also can be combined and analyzed for groups (e.g., occupational clusters) and entire communities (see Appendix G). In doing so, composite risk values are provided for groups, which, in turn, enable planners, managers, and educators to estimate health needs (see Appendix G). As one example of a group analysis, data from HRAs administered to a community group may indicate a very low level of seatbelt usage. The comparison of those data with vehicular accident mortality and injury data may emphasize the need for a seatbelt education effort directed at the assessed target audience.

Reviewing an Example

The author was responsible for the development and implementation of a statewide program for interested school health professionals (teachers, school health nurses, counselors, and administrators) to assist them in developing health promotional programming for students and professional colleagues at the school worksite. The program was sponsored by the Wisconsin State School Health Council, which cited among its objectives:

> Program participants will: (1) personally experience the Health Risk Appraisal (HRA) process; (2) review ways in which the Health Risk Appraisal process can be applied in the school setting for student health promotion; and (3) review ways in which the Health Risk Appraisal process can be applied in the school setting for adult health promotion.

This effort was a 1-day program, necessitating that the HRAs be mailed to the program participants in advance. The format for the program provided for the following components:

- An overview presentation on HRAs for students and school professionals
- Small-group advising sessions to which the participants were assigned, with continued group discussions during the lunch hour
- An afternoon session describing the results of a statewide school health promotion project that used HRAs
- Presentations addressing how to incorporate HRA formats into the school settings, along with discussions on resource availability at the national and state levels
- A panel discussion to respond to participant questions about the next steps to take personally and professionally

The program included four key ingredients:

- The stimulation of a personal investment and awareness about HRAs by having the program participants take the instrument and discuss the meaning of the results
- Provision of a health promotion example using HRAs that had been conducted and evaluated in another state
- Provision through presentations and handouts of the resource contact persons and agencies at the state and national levels
- Ample opportunities throughout the program for questions and discussion

By the end of the program, each participant had developed a personal health plan for health enhancement using the five components suggested above, as well as a preliminary strategy for next steps with students and colleagues.

Online Resources

Visit go.jblearning.com/gilmore4 for links to these Web sites.

Health Risk Appraisal
An example of a health risk appraisal.

National Wellness Institute
Testwell wellness inventory.

American Heart Association
Coronary risk profile/health risk appraisal and health risk appraisal based on the Framingham Study.

NASA Occupational Health
Health risk appraisal links.

Healthfinder
Health risk appraisal links.

University of Missouri Health Care
Health risk appraisal.

U.S. Navy
Fleet health risk appraisal.

References

Abby, D. (1986). Worksite wellness using the CDC health risk appraisal: Adaption, implementation, and evaluation. In *Proceedings of the 21st annual meeting of the Society of Prospective Medicine: Equipping the professional/protecting the consumer*. Indianapolis: Society of Prospective Medicine, 46–48.

American Cancer Society (ACS). (2011). *Active for life*. Available at: http://www.cancer.org/Healthy/MoreWaysACSHelpsYouStayWell/active-for-life-description. Accessed May 29, 2011.

Beery, W., Schoenbach, V., and Wagner, E. (1986). *Health risk appraisal: Methods and programs with annotated bibliography*. Rockville, MD: U.S. Department of Health and Human Services, National Center for Health Services Research and Health Care Technology Assessment.

Centers for Disease Control and Prevention (CDC). (2011). Ten great public health achievements: United States, 2001–2010. *Morbidity and Mortality Weekly Report, 60*, 619–623.

Commission on Social Determinants of Health. (2008). *Closing the gap in a generation: Final report of the Commission on Social Determinants of Health*. Geneva: World Health Organization.

Gilmore, G. (1979). Planning for family wellness. *Health Education, 10*, 12–16.

Gilmore, G., Dosch, M., and Hood, T. (1985). Continuing evaluation of the La Crosse Wellness Project: Longitudinal and community-based process and impact analyses. In *Proceedings of the 20th annual meeting of the Society of Prospective Medicine: A decade of survival, past, present, future*. Washington, DC: Society of Prospective Medicine, 82–85.

Gilmore, G., Dosch, M., and Hood, T. (1983). The development, implementation and evaluation of the La Crosse Wellness Project. Presented at the 19th meeting of the Society of Prospective Medicine, Atlanta, GA.

Gorsky, R. (2010). *Health risk assessments (HRAs): New technologies and implications.* Elmhurst, IL: HPN Worldwide.

Hall, J., and Zwemer, J. (1979). *Prospective medicine.* Indianapolis: Methodist Hospital of Indiana.

Hyer, G., and Melby, C. (1985). Health risk appraisals: Use and misuse. *Family and Community Health, 8,* 13–25.

McKenzie, J., Neiger, B., and Thackeray, R. (2009). *Planning, implementing, and evaluating health promotion programs,* 5th ed. San Francisco: Pearson Benjamin Cummings.

Moriarty, D. (1986). Health risk appraisal for underserved populations: An overview. In *Proceedings of the 21st annual meeting of the Society of Prospective Medicine: Equipping the professional/protecting the consumer.* Indianapolis: Society of Prospective Medicine.

Powers, S., and Dodd, S. (2003). *Total fitness and wellness.* New York: Benjamin Cummings.

Richardson, G. (1986). Health risk versus lifestyle improvement instruments. In *Proceedings of the 21st annual meeting of the Society of Prospective Medicine: Equipping the professional/protecting the consumer.* Indianapolis: Society of Prospective Medicine.

Rowley, D., Mills, S., Kellum, C., and Avery, B. (1986). Are current health risk appraisals suitable for black women? *Proceedings of the 21st annual meeting of the Society of Prospective Medicine: Equipping the professional/protecting the consumer.* Indianapolis: Society of Prospective Medicine, 50–53.

Squire, K., Gilmore, G., Duquette, D., and Riley, D. (2001). The national content revalidation of the La Crosse Wellness Inventory as a part of the La Crosse Wellness Project. *American Journal of Health Education, 32,* 183–188.

U.S. Department of Health and Human Services (USDHHS). (2010). *Healthy People 2020.* Washington, DC: Author. Available at: http://www.healthypeople. gov/2020/about/default.aspx.

Observational Self-Directed Assessments

Introduction

This chapter is all about certain health-related choices we make during our lifetime. Individually, our decisions need to be based on reasonable and accurate information, and personal observations can assist us in making appropriate lifestyle choices. Mokdad, Marks, Stroop, and Gerberding (2004) convey the importance of having individuals become aware of the actual influences on one's health (e.g., lifestyle) so they can become involved in realistic approaches to health promotion. Observational self-assessments, as described throughout this chapter, enable individuals to actively engage in realistic decision-making and health-enhancing actions. These individualized assessments are most important, given the lifestyle choices that impact on illness and health. As just one example, regarding the global impact of cancer, it is recognized as "the leading cause of death in economically developed countries and the second leading cause of death in developing countries. The burden of cancer is increasing in economically developing countries as result of population aging and growth as well as, increasingly, an adoption of cancer-associated lifestyle choices including smoking, physical inactivity, and 'Westernized' diets" (Jemal, Bray, Center, Ferlay, Ward, & Forman, 2011, p. 69).

Collectively, taking a more comprehensive population-based approach, Koh's perspective, as published in the *New England Journal of Medicine*, addresses "A 2020 Vision for Healthy People." Referring to *Healthy People 2020*, he projects, "as we prepare for the next decade, the initiative aims to unify national dialogue about health, motivate action, and encourage new directions in health promotion, providing a public health roadmap and compass for the country" (Koh, 2010, p. 1653). Following a review of some of the key features of *Healthy People 2020*, he summarizes that:

> *Healthy People* can prompt Americans to consider better ways of advancing the quantity and quality of life, healthy places and environments, health equity, and disease prevention. By nurturing a unity of purpose and a vision that can mobilize communities, *Healthy People* captures both our legacy and promise for a healthier nation. (Koh, 2010, p. 1656)

The benefits of personal observation procedures, primarily designed for the early detection of illness, are demonstrated daily. These are referred to as observational self-directed assessments (OSDAs), because an individual is encouraged to periodically observe various body regions. Several voluntary agencies provide this encouragement through their educational materials. These include the breast self-examination for women; the testicular self-examination for men; oral assessments for suspicious sensations, lumps, and discolorations; and a total body review for potential skin cancer lesions. This chapter will briefly review these procedures and provide recommendations for next steps.

Reviewing and Selecting a Strategy

Personal Observation

A *personal observation assessment* encompasses a variety of physical and mental indicators that provide an individual with a sense of his or her level of well-being. These indicators include body pulse, respiration, temperature, blood pressure, fatigue level, sensory impairment (e.g., headache, ringing in the ears, bloodshot eyes), physical impairment, and mental/emotional response. They range from a high degree of specificity and quantification (such as pulse rate) to the more general awareness of our feelings at a given moment. The intent of the personal review approach is for individuals to be involved in these types of assessment processes regularly on their own. This approach also can assist individuals in having a sense of personal responsibility for their health (Saracci, 2010; Liebmann-Smith & Egan, 2007; Squire, Gilmore, Duquette, & Riley, 2001; U.S. Department of Health and Human Services [USDHHS], 2000; Breslow, 1999; Gilmore, 1979).

As shown by Vickery and Fries (2004), the physical observations can be made quite easily and can complement medical reviews. These two physicians advocate the cultivation of an informed consumer who can undertake certain body observations and utilize specially prepared algorithms indicating what steps to take next. (For example, if a sunburn is experienced with accompanying dizziness or abdominal cramps, the individual is directed through an algorithm to consult a physician. Otherwise, home treatments are recommended for a typical sunburn.) Practical examples of important observations that can be made include owning a thermometer, knowing how to shake it down (nondigital version), and recording the exact temperature, rather than guessing that one has a fever. In observing one's weight, Vickery and Fries (2004) recommend knowing an individual's normal weight and, if weight changes occur, documenting how much and over what period of time. This change-related information combined with a time line can provide a more accurate picture of key stimuli that encourage greater food consumption.

Vickrey and Fries (2004) identify seven keys to health: exercise, diet and nutrition, not smoking, alcohol moderation, weight control, avoiding injury, and professional prevention. To the last point, Vickery and Fries (2004) state that although most prevention is personal, sometimes professional help is necessary. The following five strategies can therefore be quite important: the checkup or periodic health examination, screening for early problems, early treatment for problems, immunizations and other public health measures, and health risk appraisal.

Additionally, a detailed exploration of personal signs of health and illness has been offered by Liebmann-Smith and Egan (2007). Drawing on their years of experience as a recognized medical sociologist and medical writer (Liebmann-Smith) and medical writer (Egan), coupled with recommendations authenticated by a panel of recognized medical experts, the authors provide the consumer with an array of self-recognizable signs and symptoms to consider. They point out that their intent is not to supplant seeking medical advice, but rather to help individuals become more aware of various body signals so that appropriate responses can take place at earlier points in time. Their helpful approach uses various types of "signs" in each signal category: healthy signs; warning signs; danger signs; signs of the times (historical anecdotes); speaking of signs (quotations); significant facts (little-known facts about the body); and stop signs (ways to address the underlying issues that are generating the signals). To their credit, Liebmann-Smith and Egan, address both positive (e.g., protective factors) and negative (e.g., risk factors) signals. Additionally, the authors include a series of checklists for keeping track of the various detected signals, along with prescription and over-the-counter medicinal that are being taken.

Complementing these approaches, Saracci (2010) has provided an overview of health and well-being from an epidemiologic perspective. He addresses the important topic of empowering people, whereby people take part in decisions affecting their health. He also calls for the involvement of people in "deliberations concerning the health of the population" (p. 110). Becoming involved in health enhancement in these ways, Saracci (2010) cautions that with approximately 100,000 Web sites addressing health issues, the assurance of accuracy is paramount.

Saracci (2010) offers the following general advice for those seeking information and insight from such sources:

- Trust new findings only if they have been replicated [". . . a causal link can only be established through replicated, separate, and concordant investigations" (p. 111)].
- Trust only findings qualified by their uncertainty [". . . most often there is some margin of uncertainty in the results and black and white descriptions hide an essential part of the relevant information. Dogmatic statements should be treated with caution" (p. 112)].
- Trust findings only if placed in context, rather than in isolation.
- Trust findings only if not framed as advertisement (i.e., for decision-making, use noncommercial sources).
- Trust findings and recommendations only if concordant (e.g., cross-checking information from a variety of sources).

Early Detection Procedures

Breast Self-Examination (BSE)

Breast self-examination was first advocated by the American Cancer Society (ACS) and the National Cancer Institute (NCI) over 40 years ago. For women, beginning in their early 20s, the American Cancer Society currently recommends they:

> should be told about the benefits and limitations of breast self-examination (BSE). The importance of prompt reporting of any new breast symptoms to a health professional should be emphasized. Women who choose to do BSE should receive instruction and have their technique reviewed on the occasion of a periodic health examination. It is acceptable for women to choose not to do BSE or to do BSE irregularly. (American Cancer Society [ACS], 2010, p. 62)

Additionally, the ACS (2010) recommends that women in their 20s and 30s should have a clinical breast examination every 3 years as part of a periodic health examination. Thereafter, women aged 40 and older who are asymptomatic "should continue to receive a clinical breast examination as part of a periodic health examination, preferably annually" (p. 62). Annual mammography should begin at age 40, with the annual clinical breast examination being performed prior to mammography (ACS, 2010). Beyond the scope of this text, but important to the ongoing review of cancer screening guidelines particularly in relation to mammography, commentary on the updated breast cancer screening guidelines from the United States Preventive Services Task Force (USPSTF) is presented in Smith, Cokkinides, Brooks, Saslow, and Brawley (2010).

With an estimated 207,090 new cases of invasive breast cancer and 39,840 deaths in women in the United States projected for 2010, which is second only to lung cancer deaths in women (American Cancer Society, 2010), early detection is an important decision for a woman to make in discussion with her health care provider. The American Cancer Society process for the self-examination is presented in **Figure 12-1** and **Figure 12-2**.

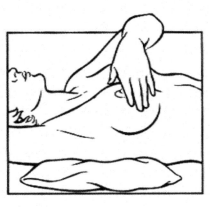
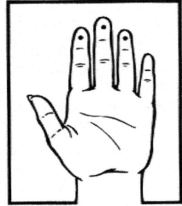

FIGURE 12-1
How to perform a breast self-examination: Preparation.

Source: Reprinted by the permission of the American Cancer Society, Inc. From www.cancer.org. All rights reserved.

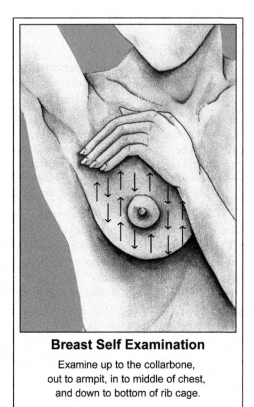

Breast Self Examination

Examine up to the collarbone,
out to armpit, in to middle of chest,
and down to bottom of rib cage.

FIGURE 12-2
How to perform a breast self-examination: Practice. Choose one pattern, do it the same way every month, and remember how your breast feels from month to month.

Source: Reprinted by the permission of the American Cancer Society, Inc. From www.cancer.org. All rights reserved.

Testicular Self-Examination (TSE)

Males are able to practice testicular self-examination. Although testicular cancer accounts for about 1 percent of all cancers in males, it is considered the most common solid malignancy in men between the ages of 20 and 34 years. In 2010, approximately 8480 new cases of testicular cancer and 350 deaths were expected in the United States (Jemal, Siegel, Xu, & Ward, 2010). In addition, it has been reported that the incidence of primary testicular diffuse large B-cell lymphoma is increasing (Gundrum, Mathiason, Moore, & Go, 2009).

The best time to do a TSE is following a warm shower or bath, when the skin of the scrotum is moist and the testicles are descended away from the body. The TSE process is as follows:

1. Examine each testicle between your thumb and fingers of both hands.

2. Find the collecting structure in the back (the epididymis). Become familiar with how it feels and do not confuse it with a lump.
3. Rolling the testicle gently between the thumb and fingers, feel for lumps.

TSEs can be performed on a monthly basis. TSE can be viewed as a type of personal health assessment for males that to some degree can encourage a sense of individual responsibility for one's health. Individuals also can be referred the *Screening Guidelines for the Early Detection of Cancer in Average-Risk Asymptomatic People* from the American Cancer Society in order to have increased awareness.

Skin Cancer Detection (SCD)

More than 2 million people in the United States were treated for basal cell and squamous cell skin cancers in 2006 (ACS, 2010). These skin cancers are highly curable. For 2010, melanoma, the most common serious form of skin cancer in the United States, was projected to be diagnosed in approximately 68,130 persons, with 8700 projected deaths (ACS, 2010). Of note, during 1990–2006, the death rate for melanoma of the skin increased in the United States (Jemal et al., 2010). The most common risk factors for melanoma include a personal or family history of melanoma and the presence of atypical or numerous moles (more than 50), in addition to risk factors for other types of skin cancer, which include excessive exposure to the sun and the use of tanning booths (ACS, 2010).

The American Academy of Dermatology (AAD) has attempted to alert the public to the increasing incidence of skin cancer and has provided a process for monthly self-examination (see **Figure 12-3**). A helpful discussion on the development of the ABCD approach and its value for consumers and health care professionals, coupled with mass screenings in the United States and worldwide, is provided by Rigel, Russak, and Friedman (2010). Sometimes clinicians also will encourage the public to be aware of "E," which refers to evolving (i.e., changing size, shape, or color). Organizations that have been engaged in these informational and screening activities have included the AAD, the ACS, and the Skin Cancer Foundation.

Oral Review (OR)

A total of 36,540 new cases of cancer of the oral cavity and pharynx and 7880 deaths were projected in the United States for 2010 (ACS, 2010). Risk factors include smoked and smokeless tobacco use and heavy alcohol consumption. The synergy between heavy smoking and alcohol use results in more than a 30-fold increased risk of cancer development. The risk of oral cancer is twice as high for males as for females. Although incidence rates have decreased since the 1980s, it has recently been reported that the "incidence is increasing for those cancers related to human papillomavirus (HPV) infection" (ACS, 2010, p. 17). A daily review of the mouth region looking for any sores, discolorations, and/or other changes, as presented in Appendix F would be advisable for youths and adults.

1 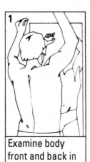	2 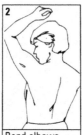	3 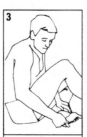	4 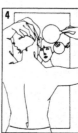	5 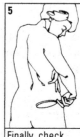
Examine body front and back in mirror, then right and left sides, arms raised.	Bend elbows, look carefully at forearms, back of upper arms and palms.	Next, look at back of legs and feet, spaces between toes, and soles.	Examine back of neck and scalp with a hand mirror. Part hair to lift.	Finally, check back and buttocks with a hand mirror.

ABCD Method

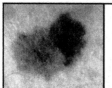

Assymetry One half doesn't match the other half.

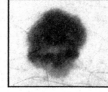

Color The pigmentation is not uniform. Shades of tan, brown and black are present. Dashes of red, white and blue add to the mottled appearance.

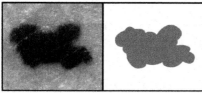

Border Irregularity The edges are ragged, notched or blurred.

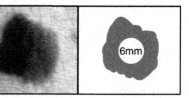

Diameter Greater than six millimeters (about the size of a pencil eraser). Any growth of a mole should be of concern.

FIGURE 12-3
Melanoma recognition and periodic self-examination for skin lesion detection.

Preparing for the Assessment

Although it is possible for consumers to contact the agencies offering the OSDA literature and request a copy for personal use, these materials usually are offered in conjunction with a program. Although dissemination based on individual request distributes the information to a wider audience more quickly, it offers fewer opportunities for clarification of the process, demonstration (many times with models), discussion, group brainstorming about how the process can be personally incorporated, and the motivational aspects that a program can offer. It is recommended that whenever possible a program opportunity be organized. It is important to remind individuals who are using these materials that they are not intended to take the place of regularly scheduled examinations or other planned health care visitations (Vickery & Fries, 2004). Instead, these materials are offered in partnership with the health care practitioner in the hope that if a particular symptom is recognized by the participant, he or she will seek follow-up assessments by the appropriate practitioner.

Conducting the Assessment

OSDAs can conveniently be built into one's lifestyle. They are meant to be quite simple procedures, typically conducted on a monthly basis. For example, BSE and TSE can be conducted monthly following a shower, at the end or beginning of each month. Skin cancer and oral reviews also can be accomplished at those times. The key to any of these procedures is practicing them at a similar time through the year so that a habit is more likely to be formed.

Although health care practitioners can offer patients individualized training in the use of these early detection procedures, time constraints may impede doing this in a routine and in-depth fashion. Group educational activities appear to work quite well in training participants with the basic assessment procedures as well as providing opportunities for group discussion (particularly so that other questions, concerns, and vantage points can be heard), resource review, and practice with models, when appropriate. The use of models with BSE training has been particularly effective in enabling participants to practice the proper palpation process. It also is possible for appropriately trained non-health care professionals to offer delimited educational experiences to certain target groups (usually with the planning assistance of health care practitioners). It is important to follow guidelines for early detection, such as using the general health detection recommendations offered through the algorithms developed by Vickery and Fries (2004), those in Appendix F, or the specific guidelines in **Figure 12-4** created by the American Cancer Society.

Cancer Site	Population	Test or Procedure	Frequency
Breast	Women, age 20+	Breast self-examination	Beginning in their early 20s, women should be told about the benefits and limitations of breast self-examination (BSE). The importance of prompt reporting of any new breast symptoms to a health professional should be emphasized. Women who choose to do BSE should receive instruction and have their technique reviewed on the occasion of a periodic health examination. It is acceptable for women to choose not to do BSE or to do BSE irregularly.
		Clinical breast examination	For women in their 20s and 30s, it is recommended that clinical breast examination (CBE) be part of a periodic health examination, preferably at least every three years. Asymptomatic women aged 40 and over should continue to receive a clinical breast examination as part of a periodic health examination, preferably annually.
		Mammography	Begin annual mammography at age 40.*
Colorectal[†]	Men and women, age 50+	*Tests that find polyps and cancer:*	
		Flexible sigmoidoscopy,[‡] or	Every five years, starting at age 50.
		Colonoscopy, or	Every 10 years, starting at age 50.
		Double-contrast barium enema (DCBE),[‡] or	Every five years, starting at age 50.
		CT colonography (virtual colonoscopy)[‡]	Every five years, starting at age 50.
		Tests that mainly find cancer:	
		Fecal occult blood test (FOBT) with at least 50% test sensitivity for cancer, or fecal immunochemical test (FIT) with at least 50% test sensitivity for cancer [‡§] or	Annual, starting at age 50.
		Stool DNA test (sDNA)[‡]	Interval uncertain, starting at age 50.
Prostate	Men, age 50+	Prostate-specific antigen test (PSA) with or without digital rectal exam (DRE)	Asymptomatic men who have at least a 10-year life expectancy should have an opportunity to make an informed decision with their health care provider about screening for prostate cancer after receiving information about the uncertainties, risks, and potential benefits associated with screening.

Cancer Site	Population	Test or Procedure	Frequency
			Men at average risk should receive this information beginning at age 50. Men at higher risk, including African American men and men with a first-degree relative (father or brother) diagnosed with prostate cancer before age 65, should receive this information beginning at age 45. Men at appreciably higher risk (multiple family members diagnosed with prostate cancer before age 65) should receive this information beginning at age 40.
Cervix	Women, age 18+	Pap test	Cervical cancer screening should begin approximately three years after a woman begins having vaginal intercourse but no later than 21 years of age. Screening should be done every year with conventional Pap tests or every two years using liquid-based Pap tests. At or after age 30, women who have had three normal test results in a row may get screened every two to three years with cervical cytology (either conventional or liquid-based Pap test) alone or every three years with an HPV DNA test plus cervical cytology. Women 70 years of age and older who have had three or more normal Pap tests and no abnormal Pap tests in the past 10 years and women who have had a total hysterectomy may choose to stop cervical cancer screening.
Endometrial	Women, at menopause	At the time of menopause, women at average risk should be informed about risks and symptoms of endometrial cancer and strongly encouraged to report any unexpected bleeding or spotting to their physicians.	
Cancer-Related Checkup	Men and women, age 20+	On the occasion of a periodic health examination, the cancer-related checkup should include examination for cancers of the thyroid, testicles, ovaries, lymph nodes, oral cavity, and skin, as well as health counselling about tobacco, sun exposure, diet and nutrition, risk factors, sexual practices, and environmental and occupational exposures.	

*Beginning at age 40, annual clinical breast examination should be performed prior to mammography.
†Individuals with a personal or family history of colorectal cancer or adenomas, inflammatory bowel disease, or high-risk genetic syndromes should continue to follow the most recent recommendations for individuals at increased or high risk.
‡Colonoscopy should be done if test results are positive.
§For FOBT or FIT used as a screening test, the take-home multiple sample method should be used. A FOBT or FIT done during a digital rectal exam in the doctor's office is not adequate for screening.

FIGURE 12-4
Screening guidelines for the early detection of cancer in average-risk asymptomatic people.
Source: American Cancer Society. *Cancer Facts and Figures 2010.* Atlanta: American Cancer Society, Inc.

Using the Results

The key to an effective OSDA early detection procedure is having the participant follow up on a particular symptom or series of symptoms. A person should be encouraged to do so for a variety of reasons:

- For certain conditions, such as breast cancer, earlier detection can lead to a greater range of treatment options (Smith et al., 2010).
- One can obtain a more complete understanding of the meaning of the symptom from the health care professional (rather than, for example, remaining in fear of what it "might" mean).
- One can have a sense of being an active participant in his or her health, addressing the health promotion dimension of self-responsibility (Vickery & Fries, 2004).

By the same token, in those instances when no symptoms are detected through the use of these assessment procedures, individuals can be encouraged to view them as more positive health-related indications at that point in time. In this sense, they can provide some positive reinforcement to the individual, obviously without supplanting the need for routine health-related examinations (one needs to continue to guard against a false sense of security).

Reviewing an Example

Three national health-related voluntary organizations are joining together for the first time to encourage members of the American public to assess their lifestyle choices and make decisions about reducing their risk of heart disease, certain types of cancer, stroke, and type 2 diabetes. The American Cancer Society, the American Diabetes Association, and the American Heart Association developed a joint educational and media effort initiated in the spring of 2004 that focused on risk factor awareness and reduction related to poor diet, obesity, physical inactivity, smoking, and lack of regular medical care (Seffrin, Stevens, & Wheeler, 2003). As one example, regarding modifiable and nonmodifiable risk factors that are common to both cancer and diabetes, it is important for people to have an increased awareness of the impacts of age, sex, obesity, physical inactivity, diet, alcohol, and smoking on these conditions (Giovannucci, Harlan, Archer, Bergenstal, Gapstur, Habel, Pollak, Regensteiner, & Yee, 2010). Along with public service announcements, Web site and toll-free telephone information dissemination efforts, and collaboration with health care organizations to develop screening guidelines, joint initiatives will be developed in local communities. As the representatives of the three organizations have stated, "through an unprecedented and historic collaboration, we will reach an unparalleled number of people with simple, shared messages of awareness and prevention that have enormous potential to save lives" (Seffrin, Stevens, & Wheeler, 2003, p. 1). Clearly, collaboration of this magnitude has the potential not only to apply substantial organizational resources to affect key lifestyle changes, but also to assess and marshal individual and community-based resources throughout the nation for sustainability.

Online Resources

Visit go.jblearning.com/gilmore4 for links to these Web sites.

Breast Cancer Information Center
Information about breast self-exams, their importance, and links to instructions about how to perform a breast self-exam.

American Cancer Society
Links with information about how to prevent certain types of cancer.

National Cancer Institute
Information on how to do a skin self-exam.

National Institute of Mental Health
A self-screening test for obsessive-compulsive disorder.

Center for Health and Well-Being, University of Vermont
Information on breast self-exams and testicular self-exams.

Everyday Choices
A collaborative public service for health assessment and action by the American Cancer Society, American Diabetes Association, and American Heart Association.

References

American Cancer Society (ACS). (2010). *Cancer facts and figures: 2010*. Atlanta, GA: Author.

American Cancer Society (ACS). (2002). *Active for life*. Atlanta, GA: Author.

Breslow, L. (1999). From disease prevention to health promotion. *Journal of the American Medical Association, 281*, 1030–1033.

Gilmore, G. (1979). Planning for family wellness. *Health Education, 10*, 12–16.

Giovannucci, E., Harlan, D., Archer, M., Bergenstal, R., Gapstur, S., Habel, L., Pollak, M., Regensteiner, J., and Yee, D. (2010). Diabetes and cancer: A consensus report. *CA: A Cancer Journal for Clinicians, 60*, 207–221.

Gundrum, J., Mathiason, M., Moore, D., and Go, R. (2009). Primary testicular diffuse large B-cell lymphoma: A population-based study on the incidence, natural history, and survival comparison with primary nodal counterpart before and after the introduction of Rituximab. *Journal of Clinical Oncology, 27,* 5227–5232.

Jemal, A., Bray, F., Center, M., Ferlay, J., Ward, E., and Forman, D. (2011). Global cancer statistics. CA: *A Cancer Journal for Clinicians, 61,* 69–90.

Jemal, A., Siegel, R., Xu, J., and Ward, E. (2010). Cancer statistics, 2010. *CA: A Cancer Journal for Clinicians, 60,* 277–300.

Koh, H. (2010). A 2020 vision for Healthy People. *New England Journal of Medicine, 362,* 1653–1656.

Liebmann-Smith, J., and Egan, J. (2007). *Body signs.* New York: Bantam Books.

Mokdad, A., Marks, J., Stroop, D., and Gerberding, J. (2004). Actual causes of death in the United States, 2000. *Journal of the American Medical Association, 291,* 1238–1244.

Rigel, D., Russak, J., and Friedman, R. (2010). The evolution of melanoma diagnosis: 25 years beyond the ABCDs. *CA: A Cancer Journal for Clinicians, 60,* 301–316.

Saracci, R. (2010). *Epidemiology: A very short introduction.* New York: Oxford University Press.

Seffrin, J., Stevens, C., and Wheeler, M. (2003). Joint communication from the American Cancer Society, American Diabetes Association, and the American Heart Association.

Smith, R., Cokkinides, V., Brooks, D., Saslow, D., and Brawley, O. (2010). Cancer screening in the United States, 2010: A review of current American Cancer Society guidelines and issues in cancer screening. *CA: A Cancer Journal for Clinicians, 60,* 99–119.

Squire, K., Gilmore, G., Duquette, D., and Riley, D. (2001). The national content revalidation of the La Crosse Wellness Inventory as a part of the La Crosse Wellness Project. *American Journal of Health Education, 32,* 183–188.

U.S. Department of Health and Human Services (USDHHS). (2000). *Healthy People 2010: Understanding and improving health.* Washington, DC: Author.

Vickery, D., and Fries, J. (2004). *Take care of yourself: The complete illustrated guide to medical self-care,* 8th ed. Jackson, TN: Da Capo Press.

PART

V

Case Studies and a Needs Assessment Simulation

The following case studies are drawn from actual needs and capacity assessments in very different settings globally. Each case study has been written specifically for inclusion in this text in order to provide greater insight into the processes and the rationale for their selection.

- Tobacco Control Assessment, Iowa
- Community-Based Health Needs Assessment, Waupaca County, Wisconsin
- Nutrition and Physical Activity Assessment Through Day Care Observation and Interview, Los Angeles County, California
- Tobacco Usage Assessment with Focus Groups, La Crosse, Wisconsin
- Nutrition and Physical Activity Assessment Through Photovoice, Monroe County, Wisconsin
- Postnatal Assessment through At-Home Observation and Interview, England, United Kingdom
- Multifaceted Community-Based Health Needs Assessment, Mid Glamorgan, Wales, United Kingdom

These studies provide in-depth examples of needs and capacity assessment strategies and the application of the findings. In addition to the case studies, a needs assessment simulation game is presented. It provides an opportunity to facilitate a needs assessment experience with a group of people so they can learn by doing.

In addressing the case studies, here are some review considerations:

1. After reading the studies, select one case to study thoroughly.
2. Consider how closely the described situation and/or setting aligns with your present or projected professional responsibilities.
3. Note the particular needs assessment strategy that was used in each instance. Review its appropriateness for the defined target audience. Discuss the pros and cons with a colleague.

205

4. Determine whether some aspects of the case study might be beneficial to you in your professional responsibilities. What changes would you make?
5. Write down the next steps you could take to assess the needs and capacities of a specific target audience or to support the needs assessment efforts of colleagues.

Up in Smoke: A Recent History of Iowa Smokefree Legislation and Public Health Outcomes

Megan Sheffer, PhD, MPH, CHES, Center for Tobacco Research and Intervention, University of Wisconsin–Madison

Christopher Squier, PhD, DSc, College of Dentistry and Global Health Studies Program, University of Iowa

Background

Iowa was an early leader in tobacco control when, in 1897, the Iowa General Assembly completely prohibited the use, sale, and possession of tobacco products in the state. However, the state's subsequent responses to the burden of tobacco-related death and disease have been less than adequate, and legislation has been obstructed or influenced by the tobacco industry and its surrogates (Crime Prevention Group, 2000). For example, in 1990 when the General Assembly amended the smoking prohibition chapter of the state law to create smokefree areas in all restaurants seating more than 50 people, legislators also added preemption language to ensure that local laws could not be more restrictive than the state code (Iowa General Assembly, 1990).

In 2000, the Iowa Attorney General issued an opinion that state law did not preempt local regulation concerning smoking in public places, including restaurants and the smokefree ordinances enacted by two Iowa cities (Iowa Legislative Services Bureau, 2001–2005; Miller, 2003). Although this opinion was subsequently voided by the Iowa Supreme Court, the persistent grassroots efforts of a community coalition led to a campaign to regain local control and, finally, to a statewide ordinance. The Iowa Smokefree Air Act was implemented July 1, 2008.

Acknowledgment: The authors acknowledge Dr. William Haynes, University of Iowa College of Medicine, and Joanna Muldoon, Iowa Department of Public Health, for their assistance in obtaining the data on Iowa hospital admissions.

Agencies Involved

In 1996, a group of concerned parents, health professionals, and prevention specialists dedicated to reducing tobacco-related death and disease in Johnson County came together as the Johnson County Tobacco-Free Coalition. The group launched a campaign for a smokefree restaurant ordinance in Iowa City under the acronym of CAFE (Clean Air for Everyone) Johnson County in 1999. The campaign featured a series of organized educational and awareness activities, community activism, and periodic assessments of community readiness.

Needs Assessment, Strategic Planning, and Activities

A significant first step in the CAFE Johnson County campaign was to conduct a needs assessment to measure the readiness of Iowa City residents for a smokefree restaurant ordinance. Using an independent consulting firm, with support from the American Cancer Society-Midwest Division, a random survey assessed the knowledge and expectations of citizens in Iowa City and the adjacent community of Coralville. The results of the assessment revealed that the communities clearly recognized secondhand smoke as a health risk and overwhelmingly supported a local clean indoor air ordinance (see Table CS1-1).

After several years of planning, strategic activity, and evaluation, a smokefree dining ordinance was enacted on March 1, 2002, in Iowa City, Iowa (Sheffer, 2007). The ordinance stipulated that smoking was prohibited in restaurants where revenue from food sales exceeded 50 percent of total gross receipts (Iowa City Council, 2002). This was the state's second smokefree restaurant ordinance; in the preceding year, the City of Ames passed a clean indoor air ordinance, but it permitted smoking in bars and restaurants after 8.30 P.M.

TABLE CS1-1
Survey on Secondhand Smoke

Percentage of respondents who believe . . .	
Secondhand smoke is a personal health risk	68.5%
Separating smokers and nonsmokers does not solve the problem	83.8%
Workers should not have to be exposed to secondhand smoke	79.5%
Restaurants that do not allow smoking inside are preferred	67.5%
Other businesses should be smokefree	88.2%

Big Tobacco Strikes Again

Despite popular support for smokefree restaurant ordinances in Iowa, eight restaurant owners from the City of Ames, financed by Philip Morris, appealed an Iowa District Court's ruling upholding the constitutionality of the Ames smokefree restaurant ordinance to the Iowa Supreme Court (Judicial Branch in the Supreme Court of Iowa [JBSCI], 2003). On May 7, 2003, the Iowa Supreme Court overturned the lower court's ruling and rendered local smokefree ordinances unconstitutional (JBSCI, 2003)!

The ruling was a major public health setback for smokefree ordinances in particular and for tobacco control in general in the State of Iowa. Undeterred, CAFE Johnson County immediately launched a new statewide campaign—CAFE Iowa—to amend the state law on preemption to regain local control.

Building Momentum for Restoring Local Control

Despite widespread community support evidenced by the needs assessment and the passage of the Iowa City smokefree restaurant ordinance by voters, local businesses continued to express fear of economic losses. Not surprisingly, such concerns tend to be propagated by the tobacco industry in an effort to obstruct and overturn local smokefree legislation. Despite the growing body of scientific evidence to dispel such propaganda, Iowa City restaurateurs persisted in claims that their businesses would be impacted differently than those elsewhere in the nation (Dresser, 1999; Glantz & Smith, 1994, 1997; Maroney, Sherwood, & Stubblebine, 1994; Hayslett & Huang, 2000; Sciacca & Ratliff, 1998).

To examine these claims, Sheffer, Gilmore, and Squier (in press) assessed the impact of the Iowa City smokefree restaurant ordinance by analyzing restaurant volatility. This measure is defined as the ratio between the establishment of new restaurants and the closing of existing ones between 1997 and March of 2003. The period represents trends 5 years prior to the passage of the ordinance and 1 year afterwards. As a control, results were compared with data from Coralville, an adjacent city with similar demographics to Iowa City that has never enacted a smokefree dining ordinance.

Figure CS1-1 shows the net change in the number of Iowa City and Coralville restaurants; net change is expressed as the difference between the relative number (percentage) of restaurants opening and closing. Between 2002 and March 2003, the ordinance period, Iowa City showed no net change in the number of restaurants. In contrast, Coralville, which never enacted a smokefree restaurant ordinance, experienced an overall loss of restaurants between 2002 and March 2003. Sheffer et al. concluded that the ordinance did not adversely impact the restaurant industry in terms of restaurant closures and in a subsequent study showed that there had been no loss of revenue (Sheffer, 2007; Sheffer et al., in press).

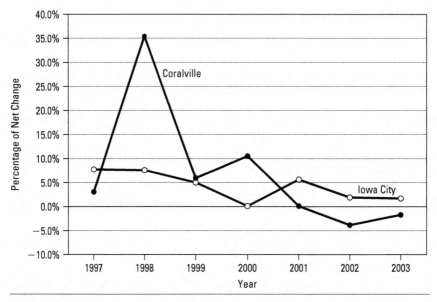

FIGURE CS1-1
Net change (percentage) of Iowa City and Coralville restaurants.

Such studies are important because they provide local data to assist citizens and policy makers in making informed public policy decisions to protect and enhance the health of their community. As the CAFE Iowa campaign progressed, politicians became increasingly receptive to the concept of a statewide Smokefree Air Act rather than repealing preemption and permitting local ordinances to be enacted city by city. On July 1, 2008, the Iowa Smokefree Air Act was enacted and is one of the strongest laws in the country, prohibiting smoking in all workplaces, with the exception of tobacco stores and casino gaming floors (Iowa Department of Public Health, 2010).

Tobacco Control Policy and Public Health Outcomes

In 2007, 1 year prior to the enactment of the Iowa Smokefree Air Act, the Iowa General Assembly raised the cigarette tax by $1.00; this marked the first increase in 16 years and raised per pack taxes to $1.36 (Lindblom, 2010). Following the implementation of these two evidence-based tobacco control interventions, the Iowa adult smoking rate and consumption of cigarette packs per capita have both sharply declined (see **Figure CS1-2**). Since 2002, the Iowa adult smoking rate has decreased 9 percent, from 23 to 14 percent (National Center for Chronic Disease Prevention and Health Promotion [NCCDPHP], 2002; Iowa Department of Revenue and Finance, 2010; Lutz, Cornish, Gonnerman, & Dietzenbach, 2010). Consumption of cigarette packs per capita

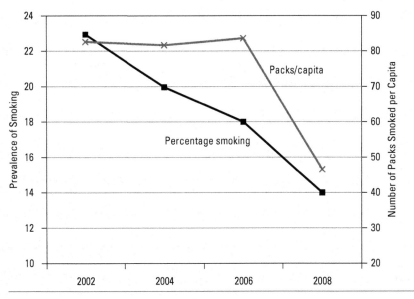

FIGURE CS1-2
Iowa adult smoking prevalence and cigarette consumption, 2002–2008.

declined from 83 to 47 percent during this time period (NCCDPHP, 2002; Iowa Department of Revenue and Finance, 2010; Lutz et al., 2010).

In a 2009 publication, the Institute of Medicine (2009) reported a decrease in myocardial infarctions (heart attacks) following the enactment of clean indoor air laws, ranging from 6 to 47 percent. In the short time the Iowa Smokefree Air Act has been in place, Iowans have experienced similar beneficial health effects. Using data submitted to the Iowa Department of Public Health from hospitals across Iowa, data on the number of monthly hospital admissions between July 2005 and June 2009 were examined for cardiovascular diseases and conditions that are caused or exacerbated by tobacco smoke and smoking (coronary heart disease, heart attacks, and stroke). The monthly hospitalizations for kidney infection and pancreatitis, conditions unrelated to tobacco use or exposure, were also examined throughout the same time period to control for variation in hospital admissions. As might be expected, the admissions for the control conditions did not increase following the implementation of the statewide smokefree legislation.

Figure CS1-3 shows that with the introduction of the Smokefree Air Act there was an average 18 percent reduction in hospital admissions, meaning that 2952 fewer Iowans were hospitalized for the single greatest cause of death in the nation—coronary (ischemic) heart disease (CHD)—compared to the average of the previous 3 years. The benefit appears to increase over time, with a more than 40 percent decrease in CHD admissions in June 2009 compared to June 2008.

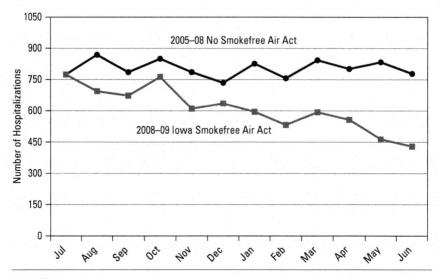

FIGURE CS1-3
Cumulative number of hospitalizations in Iowa for coronary heart disease, 2005–2009.

An average 8 percent reduction in hospital admissions for acute myocardial infarctions (heart attacks), the leading cause of death worldwide, occurred during the first year of the statewide clean indoor air law. This represents 483 fewer Iowans hospitalized for heart attacks compared to the preceding 3 years (see **Figure CS1-4**).

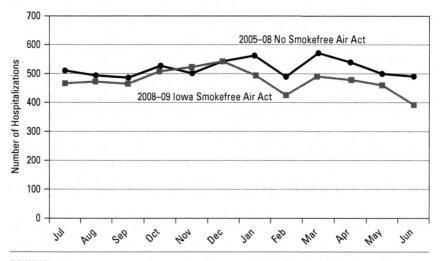

FIGURE CS1-4
Cumulative number of hospitalizations in Iowa for myocardial infarctions, 2005–2009.

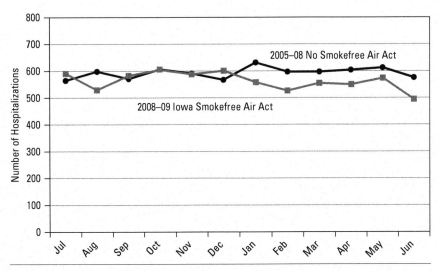

FIGURE CS1-5
Cumulative number of hospitalizations in Iowa for strokes, 2005–2009.

Similarly, as shown in **Figure CS1-5**, hospital admissions for acute cerebro-vascular disease (stroke), the leading cause of disability in the United States and the second cause of death worldwide, was reduced on average by 5 per-cent. This figure represents 373 Iowans who were not hospitalized for stroke.

Conclusion

The Iowa Smokefree Air Act provides safer workplaces and has reduced the risk of debilitative or fatal cardiovascular disease among hundreds of Iowans in just the first year of implementation. Together with the tobacco tax increase, there has been a marked reduction in prevalence and intensity of smoking in the state. Such legislation represents a major public health victory, but the danger of such success is a general belief among the public and the legislature that the task is complete and no further efforts or funding are necessary. Maintaining these health benefits requires not only adequate enforcement and protection of the laws, but the need to remain vigilant and work to maintain educational efforts and expand funding for tobacco control efforts to continue to enhance health benefits for Iowans.

References

Crime Prevention Group. (2000). Iowa Cigarette Control Law: 1897. Available at: http://medicolegal.tripod.com/iowalaw1897.htm. Accessed October 15, 2010.

Dresser, L. (1999). *Clearing the air: The effect of smoke-free ordinances on restaurant revenues in Dane County.* Madison, WI: Tobacco-Free Wisconsin Coalition.

Glantz, S., and Smith, L. (1994). The effect of ordinances requiring smoke-free restaurants on restaurant sales. *American Journal of Public Health, 84,* 1081–1085.

Glantz, S., and Smith, L. (1997). The effect of ordinances requiring smoke free restaurants and bars on revenue: A follow up. *American Journal of Public Health, 87,* 1687–1693.

Hayslett, J., and Huang, P. (2000). *Impact of clean indoor air ordinances on restaurant revenues in four Texas cities.* Bureau of Disease, Injury, and Tobacco Prevention. Texas Department of Health.

Institute of Medicine. (2009 October). *Secondhand smoke exposure and cardiovascular effects: Making sense of the evidence.* Washington, DC: The National Academies Press.

Iowa City Council. (2002). Smoking in food establishments: Ordinance number 024000. Iowa City, Iowa.

Iowa Department of Public Health. (2000). Healthy Iowans 2010: Tobacco use. Available at: http://www.idph.state.ia.us/cpp/healthy_iowans_2010.asp. Accessed January 10, 2003.

Iowa Department of Public Health. (2010). 2008 Acts, Chapter 1084, Iowa Code 142D: The Smokefree Air Act. Available at: http://www.iowasmokefreeair.gov/common/pdf/iowacode142D.pdf. Accessed October 15, 2010.

Iowa Department of Revenue and Finance. (2010 June). Cigarette and tobacco receipts report. Retrieved October 15, 2010, from http://publications.iowa.gov/9750.

Iowa General Assembly. (1990 November 19). Senate File 2069. Available at: http://search.legis.state.ia.us/nxt/gateway.dll/legarch/76ga-archive/sf/02000/sf02069/index.html?fn=document-frame.htm$f=templates$3.0. Accessed October 15, 2010.

Iowa Legislative Services Bureau. (2001–2005). Attorney General opinions requested by members of the General Assembly.

Judicial Branch in the Supreme Court of Iowa. (2003 May). No. 33/02-0415. Available at: http://www.judicial.state.ia.us/supreme/opinions/20030507/02-0415.asp. Accessed September 26, 2003.

Lindblom, E. (2010 August 3). State cigarette excise tax rates and rankings. Available at: http://tobaccofreekids.org/reports/prices. Accessed October 15, 2010.

Lutz, G. M., Cornish, D. L., Gonnerman, M. E. Jr., and Dietzenbach, K. (2010). Iowa 2009 tobacco control progress report. Available at: http://www.uni.edu/csbr. Accessed October 15, 2010.

Maroney, N., Sherwood, D., and Stubblebine, W. (1994). *The impact of tobacco control ordinances on restaurant revenues in California.* Claremont, CA: The Claremont Institute for Economy Policy Studies.

Miller, T. (2003 May). The Iowa Attorney General's report on secondhand smoke. Iowa Attorney General's Office.

National Center for Chronic Disease Prevention and Health Promotion. (2002). Behavioral risk factor surveillance system (BRFSS): 2002 prevalence data. Available at: http://www.cdc.gov/brfss. Accessed August 20, 2003.

Sciacca, J. P., and Ratliff, M. I. (1998). Prohibiting smoking in restaurants: Effects on restaurant sales. *American Journal of Health Promotion, 12*(3), 176–184.

Sheffer, M. A. (2007). An economic evaluation of the Iowa City smoke-free restaurant ordinance. Unpublished doctoral dissertation, University of Iowa.

Sheffer, M. A., Gilmore, G. D., and Squier, C. A. (in press). Restaurant Volatility and the Iowa City Smoke-free Restaurant Ordinance. *American Journal of Health Promotion.*

Public Health Needs Assessment in Waupaca County, Wisconsin: A Guide for Community Health Programs

Connie Abert, Youth Development Educator, University of Wisconsin–Extension

Linda Behm, Manager/Needs Assessment Coordinator, WCDHH, Public Health Nurse

Marilyn Herman, Family Living Educator, University of Wisconsin–Extension

Alyson Luchini, Nutrition Education Program Coordinator, University of Wisconsin–Extension

Gail Yest, WCDHH, Health Services Coordinator

Agency Overviews

Health Services Division of Waupaca County Department of Health and Human Services (Health Services) and Waupaca County University of Wisconsin–Extension (UWEX) collaborated on the last two health needs assessments, which were initiated in 2002 and 2007. The vision, and subsequently the mission, of Health Services is that "its individuals, families and communities be healthy" and "to be a leader in developing resources (prevention), assuring quality services (protection), and managing public funds responsibly." To carry out these essential purposes, Health Services sought assistance and guidance from UWEX with regard to the 5-year assessment process. UWEX, a division of the University of Wisconsin, has local faculty in each of Wisconsin's 72 counties. This faculty has extensive experience working with community partners, developing surveys, providing educational research, and facilitating partnership plans that impact their communities for change. Foundational to

UWEX is its purpose of educational outreach, which closely aligns with the purpose of prevention and protection in Health Services. Thus, Health Services and UWEX were natural partners for gathering statistical information about residents' health and designing a process for resident input on local health needs. Both Health Services and UWEX were able to present an unbiased look at the health needs of Wisconsin's citizens.

Agency Personnel, Community Partners, and Contract Services

The health services needs assessment coordinator gathered Census data, demographic data, and socioeconomic information from the literature and from other available resources in 2002. Some of these resources were dated; nevertheless, it was the most up-to-date information available. In 2007, this information came from one source: the Wisconsin County Health Rankings (Health Rankings), a publication from the University of Wisconsin Population Health Institute (Institute). The Institute also was able to supply county comparisons and trend data that could give counties a glimpse of future health patterns.

Health Services and UWEX planned the community survey in 2002 and the focus groups in 2007. The UWEX faculty provided expertise in developing the assessment tools and protocol for both the survey and the focus groups. In 2002, Health Services utilized nursing students from the University of Wisconsin–Oshkosh to disseminate the survey. The University of Wisconsin–Oshkosh performed the required statistical analyses on the survey data. In 2007, Health Services nursing staff facilitated the 14 focus groups. The Health Services needs assessment coordinator and administrative assistant then summarized focus group responses.

In spring 2002, additional input was obtained from the Waupaca County Needs Assessment Steering Committee. Members of this provisional committee included private citizens, business professionals, law enforcement, health care providers, senior citizens, mental health counselors, faith community leaders, complementary therapists, Health Services staff, and county board supervisors. The steering committee provided feedback on the tool that was used for community assessment, reviewed the data collected, and provided their personal insights to the results.

Steering committee feedback was not continued in 2007; however, the focus groups provided a similar forum for community input. In 2002, the data collection process and the comparison of resident data to similar counties in the state of Wisconsin took a large amount of time. This was accomplished in 2007 through the Institute, which was not available at the time of the previous assessment in 2002. Besides the information that was published in the Health Rankings, the Institute was available for additional statistical analysis or questions about data through a simple phone call or e-mail. The on-the-street survey tabulation expense of the 2002 survey far exceeded what was possible in 2007. By utilizing the focus group process, it was possible to narrow community health concerns with limited staff time.

Target Groups

The target group was residents of Waupaca County. Waupaca County is a rural county of slightly more than 50,000 residents neighboring the Fox Valley Area of approximately 200,000 people in Central Wisconsin. Communities range from barely 1000 to 7000 people. These areas do not have as many nonprofit groups (e.g., Boys and Girls Clubs, YMCA, afterschool programs, domestic violence shelters) or government resources as are available in the larger counties of the Fox Valley. The county is home to the Wisconsin Veterans Home, which provides elder and disability care to veterans residing in Wisconsin. The county is known for its natural environment, with many beautiful lakes and forested areas ideal for outdoor recreation and hunting. Waupaca County residents depend on agriculture, manufacturing, outdoor recreation, and tourism to provide most of their jobs and income. The 2002 demographic information revealed that the largest minority group is Hispanic residents, at 2.1 percent. The majority of residents, 97.9 percent, are Caucasian. The numbers of males and females in Waupaca County are relatively equal. The fastest growing age group is the senior population. The county has one of the highest numbers of nursing home beds per county per capita in the state of Wisconsin (U.S. Census Bureau, 2002).

Wisconsin has the highest incidence of underage drinking among high school students and binge drinking among adults in the nation (Jovagg, Moberg, Ziege, & Nametz, 2007). Waupaca County residents similarly struggle with this risk behavior. Socioeconomic concerns are evident, with 10.2 percent of the county's children under the age of 17 living in poverty. The State of Wisconsin poverty rate for children is 9.2 percent. Single-parent families in poverty are 21.8 percent of Waupaca County's families. Median earnings for a female, full-time, year-round employee are $22,149. Median earnings for male, full-time, year-round employees are $13,000 higher than those of female wage earners. The median income in Waupaca County is $3000 less than the Wisconsin average and $4000 less than U.S. median income. Social disruption is represented by factors such as single-parent families, with the region having the highest percentage of single-parent families in Wisconsin. As many as 30.5 percent of these single-parent households have children younger than 18 years of age and 37 percent of those children are younger than 5 years of age. In Waupaca County, 82.7 percent of county residents have a high school diploma or higher. The national rate is approximately 10 points lower; however, Wisconsin is about two (85 percent) points higher (Athens, Taylor, Booske, Kempf, & Remington, 2007).

Financially, Waupaca County residents suffered from the economic downturn in mid-2000, but it was comparable to other counties around the state of Wisconsin. For example, community discussions revealed that food banks saw their numbers almost triple during the recession. However, as mentioned earlier, not as many resources are available in Waupaca County as there are in more densely populated counties in the state.

Many of these demographics remained constant during both the 2002 and 2007 needs assessments. The Hispanic population increased slightly. The statistical poverty rate for children varied slightly in Waupaca County; however, some of the local schools experienced significant increases in the number of free and reduced lunches served. Because the needs assessment reflects the influences and different aspects of the community, the picture it paints is essential for a realistic look at resident's health.

Collection of Statistical Data

The county health departments in Wisconsin are mandated by state statute to conduct a local health needs assessment every 5 years. Using published statistics, including morbidity and mortality data, as well as qualitative information from residents, it serves to clarify community health concerns, identify priority needs, and uncover potential resources. Public health has an important role in the health of our community; however, it is a fairly invisible role as custodian of the health needs assessment process. Because public health's primary purpose is prevention and UWEX's core purpose is educational outreach, the needs assessment is essential for guiding program efforts for both departments. In an era of rapidly changing economics and increasingly limited resources, it is critical to prioritize local needs and programs that use public health and education funds.

As mentioned earlier, statistics that influenced health in 2002 were gathered from approximately 14 different sources; in addition, it was very difficult and time consuming to compare Waupaca County with similar or surrounding counties to determine trends in residents' health. In 2007, the University of Wisconsin Population Health Institute gathered statistics from similar sources and compiled county statistics and rankings. The Health Rankings are built on the model of population health improvement (Athens et al., 2007; Kindig & Stoddart, 2003). They are designed to summarize the current health of county residents and to identify key factors or determinants of future health. In this model, health outcomes are considered the results of health determinants. Both are affected by policies or interventions and programs. Counties and community partners can significantly improve health outcomes by improving the health determinants or specifically adopting appropriate programs, policies, and laws that would influence large numbers of people. For example, the Wisconsin legislature passed in 2009 and enacted in 2010 a law that requires public places in Wisconsin to be smokefree (Wisconsin State Legislature, 2009). This law will improve air quality for all residents in public places.

Health Determinants

Health determinants, the things that make people healthy, are not completely under the control of the individual or the community. Many factors combine to affect health. Whether people are healthy or not can be determined by their physical environment and circumstances. To a large extent, factors such as where we live, the state of our environment, genetics, life choices, our income, our education level, and our relationships with friends and family all have considerable impact on our health. More commonly considered factors such as access and quality of outpatient health care services often have less impact than we would expect (Athens et al., 2007). The comprehensive context of people's lives is what determines their health.

Though the terminology may differ, many sources agree that health is determined by four major categories of health determinants: behaviors (40 percent of total health); socioeconomic factors (40 percent); physical environment (10 percent); and health care (10 percent) (Athens et al., 2007). These personal, social, economic, and environmental factors determine the health status of individuals and our population in general. Within each of these four major categories are multiple components. It is difficult to consider all of the specific determinants of a population's health, so a finite number were selected by the Institute for inclusion in the Health Rankings. The health determinants examined were selected based on priorities identified in the Wisconsin State Health Plan and availability of data at the county level (Peppard et al., 2003; Wisconsin Turning Point Transformation Team, 2002).

Health rankings and their determinants are especially important at the county level because they serve as predictors of future health. There are 72 counties in Wisconsin, yet there are 73 rankings. Milwaukee, the largest city in the state of Wisconsin, is considered an entity with the other counties (Athens et al., 2007). Waupaca County, with regard to each health determinant and its components, was compared to regional and state averages by the Institute. Lower rankings are healthier indicators. In 2008, Waupaca County ranked 49th of 73 for overall determinants of health (Taylor, Athens, Booske, O'Connor, Jones, & Remington, 2008). This was up from 56th in 2007 (Athens et al., 2007). This raised Waupaca County from the bottom quartile in 2007 to the lower-middle quartile in 2008. It will be significant if this trend can continue over time.

Health Outcomes

Health outcomes are simply the result of the composite of health determinants. It is particularly noteworthy if health outcomes improve with sustained improvement in determinants of health, which will indicate residents' progress toward better health. Health outcomes are often reported in terms of mortality statistics, such as life expectancy and years of potential life lost. These statistics are relatively easy to track. However, most models of individual and population health do not merely include measures of longevity, but also quality of life or general health status. For this reason, the Wisconsin County Health Rankings contain an outcome component that weights quality of life with length of life. The health outcomes weighted equally are based on mortality, expressed in years of potential life lost (50 percent), and general health, expressed in terms of how people rate their overall quality of health (50 percent) (Athens et al., 2007).

Years of Potential Life Lost (YPLL) is a measure of mortality and years of potential life lost prior to age 75. It is a measure that accounts for the age at which a person dies. Persons who die at a younger age are considered to have lost potential years of life. For example, a person who dies at age 65 has lost 10 potential years of life. An individual who dies at age 50 will have lost 25 potential years of life. Waupaca County has maintained a rank in the mid-40s (of 73) for YPLL, which is the lower-middle quartile (Taylor et al., 2008). YPLL is a widely used measure of premature mortality. It enables Waupaca County to investigate further into the causes of death and target resources at high-risk areas when funding is available.

General health status is the personal report from residents of their level of health. Data were based on responses to a telephone survey that asked the question, "In general, would you say your health is excellent, very good, good, fair or poor?" Waupaca County has consistently ranked around 60 (of 73) in the category of general health status. The 2008 rank of 66 kept this outcome component in the bottom quartile (Taylor et al., 2008). People reporting fair or poor health provides an estimate of health-related quality of life or illness.

Wisconsin County Health Rankings

Whether it is the 2004 Wisconsin County Health Rankings or the 2008 Wisconsin County Health Rankings, the name seems to imply that the report represents just 1 year of data. However, The rankings are actually compilations of statistical information from multiple sources from 1999 to the present. Produced by the University of Wisconsin Population Health Institute, their purpose is to summarize the current health of individual county populations and the distribution of factors that determine future health (Athens et al., 2007).

As health determinants improve, health outcomes should also improve. In 2008, there was a dramatic improvement in the Waupaca County health determinant ranking: 56th of 72 in 2007 (Athens et al., 2007) and 49th of 73 in 2008 (Taylor et al., 2008). Although the county's health outcomes do not yet reflect this change, improvements in health within the general population often lag behind individual health determinant statistics. The programs and interventions enacted by Waupaca County NuAct, and discussed in the following section, "Utilization of the Needs Assessment," could contribute to improved health determinants and outcomes in the future.

No county ranks highest in one aspect of the rankings and lowest in another. For example, one county may rank well (4th) in a determinant, but worse (38th) in outcomes. Because their determinant rank is better than their outcome rank, one may see an improvement in future health outcomes. The lag could be a result of recently instituted policies and programs that have not shown anticipated improvements in community health. Similarly, a poor rank in health determinants may experience declining population health outcomes in the future.

Although mandated by state statute, the community needs assessment process can serve to deliver a realistic representation of local health. Not only does the assessment reveal what residents say they need, but also verifies needs via statistical means. As partners in the health improvement process, either through the survey or the focus groups, community members are able to see positive changes in health outcomes as coming through their own hands and by their own efforts. Taking ownership of community health issues is assuredly one giant step toward a better-informed, healthier community.

The Wisconsin County Health Rankings are based on the University of Wisconsin–Madison Population Health Institute's model of health improvement (see **Figure CS2-1**).

Input from Community Residents

In spring and summer of 2002, Waupaca County residents were asked to participate in the community needs assessment survey (see **Figure CS2-2**). Because Waupaca County is a popular tourist location, particularly in the summer months, extra care was taken to ensure that subjects contributing data to the survey database were Waupaca County residents. Steps were also taken to minimize the likelihood of participants completing more than one survey. A statement was included at the top of the survey instrument that stated, "Please do not complete this survey if you have done one before or if you are *not* a resident of Waupaca County."

The Waupaca County Community Survey did not allow for identification of individual participants. Although community of residence and specific demographic information were elicited, no names or other identifying characteristics were a part of this survey. Client demographic data included gender, age, marital status, annual household income, education level, languages spoken, ethnicity, as well as community of residence.

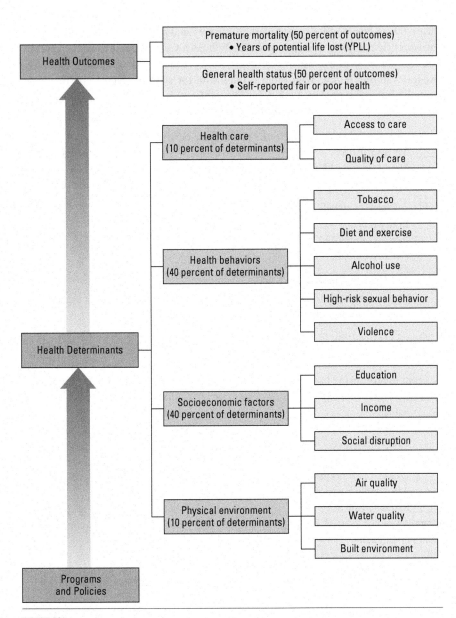

FIGURE CS2-1
Model of health improvement.
Courtesy of University of Wisconsin Population Health Institute. *County Health Rankings 2010.*

Please take a few minutes to complete this survey and give us your opinions about the issues that concern you the most. The Waupaca County Department of Health and Human Services will use this information to plan for the development of future programs in the county. Your input is important for all of us. Thank you for your contribution to this project. *Please do not complete this survey if you have done one before or if you are not a resident of Waupaca County.*

1. Please place a check (√) next to the community in which you live:

_____ Marion 10.5%   _____ Clintonville 17.9%   _____ Manawa 8.3%

_____ New London 11.6%   _____ Weyauwega 10.4%   _____ Fremont 8.8%

_____ Waupaca 19.4%   _____ Iola 7.8%   _____ Other 5.5%

2. Please check (√) whether you live:

_____ In town 57.1%

_____ In the country 42.1%

_____ No answer 0.8%

3. Please check (√) whether you are a:

_____ Seasonal resident 2.5%

_____ Year-round resident 97.5%

4. How long have you lived in the above-named community? _____
All my life

5. From the following list, check (√) the *four major strengths* of your community.

_____ Low crime rate 2   _____ Church

_____ Safety   _____ Low taxes

_____ Child care   _____ Recreation

_____ Family-oriented   _____ Friendly people 1

_____ Conveniently located services _____ Arts

_____ Quality of schools 4   _____ Economic stability

_____ Affordable housing   _____ Transportation

_____ Rural setting 3   _____ Other strengths (please specify)

Churches

Family orientation

Safety

6. From the following list, please check (√) the *three most important factors* that improve the quality of life in a community.

_____ Good jobs and a healthy economy 1   _____ Strong family life

_____ Parks and recreation   _____ Good place to raise children

_____ Quality, affordable housing   _____ Religious or spiritual values

FIGURE CS2-2
Waupaca County community survey.

Courtesy of Connie Abert, UW–Extension Youth Development Educator (primary author); Linda Behm, WCDHH-Public Health Nurse Manager/Needs Assessment Coordinator; Marilyn Herman, UW–Extension Family Living Educator; Alyson Luchini, UW–Extension Nutrition Education Program Coordinator; and Gail Yest, WCDHH–Health Services Coordinator.

_____ Low death and disease rates
_____ Good transpiration services
_____ Medical care
_____ Low crime rate/safe neighbors **3**
_____ Good schools **2**
_____ Arts and cultural events
_____ Healthy lifestyle

_____ Clean environment
_____ Access to health care
_____ Disability services
_____ Preventative healthcare
_____ Shopping/competitive prices
_____ Other factors (please specify)

7. From the following list, please check (√) the *three health problems* you feel have the greatest effect in your community.

_____ Motor vehicle accidents **3**
_____ Rape/sexual assault
_____ Lack of access to mental health care
_____ Inactivity
_____ Homicide
_____ Child abuse/neglect
_____ Teen pregnancy
_____ Domestic violence
_____ Hunger
_____ Physical problems of aging **2**
_____ Drug abuse **4**
_____ Alzheimer's/dementia

_____ Sexually transmitted infections
_____ Infectious diseases
_____ Poor diet/nutrition
_____ Alcohol abuse **1**
_____ Lack of access to health care
_____ Chronic diseases (cancer heart disease, diabetes) **5**
_____ Firearm-related injuries
_____ Poor housing
_____ Tobacco use **6**
_____ Homelessness
_____ Other (please specify)

8. Please check (√) the *five most serious problems or needs* in your community.

_____ Poor parenting skills
_____ Single parent families
_____ Lack of affordable day care
_____ Shortage of food
_____ Lack of recreation activities
_____ Gangs
_____ Problems with schools
_____ Lack of legal aid
_____ Lack of support for caregivers
_____ Poor or low wages **2**
_____ Jobs are seasonal or part-time
_____ Unemployment
_____ Lack of job training
_____ Employment for disabled
_____ Chronic disease
_____ Communicable disease
_____ Poor air quality

_____ Poor water quality
_____ Inadequate health insurance
_____ Poor diet/food choices
_____ Lack of physical activity
_____ Lack of services for elderly to remain in own home
_____ Child abuse
_____ Gambling abuse
_____ Adult alcohol abuse **4**
_____ Adult tobacco use
_____ Adult drug use
_____ Domestic violence
_____ Elder abuse
_____ Age discrimination
_____ School truancy/dropouts
_____ Youth crime/violence
_____ Adult crime/violence

(continued)

_____ Poor housing conditions
_____ Lack of transportation
_____ Minority discrimination
_____ High rents/mortgages
_____ High property taxes **1**
_____ Money problems
_____ Financial elder abuse
_____ Scams
_____ Credit problems
_____ Services for 3–5 year olds
_____ Services for elderly
_____ Services for physically disabled
_____ Better transportation services

_____ Lack of information about avail-
    able services
_____ Services are not accessible
_____ Lack of smoking cessation re-
    sources
_____ Inability to get healthcare in own
    county
_____ Youth alcohol use **3**
_____ Youth tobacco access
_____ Teenage pregnancy
_____ Gang activity
_____ Youth drug use **5**

9. From the list in Question 8, please list the *problem or needs* you and your family have experienced in the last year.
   1. High taxes
   2. Poor/low wages
   3. Money problems
   4. Unemployment
   5. Lack of recreational activities
   6. Inadequate health insurance
   7. Problems with schools
   8. Youth alcohol use
   9. Lack of information about available services
   10. Lack of physical activities

10. Where did you get help handling the problems listed on the previous page? Check (√) all that apply.

_____ Family **1**
_____ Support groups
_____ Private agency
_____ Schools
_____ Job service
_____ Hospital
_____ Local government
_____ Neighbors/friends **2**
_____ Physician **5**
_____ Church **3**

_____ Law enforcement
_____ Extension office
_____ Technical college
_____ State agency
_____ Co-workers
_____ Housing authority
_____ Health and Human Services **4**
_____ County agency
_____ Employee assistance program
_____ Other (please specify in Question 11)

FIGURE CS2-2
Continued.

11. If you did not receive help in handling these problems, please check (√) all that apply.

_____ I handled it myself **1**   _____ I didn't have transportation

_____ I didn't know where to go **2**   _____ I couldn't afford the service **5**

_____ I was placed on the waiting list   _____ I didn't qualify **3**

_____ The hours weren't convenient   _____ I was told they couldn't help me **4**

_____ I was not satisfied with the ser-   _____ Other reasons (please specify)
vices offered

12. What other services or programs would be helpful to you, your family or your community?
1. Youth activities
2. Exercise/physical activity/recreation programs
3. Transportation
4. Health care/insurance
5. Day care/parenting/family help/jobs/job training

13. What services(s), provided by the Waupaca County Department of Health and Human Services, would you and your family not want to be without?
1. Elder services/senior citizen programs/nutrition programs
2. WIC/immunizations
3. Health services/county nurse/communicable disease control
4. What do you offer?
5. Medical assistance/financial help
6. Social services (including juvenile programs)/food stamps/Badger Care
7. Mental health services/hospice

The following questions are about your healthcare needs.

14. When did you last receive healthcare?

_____ In last year **65%**   _____ No health care **1%**

_____ In last month **14%**   _____ No answer **11%**

_____ In last week **9%**

15. How do you pay for healthcare? Please check (√) all that apply. (*Note:* Respondents could check more than one response.)

_____ Receive no healthcare unless it's   _____ Indian Health Service **0.3%**
an emergency **3.9%**   _____ Healthy Start **1.5%**

_____ No insurance **5.6%**   _____ Pay for my own insurance **13.0%**

_____ Insurance through job **55.9%**   _____ Badger Care **3.3%**

_____ Pay cash **16.0%**   _____ Veteran's Administration **2.4%**

_____ Medicare **22.0%**   _____ Self-employed/high deductible **2.5%**

_____ Medicare supplement **11.7%**   _____ Other (please specify)

Out-of-pocket/cash
Parents
Champus/tri-care

(*continued*)

16. In the last 12 months, have you or your family been unable to get any of the following services you needed?

_____ Mental health/counseling **5**	_____ Dental services **1**
_____ Physical therapy **9**	_____ Housing **12**
_____ Eye care **2**	_____ Annual physical **7**
_____ Pap test **3**	_____ Mammogram **4**
_____ Drug or alcohol services **11**	_____ Help to stop smoking **6**
_____ Caregiver support services **10**	_____ Nutrition services **10**
_____ Supportive services in my home **12**	_____ Other (please specify) **8**

Prescriptions
Routine medical care (job doesn't cover or wages are too low to buy)

17. What services do you need access to the most?
Medical care
Dental care
Eye care
Annual exam
Mental health services/counseling

18. Which of the following therapies have you or your family used in the last 12 months:

_____ Acupuncture/acupressure	_____ Homeopathy
_____ Herbal medicine **4**	_____ Reflexology
_____ Massage **3**	_____ Nutrition therapy **6**
_____ Meditation	_____ Yoga
_____ Spiritual healing	_____ None **1**
_____ Tai Chi	_____ Other (please specify) **5**
_____ Chiropractic realignment **2**	

Exercise
Physical therapy

The last group of questions is about your home and family life.

19. Approximately how many hours per week do you spend doing the following? Place the appropriate number in the space provided: (1) None; (2) 1–5 hours; (3) 6–10 hours; or (4) More than 10 hours.

_____ Working	_____ Playing video games
_____ Watching television	_____ Reading
_____ Volunteering (other than work)	_____ Using computer
_____ Exercising	_____ Attending school/training

FIGURE CS2-2
Continued.

_____ Socializing

_____ Visiting friends

Sports/outdoor activities

With family

Gardening

Crafts

Helping others

Church

Artistic skills

_____ Please specify other ways you like to spend your time:

20. What recreation activities would you and your family use if they were available in your community?

Swimming pool

Health/fitness/community center/YMCA

Hiking/biking trails

21. Please respond to the following statement: "I would be willing to pay more for…" Please check (√) all that apply.

_____ Schools 3

_____ Health care 7

_____ Community beautification 8

_____ Recreational facilities 1

_____ Police 6

_____ Elderly services 6

Cut taxes

Transportation

Day care (include second-shift workers)/community pool

_____ Youth services 2

_____ Parks 4

_____ Church-based activities 5

_____ Other community needs (please specify) 9

22. If you or someone in your home has a disability, please check (√) all the categories that apply.

_____ Blindness/vision impairment 3

_____ Other physical disability 1

_____ Learning disability 5

_____ Inability to read/write English well 6

Joint problems (including arthritis, RA)

Breathing difficulty

Diabetes/old age/seizures/difficulty walking

_____ Deafness/hearing impairment 2

_____ Mental disability 4

_____ Other disability (please specify) 4

23. Please indicate services you need, related to these disabilities, which you are *not* able to get:

Mental health services

Eye care

Transportation/dental care

(continued)

24. Why have you been unable to get these services?
Not in the area
Too expensive/no money
Over limit
Funding unavailable
Waiting lists

Please answer these last questions so we can see how different people feel about these local health issues. Thank you for helping to identify our needs in Waupaca County.

25. Your gender:
_____ Male 36.5%
_____ Female 63.5%

26. Marital status:
_____ Single 19.5%
_____ Married 63.1%
_____ Widowed 9.9%
_____ Divorced 7.6%

27. Your age:
_____ Under 18 years 4%
_____ 18–25 years 8.8%
_____ 26–39 years 18.2%
_____ 40–54 years 32.9%

_____ 55–64 years 15.0%
_____ 65–75 years 11.2%
_____ 76–85 years 8.0%
_____ 86 years and over 1.9%

28. Annual household income:
_____ Less than $10,000 9.2%
_____ $10,000–$19,000 14.5%
_____ $20,000–$29,000 15.3%
_____ $30,000–$49,000 25.7%

_____ $50,000–$74,000 20.0%
_____ $75,000–$99,000 10.2%
_____ $100,000 or more 5.1%

29. How many people live in your household?
See attached information

30. Your highest level of education: (*Note:* Response information placed in an attachment to the original report.)
_____ Less than high school 10.5%
_____ High school diploma/GED 37.1%
_____ College credits 19.0%
_____ College degree 22.7%

_____ Master's Degree 7.1%
_____ PhD 0.5%
_____ Other (please specify) 3.0%

FIGURE CS2-2
Continued.

31. Ethnic group you most identify with:

_____ White/Caucasian **1**   _____ Asian/Pacific Islander **4**

_____ Hispanic/Latino **5**   _____ Native American **2**

_____ African American/Black **3**   _____ Other (please specify) **American**

32. Languages spoken in your home:

_____ English **72.0%**   _____ Hmong **0.0%**

_____ Spanish **1.7%**   _____ Other (please specify) **26.3%**

German mentioned most frequently

The Waupaca County Community Survey was simply a data collection tool for the project, which gathered information about community needs and strengths, quality of life factors, use of personal time, service program needs, health care resources, use of complementary therapies, and recreational activity preferences, needs, and utilization. All data were reported as aggregate data.

Participants were asked to check off responses and fill in the blanks. Space was also provided for respondents to elaborate on most questions, if needed. The average time required to complete the survey was about 10 minutes. Qualitative and quantitative analyses of the data were performed by graduate students at the University of Wisconsin–Oshkosh.

In April and May of 2002, needs assessment workers went to the seven largest cities, towns, and villages in Waupaca County to collect survey data. Survey sites were located at grocery stores, community pools, drug stores, local businesses, libraries, gas stations, and restaurants. The survey locations were identified by UWEX and townspeople as places where a diverse population of community residents could be surveyed. Workers manning the stations asked people to complete the survey instrument. Surveys, pens, clipboards, and, whenever possible, chairs were provided to participants. When assistance was needed, workers read the questions to participants or filled in the blanks with answers the participants provided. Most often, participants completed the surveys on their own with no help from the workers. Participants were reminded not to put their names on the surveys and were confirmed to be Waupaca County residents before they began.

By phone or in person, local officials were also invited to complete surveys. In April, May, and June of 2002, town meetings were held in each of the communities previously identified. The purpose of the town meetings was to gather survey information from interested individuals who had not yet had an opportunity to complete a survey. Signs and invitations were posted in a variety of public locations, local newspapers, and newsletters. Advertising was prepared well in advance for each community meeting. Overall, these meetings were poorly attended, but it was important to the design team to offer an opportunity for general public participation.

Waupaca County residents completed 1021 community surveys. Of those completing the survey, 57.1 percent described themselves as living in town; 42.1 percent lived in the country or a rural area of the county; and 97.5 percent of respondents were year-round residents.

Respondents identified those features that most improve the quality of life in our community. In order of importance, those features were (1) good jobs and a healthy economy, (2) good schools/education, and (3) low crime and safe neighborhoods. These can easily be correlated to socioeconomic, environment, health behaviors, or health care determinants.

When asked how respondents dealt with problems in the community, they indicated they went to friends, family, and neighbors first. After this, they sought out churches, health and human services, and their physicians as resources. When they were not able to get help, the reasons cited were, in order of importance, (1) I handled it myself, (2) I didn't know where to go, (3) I didn't qualify, (4) I was told they couldn't help me, and (5) I couldn't afford the services.

Despite financial concerns, residents indicated that they would be willing to pay more for recreational facilities, youth services, schools, and parks. Consistently, youth activities and exercise/physical activity/recreation programs were mentioned as services or programs in the community that were helpful to respondents, families, and communities. The most frequent responses to the question "What recreation activity would you and your family use if they were available in your community?" were (1) swimming pool, (2) health/fitness/community center/YMCA, and (3) hiking/biking trails.

County residents identified the following services, specifically provided by the Health and Human Services Departments, that they would not want to be without: (1) elder services/senior citizen programs/nutrition program; (2) WIC/immunizations; and (3) health services/county nurse/communicable disease. The fourth most frequent response to this item was "What do you offer?" Also identified as essential services to respondents were (5) medical assistance/financial help, (6) social services (including juvenile programs, food stamps, and Badger Care), and (7) mental health/hospice.

With regard to health care, 65 percent of respondents indicated that they had received health care in the last year. The majority of respondents' (55.9 percent) health care was paid for by insurance offered by an employer; 22 percent of respondents received Medicare; 13 percent paid their own insurance; 16 percent paid cash for medical care; 5.6 percent were uninsured; and 3.9 percent indicated they received no health care unless it was an emergency.

When asked what services they need access to the most, respondents identified (1) medical care, (2) dental care, (3) eye care, and (4) annual exams. In a related question, participants were asked which services they had not been able to access in the last 12 months. The five most frequent responses were (1) dental services, (2) eye care, (3) Pap test, (4) mammogram, and (5) mental health/counseling.

The three health problems having the greatest affect on the Waupaca County communities were identified as: (1) alcohol abuse, (2) physical problems of aging, and (3) motor vehicle accidents. Other frequently identified problems included drug abuse, chronic diseases, and tobacco use. The five most serious problems identified by Waupaca County residents were (1) high property taxes, (2) poor or low wages, (3) youth alcohol use, (4) adult alcohol use, and (5) youth drug use.

In 2007, UWEX assisted Health Services in developing a presentation and questions that would gather qualitative information needed to deepen the quantitative data from the Institute. UWEX detailed facilitation steps for the public health nurses who would be presenting and facilitating community focus groups. Health Services and UWEX identified organizations in each community in the county that would be willing to participate in a needs assessment focus group. The groupings were composed of community leaders and encompassed various age groups represented in the county demographics. Leaders of the identified organizations were contacted by the health needs assessment coordinator. Fourteen organizations from around the county agreed to allow time at one of their meetings for Health Services to facilitate a focus group about local health concerns.

The instrument used with the presentation proved to be more time consuming than most community groups could allow. Because most groups could only allot 20 to 30 minutes of meeting time for the needs assessment, the needs assessment questions were simplified, but collected the same information. The focus group process involved introductory remarks from the Health Services facilitator (nurse), which included an explanation of the needs assessment process, the participants' role in determining health priorities, and Health Services role in county health. Participants were then asked to take a few moments to respond to the question: "What do you think are the most important health concerns in your community?" Participants listed as many concerns as possible in the approximate 5 minutes allotted. These written responses were collected, and a public health nurse then grouped and posted all responses on a poster board. While sorting the responses, the health needs assessment coordinator advanced to the next question: "What do you think needs to be available to make a healthier community?" or "If you had a magic wand and, with one wish, you could improve the health of the residents of Waupaca County, what would you do?" These responses were then collected and grouped. The final step in the process was to have participants vote on their top three to five choices of all the health needs posted earlier on the board. The number of votes was determined by the number of items posted. If there were 11 or fewer items, only three votes were permitted per participant. If there were more than 11 items, 5 votes would be allowed by each focus group participant. An individual was not permitted to place more than one vote on the same need. The three categories receiving the most votes became the highest health priorities identified by the group. A group decision, rather than an individual decision, was at the heart of this data collection process. The focus groups were inclusive of every community in the county, with participation from a wide range organizations, including service organizations, business associations, ministerial clusters, and young mothers' support groups.

In response to the question, "What do you think needs to be available to make a healthier community?" the most frequent replies included: education/ seminars, health care/access to care, walking trails/exercise opportunities, and local physicians. Respondents emphasized personal responsibility in the need for education and exercise. Respondents also indicated significant concern regarding the need for appropriate, accessible health care in their communities. In response to the question, "If you had a magic wand and, with one wish, you could improve the health of Waupaca County residents, what would you do?" the most frequent answers included smoking-related issues: no smoking in restaurants/bars, smoking cessation programs for all smokers, and smoking bans in communities. This was before the state implemented legislation for smokefree public places in 2010 (Wisconsin State Legislature, 2009). Additional responses to the question included affordable health insurance for all, health care for all, and education about healthy lifestyles.

These focus group questions were asked in order to gather citizens' perspectives on the county's greatest health needs and what they thought might improve the health of county residents. The public health nurses utilized the focus group process to gather qualitative information that was then added to the statistical information gathered from the UW Population Health Institute to enable a more in depth account of local health.

Comparison of Statistical Needs Assessment Results

The 2002 Waupaca County Needs Assessment revealed the following as priority concerns: alcohol use in adults and youth; tobacco use in adults and youth; overweight, obesity, and lack of physical activity; access to primary and preventive health services; mental health/mental disorders; adequate and appropriate nutrition; social and economic factors. The survey was informative but not as informative about specific health needs as the designers had anticipated.

As is the case with most communities, the problems identified by Waupaca County residents touched nearly all of the health priorities in *Healthiest Wisconsin 2010* (Wisconsin Turning Point Transformation Team, 2002). Therefore, to be effective and make an impact, Health Services and UWEX knew that prevention dollars and educational programs had to focus on those areas where outcomes could be produced that would result in improved health. Alcohol and tobacco use have had a significant negative impact on the Waupaca County population for many years. Statewide and community prevention efforts are in place for both these health risks. County leadership felt that based on the current information the prevention dollars available should be spent to support reducing the priority health risk of obesity.

In 2008, more detailed statistical data were available from the University of Wisconsin–Madison Population Health Institute for the Waupaca County Needs Assessment. Health determinants of (a) no health insurance (61), a health care health determinant; (b) motor vehicle crash-related ER visits–on road (59), a health behavior health determinant that is a proxy for alcohol use while driving; (c) nitrate levels in water (63), a physical environment health determinant; and (d) radon risk (72), a physical environment health determinant. Waupaca County ranked in the bottom quartile (56–73) for these four health determinants (Taylor et al., 2008).

The focus group results that correlated with the Healthiest Wisconsin 2010 Health Priorities (Wisconsin Turning Point Transformation Team, 2002) were related to the following health determinants:

- Access to primary and preventive health services
- Alcohol and other substance use and addiction
- Environmental and occupational health hazards

Several other health determinant factors have a significant impact on the health outcomes of residents of Waupaca County. The county scored in the lower-middle quartile on the following: (a) did not receive needed health care (54), an access to care health determinant; (b) no recent dental visit (48), an access to care health determinant; (c) fewer than five fruits and vegetables a day (51), a health behavior determinant; (d) cigarette smoking (54), a health behavior health determinant; (e) divorce (51), a socioeconomic health determinant; and (f) houses with increased lead risk (53), a physical environment health determinant (Taylor et al., 2008).

Healthiest Wisconsin 2010 Health Priorities (Wisconsin Turning Point Transformation Team, 2002) related to these issues, not listed previously, are:

- Adequate and appropriate nutrition
- Social and economic factors that influence health

As expected by the health improvement model, the rankings of current health outcomes and current health determinants are closely related.

It is apparent that access to health services, at all levels, is an issue for Waupaca County residents. Both the published statistics and the community survey bore out the need for greater availability of medical and dental services, closer to home, at an affordable price. An opportunity for affordable health insurance was cited as being key to this access.

Motor vehicle crash data is a proxy for alcohol use while driving, because alcohol is a factor in a large percentage of motor vehicle crashes. Waupaca County has yet to reach a level of success in dealing with alcohol issues in the population. Cultural acceptance within the state and the region's status as a tourist destination make it difficult to effectively deal with alcohol issues.

Issues related to the physical environment are significantly contributing to residents' poor health. In 2003, the overall physical environment health determinant rank was 46 of 72 (Peppard, Kindig, Riemer, Dranger, & Remington, 2003). In 2007, it was 64 of 72 (Athens et al., 2007). In 2008, it was 67 of 73 (Taylor et al., 2008). Nitrate levels in water, houses with increased lead risk, and radon risk have been the largest contributors to the county's poor showing in this area. Education campaigns, including media strategies and public forums, to inform people of how to lower their risks of exposure to these three threats, will be a strategy health services can implement to help reduce the prevalence of these issues and contribute to more positive health outcomes for our residents in future years.

Cigarette smoking continues to be a key issue for Waupaca County residents. Although smoking rates have improved, the county still ranks in the lower-middle quartile (53 of 73) (Athens et al., 2007). Waupaca County continues to exceed the state rate of smokers, and the smoking rate is almost double the target rate of 12 percent. Cigarette smoking remains the single most prevalent cause of death in Wisconsin and the United States, contributing to more deaths than alcohol, drugs, and motor vehicle accidents. This is a modifiable health determinant, and support for Smoke Free Wisconsin legislation could improve this health outcome significantly.

Adequate and appropriate nutrition for Waupaca County residents is an ongoing concern. Food insecurity continues to increase in the population. Another modifiable health determinant—nutrition—plays a statistically significant role in a healthier population, but it should not be viewed as an isolated issue. Socioeconomic concerns play strongly into the nutritional status of families. With a shortage of resources in general, families have a shortage of resources for food. This may be especially true in single-parent, female head of household or divorced households where incomes are usually lower. With fewer resources, people tend to consume fewer fruits and vegetables and more foods with lower nutritional value. Adults in food-insecure homes, especially women, are at increased risk for being obese, partly due to the choice of low-cost foods that are higher in sugar, fat, and calories. Adults and children in food-insecure homes and divorced or single-parent homes experience more adverse health effects such as depression, chronic disease, and other poor levels of overall health. Food insecurity is a critical piece of the overall health puzzle and needs to be dealt with aggressively. Greater access to supplemental food programs (e.g., church suppers, food pantries, FoodShare) will help in reducing food insecurity in Waupaca County.

Waupaca County Strengths

Although Waupaca County had some improvements in health outcomes in 2008, its rankings are still in the 60s (Taylor et al., 2008). Probably the most significant change has come in the health behavior determinant ranking, where, for the first time since at least 2004, the county improved from 56th to 50th of 73 (Peppard, Kempf, Dranger, Kindig, & Remington, 2004; Taylor et al., 2008). The health determinant ranking of 50 is significant, because it is a predictor of future health. Health determinant changes lag behind overall outcomes in that it takes some time for individuals' improved health behaviors to impact their overall health. So, although the county's health outcome ranking improved only slightly, the effects of interventions on overall health may yet to be seen. It is necessary to give emphasis to deaths due to heart disease or cancers; however, we should keep in mind that factors such as tobacco, diet, activity, and alcohol are substantial contributors to these deaths. Thus, we are considering determinants of health as those personal behaviors and choices that contribute to health or illness in our Waupaca County population. As the Institute has pointed out, they can reduce premature deaths.

Waupaca County is seeing some improvement in lowering the obesity rate, which is not the case across the state. The greatest change has come in the area of physical activity. Waupaca County residents took the county from the lower to the middle quartile range in this health determinant category. Physical inactivity and nutrition are two health behavior determinants that are modifiable. They are strongly influenced by individual choices that can be influenced by programs and policies. These two determinants bear a direct correlation to the amount of hypertension, heart disease, cancer, and diabetes that is evident in our population. Interventions that reduce weight and increase activity will bring about reductions in these chronic health problems and serve to usher Waupaca County into a higher level of overall health in the years to come (Athens et al., 2007).

Primary, secondary, and tertiary prevention strategies will be needed to continue this improvement. This means prevention, early diagnosis, treatment, and rehabilitation strategies will also be necessary. These are the means toward a healthier Waupaca County.

How Needs Information Was Utilized

In 2002, after the needs assessment process was finished, Health Services and UWEX designed a strategic planning process that would address the health concerns identified. The planning process involved a comprehensive group of stakeholders. Participants recognized existing efforts that were important to continue, such as the Waupaca County Tobacco-Free Coalition, alcohol compliance checks, and the WIC program, but they also recognized gaps in programs, support, and policies. These partners in the strategic planning process chose to create a new organization, NuAct-Nutrition and Activity Coalition. A committee structure was developed with strategies to address priority concerns that attribute to childhood obesity. As the work of this coalition continued and the 2007 assessment was completed, additional stakeholders were engaged and new efforts were initiated to address more recently identified health priorities. Current prevention dollars and targeted grants ($470,000) are utilized to support NuAct's efforts. The initiatives that are supported by or that originated from this coalition are described next.

NuAct News and Notes (Quarterly Report) and NuAct Web Site

The NuAct News and Notes quarterly report and the NuAct Web site provide information to all coalition members and subscribers about program impacts, outreach, current resources, educational materials, and partnering opportunities.

School Wellness Plans

School wellness plans were developed by committees at each of the seven school districts in Waupaca County. The federal government encouraged schools to undertake wellness initiatives. Schools offering free and reduced lunches were asked to develop comprehensive wellness plans and have these plans adopted by their school boards. NuAct provided workshops, resources, and support for development of the plans.

Safe Routes to School

NuAct collaborates with the East Central Regional Planning Commission, which facilitates a regional grant for Safe Routes to Schools. The goal of the Safe Routes to Schools program is to encourage students, K–8, to walk or bike to school. For many children, a major obstacle to walking and biking to school is lack of safe facilities, such as sidewalks, crosswalks, signage, and safe crossings. Safe Routes to School provides schools, students, and their parents with education and an opportunity to participate in a bike day in the spring and a walk day in the fall. Incentives for participants were also supplied as a part of the county and regional effort. Five school districts in Waupaca County sent Safe Routes to Schools information home with students and participated in incentive programs.

Community Trail Initiatives

NuAct developed and published a map called Explore and Discover Waupaca County. This map marks canoeing routes and walking, biking, cross-country skiing, and horseback riding trails. All these outdoor activities are local and free. The map also promotes special community activities that involve walking, running, or biking. This initiative has helped trail groups complete drawings of their community trail system and apply for grants. One of the grants received to develop their trail system equaled $278,000.

Active Schools

This CDC grant came from a collaboration between the Wisconsin Department of Public Instruction and Department of Health Services to improve children's health by increasing physical activity to the recommended 60 minutes per day and choosing healthier eating habits. NuAct is utilizing this $8000 grant to promote wellness and increase physical activity opportunities for schools and communities through service learning. Teachers will receive professional development about service learning and then utilize service learning to improve wellness and physical activity choices for students in their school/community.

Nutrition, Health, and Wellness Speakers Bureau

A list of local and regional speakers, their specialties, and their fees was organized and posted electronically on the Web site as a resource for businesses and organizations. The resource list was used most by NuAct partner and Working on Wellness business sites.

Community/School/Business Wellness Project Grants

NuAct offers $500 to $5000 in grants to encourage new efforts in training, health promotion, community enhancements, and wellness programs.

Working on Wellness (WOW)

NuAct received two wellness promotion grants. One was a Healthier Wisconsin Partnership grant from 2006–2009 for $150,000. The other was from 2010–2011 from the Wisconsin DHS for $25,000. In 2006–2009, the Medical College of Wisconsin worked with NuAct on a two-phase project for self-employed/uninsured individuals and for human resource contacts in local businesses. The self-employed/uninsured businesses were provided health risk assessments and health coaching with educational materials. The businesses utilized the Wisconsin Worksite Wellness Toolkit and then received grant money to implement toolkit strategies, such as educational sessions or workshops (e.g., fitness, smoking cessation), for their employees. In 2010–2011, NuAct adapted the toolkit for smaller businesses to utilize for their employees, better health. These will again be businesses that cannot offer health care insurance for their employees.

Women's Heart Truth Grant

A $20,000 grant from the American Heart Association has enabled NuAct to offer health risk assessments and heart healthy eating, stress management, and activity programs to women with limited resources and to working women ages 30–80. Waupaca County has the highest rate of women's death caused by heart disease in Wisconsin.

Agrisafe Network

NuAct attained membership and certification training in Agriculture Occupation Health Issues as a resource for the agricultural self-employed.

Community Garden Grant

This was a CDC grant for $30,000 to sustain and develop current and new community gardens in Waupaca County. It provides community members of all ages with fresh vegetables through local food pantries, senior centers, community meals programs, and UWEX food preparation/preservation workshops.

AmeriCorps Farm to School Program

A state-supported effort through Wisconsin DATCP connects school food service, local farm markets, community volunteers, and school classrooms in an effort to improve student consumption of local fruits and vegetables and expand utilization of local agriculture.

Wisconsin Nutrition Education Program (WNEP)

In 2008, the UWEX Family Living Educator applied for WNEP after nutrition and availability of healthy foods were identified as health concerns. WNEP is a UWEX nutrition education program that helps families and individuals with limited resources choose healthful diets, purchase and prepare healthful food, handle food safely, and become more food secure by spending their food dollars wisely. Families or individuals who receive food stamps (FoodShare) or who are eligible to receive food stamps can participate in WNEP. Within the first year, Waupaca WNEP formed strong partnerships with CAP Head Start, CAP Skills Enhancement, CAP Women's Support Group, the ADRC, Senior Nutrition Sites, Healthy Beginnings, WIC, and the Waupaca Job Center. By the second year, strong partnerships had been formed with the Clintonville, Weyauwega, and New London school districts; the Waupaca and Weyauwega food pantries; and the Marion Family Resource Center. At the end of its second year in Waupaca County, the WNEP coordinator had made 3345 direct educational contacts (nutrition programs) and 4180 indirect teaching contacts (newsletters).

Seal a Smile

The Seal a Smile program provides sealants for elementary students. Because Dental Care is not easily accessible in Waupaca County, this program was offered by the state of Wisconsin to provide dental care for those who find it difficult to receive services locally.

References

Athens, J. K., Taylor, K. W., Booske, B. C., Kempf, A. M., and Remington, P. L. (2007). *2007 Wisconsin county health rankings full report*. University of Wisconsin Population Health Institute. Available at: http://www.pophealth.wisc.edu/uwphi/rankings2007.htm. Accessed December 1, 2010.

Jovagg, A., Moberg, D. P., Ziege, A., and Nametz, P. (2007 September). *Impact of alcohol and illicit drug use in Wisconsin*. University of Wisconsin Population Health Institute. Available at: http://uwphi.pophealth.wisc.edu/progEval/impactOfAlcoholAndIllicitDrugUse.pdf. Accessed December 1, 2010.

Kindig, D., and Stoddart, G. (2003). What is population health? *American Journal of Public Health*, 93, 380–383.

Peppard, P. E., Kempf, A., Dranger, E., Kindig, D., and Remington, P. L. (2004). *Wisconsin county health rankings*. Wisconsin Public Health and Health Policy Institute. Available at: http://uwphi.pophealth.wisc.edu/pha/wchr/2004/rankings.pdf. Accessed December 1, 2010.

Peppard, P. E., Kindig, D., Riemer, A., Dranger, E., and Remington, P. L. (2003). *Wisconsin county health rankings*. Wisconsin Public Health and Health Policy Institute. Available at: http://uwphi.pophealth.wisc.edu/pha/wchr/2003/rankings.pdf. Accessed December 1, 2010.

Taylor, K.W., Athens, J. K., Booske, B. C., O'Connor, C. E., Jones, N. R., and Remington, P. L. (2008). *Wisconsin county health snapshots*. University of Wisconsin Population Health Institute. Available at: http://www.pophealth.wisc.edu/uwphi/rankings2008.htm. Accessed December 1, 2010.

University of Wisconsin–Extension. Community Youth Topics. Available at: http://waupaca.uwex.edu/4-h-youth-development/community-youth-topics. Accessed June 28, 2011.

U.S. Census Bureau. (2002). Waupaca County, Wisconsin Fact Sheet: American Fact Finder. Available at: http://factfinder.census.gov/servlet/ACSSAFFFacts?_event=ChangeGeoContext&geo_id=05000US55135&_geoContext=&_street=&_county=waupaca&_cityTown=waupaca&_state=04000US55&_zip=&_lang=en&_sse=on&ActiveGeoDiv=&_useEV=&pctxt=fph&pgsl=010&_submenuId=factsheet_1&ds_name=ACS_2009_5YR_SAFF&_ci_nbr=null&qr_name=null&reg=nullpercent3Anull&_keyword=&_industry=. Accessed December 1, 2010.

Wisconsin State Legislature. (2009). Wisconsin Act 12. Available at: http://legis.wisconsin.gov/2009/data/acts/09Act12.pdf. Accessed December 1, 2010.

Wisconsin Turning Point Transformation Team, Wisconsin Department of Health and Family Services. (2002 April). *Healthiest Wisconsin 2010: A partnership plan to improve the health of the public, Executive Summary*. Available at: http://www.dhs.wisconsin.gov/statehealthplan/shp-pdf/pph0275execsumm.pdf. Accessed December 1, 2010.

Assessment Strategies for a Nutrition and Physical Activity Promotion Project for Licensed Child Care Centers: Los Angeles County Continuing Project

Jennifer Gamberini, BS, Community Health Preceptee, University of Wisconsin–La Crosse

Tabitha Hackett, BS, Graduate MPH Program Preceptee, University of Wisconsin–La Crosse

Eleanor Long, MSPH, Maternal, Child, and Adolescent Health Programs, Los Angeles County Public Health Department

Introduction

California is often a leader in innovative health policy. Existing nutrition and physical activity standards for licensed child care do not reflect current knowledge and recommendations. An example of an existing nutrition standard is seen in the United States Agricultural Department's (USDA) Child and Adult Care Food Program (CACFP). This program allows for federal reimbursement to child care centers serving nutritious meals to low-income children. However, the program's standards are over 30 years old and are based on meal patterns rather than current, evidence-based nutritional standards. In 2009, California attempted to address this issue with Assembly Bill 627, which would have updated health and nutrition standards in licensed child care centers. The bill was vetoed by the governor after passing both houses of the legislature.

In Los Angeles County more than 20 percent of children ages 3 to 4 years old are classified obese (Los Angeles County Department of Public Health, Office of Health Assessment and Epidemiology, 2009). This statistic is of concern to professionals, especially as the percentage continues to climb. In addition, nearly 40 percent of children under age 5 spend their day in child care centers (Whaley, 2009). Child care centers, in this study, exclude child care within homes. Child care center settings present an environment to establish healthy eating behaviors and attitudes early in life, and thus address the behaviors leading to obesity.

Those who are obese as children are at high risk for becoming obese adults and, consequently, at high risk for developing chronic health problems (Daniels, 2006). Few states have attempted to improve child health through implementing nutrition and physical activity standards within licensed child care facilities (Benjamin, Cradock, Walker, Slining, & Gillman, 2008). Assessments will be made in the poorest neighborhoods of Los Angeles County. Insights from these assessments will reflect the resources that the centers have and the resources that the centers need to improve the nutrition and physical activity environments for children. This information will guide policy development.

Purpose

As mentioned previously, California had considered legislation to address childhood obesity (AB 627). Because the legislation failed to pass, advocates refocused on reviewing current child care standards in hopes of eventually revamping the bill. Delaware was found to be the only state to have new guidelines for licensed child care centers regarding nutrition and physical activity requirements. The guidelines were examined to determine the extent to which they could be replicated in California.

Data from the Women, Infant and Children (WIC) program revealed high rates of obesity in Los Angeles preschoolers. WIC also conducted an observational study of licensed child care facilities in the county that showed a wide variation of food served in Los Angeles child care (Whaley, 2009). Findings confirmed that this was an area of high need with significant opportunity for intervention and impact.

Support for the implementation of guidelines developed as research continued. Although it was unmistakably important to focus on the role that schools play in affecting the health of children, it was also important to recognize that many children entering kindergarten are already overweight with unhealthy lifestyle habits. A limited number of interventions have targeted this population, further encouraging the assessment of preschools (Ward, Hales, Haverly, Marks, Benjamin, Ball et al., 2008).

Child care centers are being evaluated to determine a baseline that reflects current nutrition and physical activity practices. Strengths and weaknesses of the centers will be identified, conveying a measurement of their current capacity. By observing the centers twice, once at the beginning of the study and once at the end, changes can be measured. Assessing the results of the intervention will declare its effectiveness. In presenting this evidence to lawmakers, we may prompt improved child care legislation.

The Los Angeles County Department of Public Health is the lead on this childhood obesity prevention project. Maternal, Child and Adolescent Health (MCAH) programs are working with a series of both undergraduate and graduate public health interns to conduct the study. Interns serve as a major contribution to the study. In addition, several stakeholder organizations are partnering on the project:

- *Los Angeles County Department of Public Health, Maternal, Child, and Adolescent Health Programs (lead agency).* This division of the Public Health Department works to address a multitude of issues involving its population.
- *California Food Policy Advocates.* Statewide public policy and advocacy organization dedicated to improving the health and well-being of low-income families.
- *University of North Carolina–Chapel Hill.* Consultant and developer of assessment tools.
- *Los Angeles County Office of Child Care.* Provided database of licensed centers.
- *Crystal Stairs.* A resource and referral agency that encourages participation in the study and will provide training space.
- *Community and Family Resource Center.* A resource and referral agency that encourages participation in the study.
- *Charles Drew University of Medicine and Science.* Will provide statistical support and financial support for $25 incentives and mileage reimbursement.
- *First Five LA.* Will supply copies of "Sesame Street" curriculums for use at the end of the project.
- *Nemours (Delaware-based health and prevention services).* This partner allowed reprinting of its document "Best Practices for Healthy Eating: A Guide to Help Children Grow Up Healthy," which is the basis of the recommended standards. It will be distributed to centers in both intervention groups and to the control group at the end of the project.

The University of North Carolina–Chapel Hill is allowing the team to use its validated assessment tools and is consulting on the project. Its Environment and Policy Assessment and Observation Instrument (EPAO) has been adapted for the 4-hour observation. The Nutrition and Physical Activity Self-Assessment for Child Care (NAP SACC) (Ammerman, Benjamin, Sommers, & Ward, 2007; Benjamin, Neelon, Ball, Bangdiwala, Ammerman, & Ward, 2007) is completed by center directors.

Target Groups

Because the population and size of Los Angeles County is so large, the area is divided into eight geographic service planning areas (SPAs) for purposes of health care planning. This study focuses on SPA 6, a south-central region of Los Angeles County with the most alarming statistics. SPA 6 has the highest rates of obesity, inactivity, and poverty in Los Angeles Country (Los Angeles County Department of Public Health [LACDPH], 2009). The community faces crime and unsafe recreational environments. The area lacks adequate parks and sidewalks. Barriers to a healthy lifestyle also include limited access to nutritious food. Lack of adequate education caps this collection of characteristics, influencing engagement in potentially risky behaviors.

This region has the highest percentage of children in the county. The team has access to many child care facilities and can evaluate conditions where disparity is the greatest.

Observation Assessment Methodology

It was determined that an observational study, including two levels of intervention and a control group, would be effective in gathering the needed information to reform legislation. An extensive literature review identified the toolkit and the measurement instruments. This saved time and resources that would have been spent developing and testing such products.

Secondary Data Review

A full year, from 2008–2009, was spent reviewing all studies that involved child care settings. It was found that two instruments developed by the University of North Carolina–Chapel Hill could be used by the project. The EPAO and the NAP SACC had been tested and normalized to assess the nutrition and physical activity environments in child care settings. It also was found that Delaware had used these instruments in a study of child care practices leading up to its legislation.

The EPAO will be conducted by trained observers. It has 87 items, including a document review. Among the components to be evaluated are fundraising policies, menus, parent/staff handbook, and playground safety. The document review allows for information to be gathered outside of the day of observation, specifically an analysis of foods listed on the menu for the entire week. The EPAO was pilot tested to ensure that the questions were understandable. Slight revisions have been made for clarity. Because observations will be conducted by unpaid graduate and undergraduate interns, the observation time has been shortened from 8 to 4 hours, and it includes only lunch, not lunch and breakfast.

Maternal, Child and Adolescent Health Programs staff partnered with a representative from California Food Policy Advocates to examine materials that could be used during the intervention process. The Nemours resource kit, which reflects the standards in the Delaware legislation, was selected after unanimous agreement that it was the most appropriate.

This study will measure the effects of providing nutrition and physical activity information and training. The study will determine barriers to implementing these recommendations. In addition, it will provide information regarding the amount of support needed to motivate policy changes within child care centers.

Recruitment involved an initial mailing, providing information to each licensed child care facility within the targeted area. An invitational letter was signed by the Director of Public Health, Dr. Jonathan Fielding. Also enclosed were a project brochure and a written project description. Phone calls were made to follow-up with all centers that received the mailing, attempting to enlist as many participants as possible and maximize sample size. Through phone conversations, interns verified that all three of the inclusion criteria were met: that the child care center (1) served children ages 3 to 5 years, (2) provided lunch, and (3) was not designated as a Head Start facility. Confidentiality was reviewed over the phone, and informed consent was officially obtained on-site from directors. A goal was set to observe 120 licensed child care centers in order to collect sufficient data to achieve 95 percent statistical significance.

The assessment consists of three components: the EPAO, the NAP SACC, and key informant interviews. The EPAO tool focuses on nutrition and physical activity practices and policies within the child care sites. Observations are made by pairs of observers, who are trained until 85 percent interobserver reliability is achieved, because questions may be subjective in nature. Each member of the observation team makes independent assessments. Then the team reconciles their findings and produces one set of agreed-upon measurements.

The NAP SACC instrument collects similar information, but from the director's viewpoint. Key informant interviews collect information from the viewpoint of the directors as well. Predetermined, open-ended questions are prompted by the observers in a face-to-face interview. It is used to document existing resources and perceived barriers for implementing better nutrition and physical activity practices and policies. The key informant interview also gathers data reflecting existing and desired training topics.

The EPAO observation includes the following:

- Date, time period, weather
- Documentation of food: what was served, how it was served, and how the children responded
- Staff interaction with children during meals and physical activity

- Staff consumption of food/drinks in front of children
- Television/computer/screen time
- Water availability
- Center environment: indoor/outdoor play equipment, differentiating between portable and stationary
- Number of physical activity and nutrition posters and books

The EPAO document review includes the following:

- Comparison of the menu with the actual foods and beverages served
- Documentation of total weekly food servings by category (e.g., fruits, vegetables, whole grains)
- Nutrition and physical activity policy review
- Parent and staff training documentation

The initial assessment phase is being conducted over a 9-month period, from August 2010 until May 2011. The second and final assessment phase will mimic the first, from August 2011 through May 2012. The assessment will provide a comprehensive overview of the nutrition and physical activity environment. Examples of nutrition measurements include frequency of offering whole grains, processed meats, fresh and syrup-free canned fruits, and colorful vegetables and the availability of drinking water. Average number of minutes of physical activity and screen time (television, computers, and video games) also will be measured, in addition to noting play area size and safety.

The intervention phase of the study will involve randomizing the enrolled child care centers into three groups: a control group and two intervention groups. The control group will continue with its standard programs without receiving nutrition or physical activity information or training. The intervention groups will receive either the nutrition or physical activity information alone or with training. The tools to be provided will be research-based standards pertaining to nutrition and physical activity. Training will teach center directors and their staff the information and encourage them to set goals to improve practices. The control group will receive the intervention tools with training at the end of the project. Analysis of this intervention will resolve the issue of whether training is required to motivate change within the targeted population.

Future Directions

At the time this case study is being written, the first set of observations are in process. Early findings suggest that many schools are feeding children low levels of nutritious food and are not providing adequate amounts of physical activity. Interviews with directors indicate that trainings would be welcomed.

The data gathered from this study will be used to support legislation that will improve nutrition and physical activity requirements in licensed child care centers. In addition, this study will leverage the increased attention now focused on the nutrition of children younger than age 5. In 2009, the WIC Program made significant changes to its food package and client education strategies. In 2010, First Lady Michelle Obama launched "Let's Move," which has sponsored numerous events and garnered significant national media attention, especially towards the nutrition of children younger than 5 years. The timing is optimal to align messages, implement policy changes, and improve the nutrition environment for young children across Los Angeles County.

References

Ammerman, A. S., Benjamin, S. E., Sommers, J. K., and Ward, D. S. (2007). *The Nutrition and Physical Activity Self-Assessment for Child Care (NAP SACC) environmental self-assessment instrument.* Division of Public Health, NC DHHS, Raleigh, NC, and the Center for Health Promotion and Disease Prevention, University of North Carolina–Chapel Hill. Revised May 2007.

Benjamin, S. E., Cradock, A., Walker, E. M., Slining, M., and Gillman, M. W. (2008). Obesity prevention in child care: A review of U.S. state regulations. *BMC Public Health, 8,* 188–197.

Benjamin, S. E., Neelon, B., Ball, S. C., Bangdiwala, S. I., Ammerman, A. S., and Ward, D. S. (2007). Reliability and validity of a nutrition and physical activity environmental self-assessment for child care. *International Journal of Behavioral Nutrition and Physical Activity, 4*(29), 1–10.

Daniels, S. R. (2006). The consequences of childhood overweight and obesity. *The Future of Children, 16*(1), 47–67.

Los Angeles County Department of Public Health (LACDPH). Office of Health Assessment and Epidemiology. (2009 June). *Key indicators of health by service planning area.* Los Angeles: Author.

Ward, D. E., Hales, D. P., Haverly, K. M., Marks, J. P., Benjamin, S. P., Ball, S. M., et al. (2008). An instrument to access the obesogenic enviroment of child care centers. *American Journal of Health Behavior, 32*(4), 380–386.

Whaley, S. G. (2009). *It's 12 o'clock . . . What are our preschoolers eating for lunch? An assessment of nutrition and the nutrition environment in licensed child care in Los Angeles County.* Los Angeles: Public Health Foundation Enterprises, WIC, Child Care Food Program Roundtable, and California Food Policy Advocates.

Using Focus Groups to Assess Tobacco Usage in Pregnant and Postpartum Women

Keely Rees, PhD, CHES, Associate Professor of Community Health Education, University of Wisconsin–La Crosse

Overview of Organizations

This study details a collaborative approach that sought to assess the concerns, issues, and needs related to current and previous tobacco use in pregnant and postpartum women in a tri-state region in the Midwest. Many health organizations in the Coulee region—which includes communities in southwestern Wisconsin (e.g., greater La Crosse metropolitan area), southeastern Minnesota (Houston and Winona), and parts of northwestern Iowa—are working together in the area of tobacco prevention, control, and policy (Trout Unlimited, 2005). The La Crosse County Health Department (LCHD) continues to work to prevent tobacco use and assist with cessation measures. Two major health and medical systems in La Crosse—Gundersen Lutheran and Franciscan Skemp Mayo Health Systems—provide numerous programs and resources for tobacco control. La Crosse Area Health Initiative (LAHI) is a coalition that works with a wide variety of tobacco outreach, policies, and initiatives. In addition, many other health and nonprofit organizations (e.g., the American Cancer Society, the La Crosse Medical Health Science Consortium, which is composed of five organizations: Western Technical College, University of Wisconsin–La Crosse, Gundersen Lutheran Health System, Franciscan Skemp Mayo Health System, and Viterbo University) are working in areas of tobacco use and control. While working with numerous other entities in the community, LCHD prioritized monies from the March of Dimes to assess the needs of pregnant and postpartum women in their plight to quit and stay quit from tobacco. The leading organizations in this assessment included the University of Wisconsin–La Crosse; the La Crosse County Health Department; and the Gundersen Lutheran Health System.

Target Groups and Key Personnel Involved

With numerous organizations working to provide smoking-cessation services in the Coulee region, the LCHD deemed it necessary to better understand the needs of a subgroup within the population: pregnant and postpartum women using tobacco products or trying to quit/stay quit. Regular evaluation of services enables agencies to determine worth and effectiveness of the services provided. Earlier research and evaluation had indicated that pregnant and postpartum women were not typical consumers of cessation programs and quit lines. As stated earlier, the purpose of this needs assessment was to explore the concerns, issues, and needs women have during pregnancy and postpartum related to their current and previous tobacco/smoking behaviors.

This project was a continuation study (funding from the March of Dimes through the La Crosse County Health Department) to better assess and determine the types of resources needed in the Coulee region for women to quit using tobacco and maintain that status during their pregnancy and postpartum time periods. The March of Dimes (funder) has a vested interest in reducing the number of smoking women from prenatal to postpartum stages to better improve the health outcomes of newborns and thus wants to identify better ways to provide services to assist women in quitting tobacco (March of Dimes, 2007, 2008).

Focus groups were deemed most appropriate to garner in-depth, exploratory information from a group of women that may otherwise not respond to or be reached for survey methodologies. Secondary research by the research team (organizations that were currently working with clients from the region) and research team meetings were conducted in the spring in order to delineate the sample. Participants were those women who were pregnant or up to 6 months postpartum, current tobacco users or those trying to quit/stay quit, living in the Coulee region (communities within La Crosse County), and 18 years of age or older. The rationale for conducting focus groups versus interviews emerged from previous research by the March of Dimes and the services that LCHD had provided in the last 2 years. LCHD experienced lower numbers of pregnant/postpartum women participating in quit lines and educational programs and felt that these women would not be inclined to come in for individual interviews. The research team also determined that the budget would be better suited for the focus group process.

Focus groups were to be held throughout the summer and early fall to allow for enough women to participate and have equal access to the groups. Flexible days/times were set to account for working women, stay-at-home parents, and shift workers. The focus groups were held at a nonmedical setting in a centralized location on a La Crosse City bus route. The focus group technique allowed questions to be open-ended and geared toward participants' attitudes, feelings, and ideas regarding smoking and what types of resources they use, want/need, and benefit from in the Coulee Region.

The research team included Keely Rees, PhD (Associate Professor, Health Education and Health Promotion at the University of Wisconsin–La Crosse), Paula Silha (Certified Health Education Specialist, La Crosse County Health Department), Brenda Rooney, PhD (Epidemiologist and Medical Director of Community and Preventive Care Services at Gundersen Lutheran Health System), and Bachelor of Science in Community Health Education candidates from the University of Wisconsin–La Crosse, who served as research assistants throughout the project: Cortney Draxler, Amy Flock, Norissa Miller, Katie Jo Scholl, Kari Jacoby, and Gina Nielsen.

The main objective for this research project was to develop an exploratory process for generating attitudes, feelings, and behavioral patterns related to the women's tobacco usage prior to pregnancy, during pregnancy, and postpartum. Identification of demographic information, social support, and tobacco resources they have used was the secondary objective.

Needs Assessment Process

Institutional Review Board (IRB) procedures were approved and followed at four of the organizations (University of Wisconsin–La Crosse, LCHD, Gundersen Lutheran Health System, and Franciscan Skemp Mayo Health System). Researchers met regularly during the early spring and summer to set up focus groups for July through October.

The marketing and promotion of the focus groups was critical for reaching the target population. Researchers worked with a variety of health organizations and marketing outlets to try to garner as much interest as possible. Participants were garnered from Coulee region (La Crosse, Holmen, Onalaska, and West Salem in Wisconsin and Winona and La Crescent in Minnesota) health care settings (Franciscan Skemp Mayo Health System, Gundersen Lutheran Health System) and the La Crosse County's WIC program and through advertisements placed in community newspapers (La Crosse, Holmen, Onalaska, Winona) and fliers placed at establishments geared towards pregnant women (Once Upon a Child, child care centers) and general public areas (Kwik Trip gas stations, Goodwill, Festival Foods). Promotional materials indicated the purpose of the discussion groups, the incentives for participating, and instructions on how to sign up for a discussion group. The participants would then call a number at the LCHD. The women were screened over the phone to ensure that they fit the protocol requirements (18 years and older; any race/ethnicity; currently pregnant or up to 6 months postpartum, having used tobacco prior to pregnancy, during pregnancy, or postpartum or currently quitting or quit). Paula Silha and the research assistants would then follow-up with and assign the participants a date and time and describe the procedures. Participants had numerous dates, days, or times from which to choose to best accommodate their schedules. They were informed of the time commitment (approximately 2 hours) and the incentives they would receive (free childcare provided at each session and a free meal was provided for participants and their children; each participant also received a $20 Kwik Trip gas gift card and a $20 Festival Foods gift card, and a bus token, if needed). Reminder calls were conducted the week and day before the participant's scheduled discussion group.

An informal, nonmedical setting was used to allow the women to feel accommodated and at ease. Three different approaches were used to record the focus group responses: an audio-only recording device, flip charts for theme responses, and pencil/paper for backup to the audio recorder. The team met three times to conduct focus group training and to work through logistical issues (e.g., food, childcare, reminder calls). University of Wisconsin–La Crosse Community Health Education candidates served as recorders and childcare attendants and assisted with set-up and clean-up. Keely Rees served as the focus group facilitator; Paula Silha and Brenda Rooney assisted with thematic recordings. All researchers and assistants were dressed business casual, wore informal (noninstitutional) nametags, and remained open and welcoming.

Participants were greeted and given meals. They placed their children in childcare, if necessary. They completed an informed consent form to review and sign (a sample consent form is included at the end of this case study), and were given a place card to put on the table in front of them to indicate their participant number. Facilitators discussed the study objectives and expectations with the participants. To ensure confidentiality, the following measures were taken:

- Codes (e.g., P#1 for participant 1) were used to identify the participants in the written documentation.
- Participants did not give out their names but rather used a participant number when speaking and only shared what they are comfortable discussing in terms of their demographics.
- All raw data are locked in the researchers' file cabinet in a locked office area.
- Only the researchers have access to the raw data, and the data are reported using participant codes (e.g., Case #1, P#2).

The women were placed along long tables so that they were comfortable, could eat casually, and feel like they were part of a group. In the first 10 to 15 minutes of the session, the facilitators mingled with the participants, assured the participants that their children were safe and being fed, and worked to create an emotionally safe environment for the women to begin the discussion. Questions were open-ended and geared toward participants' attitudes, feelings, and ideas regarding smoking and what kinds of resources they use, still want/need, and benefit from in the Coulee region. For each focus group session, the facilitator asked the following questions regarding the participants' background:

1. Can you share with us your age and ethnicity/race?
2. Describe your pregnancy history (i.e., live births, miscarriages).
3. Describe your current occupation.
4. Tell me about your family structure (i.e., family members in household, other children).
5. Describe your smoking status (how long, when, quit for how long?).

Participants were asked the following questions regarding their tobacco use:

1. When did you begin smoking?
2. Describe how you feel before wanting or using tobacco.
3. Describe your attempts in quitting.
4. How did you feel about those attempts?
5. Did you start again and how soon? How did this make you feel?
6. Tell me what you know about smoking risks.
7. Tell us about how you have tried quitting (what method you used).
8. Describe the resources you would like in the community to help you quit/stay quit.
9. Describe the social support you have in your home/community.
10. What else can you share about your experience with tobacco use during pregnancy?

At the completion of the discussion, women were asked to sign an LCHD roster saying that they had received their monetary incentives and were provided a list of smoking-cessation resources, including information on classes, quit lines, and quit aids. Researchers and assistants all stayed for a 30- to 45-minute debriefing and evaluation of next steps after each focus group session. A total of three focus group sessions were completed, one in July and two in October. Research assistants and recorders listened to the audio-recordings, pencil/paper recorders transcribed their notes onto computer, and thematic recorders transcribed their notes to hard copy. The primary researcher analyzed the data using NVivo 7 software (NVivo, n.d.).

Needs Identified by the Assessment

Themes that were prevalent among the three focus groups included *smoking age*, *smoking habits*, and *desire for support in quitting*. Demographically, most of the focus group participants were single, non-Hispanic whites of low socioeconomic status. Significantly, most were smokers prior to pregnancy, starting in their early preteen and teenage years. Most smoked one-half to one pack of cigarettes per day and smoke to ease stress, alleviate boredom, and cope with taking care of children all day. The knowledge they shared about smoking was not at a high level; they could recite factoids about tobacco risks for them and their children.

With regards to the *type of help they would like in quitting*, the theme emerged that the participants want nonclinical smoking-cessation settings; live people leading the groups (verses a hotline to call); and a larger number of supportive, smokefree environments (e.g., youth centers, restaurants, churches). Central locations that are easy to reach and that had childcare available were also issues they all thought were important to their attending.

The women varied in their stage of pregnancy (1½ months to 9 months) to not currently pregnant but having had children in the past 1 to 18 years. Participants also spent time describing their tobacco habits. Sixty percent of the participants had *begun smoking* in their preteen and teen years ($n = 9$; see **Table CS4-1**).

Participants' stories about their *smoking habits and their knowledge* about the effects of smoking were very telling of their lives, cultural barriers, and other stressors in their lives. Following are a few excerpts:

Focus Group 1, P#2

I don't know when I started, um, but with my 6-year-old I smoked during the pregnancy 'cause I was going through a rough time. Um, I did go in at 33 weeks but they had to stop the contractions because um with me smoking, it didn't, um how should I say it, um, his kidneys weren't fully developed, because of smoking, and um, I still didn't quit because I was going through stress so they stopped the contractions and I gave birth to him and now here I am again smokin' and I'm pregnant again, and I just can't stop smoking cause it's when I drive. When I drive is when I smoke, otherwise I don't smoke. When I drive is when you'll see me smoking. And I can't stop drivin'. That's how I get to work and back.

TABLE CS4-1
Age Women Began Smoking

n	Age (in years)
1	9
1	11
3	12
1	14
3	15
1	22
5	Not reported

Focus Group 1, P#2

Everybody keeps everything confidential? Mine was abuse. Um, I went through abuse every since I was a child, tried counseling, counseling didn't work for me 'cause all it is is just somebody to talk to, so, like I said before and I'll say it again, the only person I have to talk to is my son. I won't talk to anybody else 'cause I don't trust anybody else. You say something to somebody, they have to go tell somebody, and then you're getting your butt whooped even worse. I don't say nothing. But, the reason I started smokin' was abuse. The reason why I smoke now is just because I'm used to it now.

Focus Group 1, P#4

I started smoking when I was about 8 or 9, ya know, 'cause I had to go to the store and get the cigarettes for my mom and dad. Um, when I was pregnant with A****, I smoked for the first 3 and a half months then I got locked up, and I didn't get out of prison 'til she was 16 months old so I didn't smoke that whole, whole time. And then the day I got out, the first thing I did was lit a cigarette. Um, I swear I crave cigarettes when I'm pregnant, and I've brought this up to my doctor 'cause I feel like I have to smoke every 5 minutes. I don't know, I've tried to cut back, I've tried like everything, but I'm sorry. And I'm a weed smoker, so, and then after I smoke a blunt I have to smoke a cigarette.

Focus Group 1, P#5

I was kind of a weird smoker because I kind of became a closet smoker because I had some heart problems, like, 4 years ago I had heart surgery, and so, I had thought that I had quit, and I couldn't go back and tell my doctor that I was smoking, so I had to cover it up, so I had gotten out of the habit of smoking in my car, out of the habit of smoking at work, I was just smoking like at home where no one else could know. So I thought if I could go all day long at work without having a cigarette, including travel time, cause I'm not smoking in my car, why can't I just quit? It just got to the point where it was like this is just stupid, you know? And it's not good for my heart, and taking X-rays, I see what it does to people, ya know, I mean we're actually looking at lungs, with the digital imagery we can actually peel off layers and it's just awful, it's just gross.

Focus Group 2, P#3

I started smoking at age 14 because I thought it was cool; everyone was doing it. I stopped with the older three, smoked more with the younger. Now I smoke two packs a day, don't drink. Cigarettes help keep me calm, and I don't think it would be hard to quit but haven't put effort into stopping.

Focus Group 2, P#4

I started smoking at 11 years old because of my peers. I stole cigarettes from my parents. In high school I smoked half a pack then to a full pack. During my pregnancy I cut back to half a pack. Tried the patch, but no success.

Focus Group 2, P#5

I started smoking last year. I stopped weed then turned to cigarettes. My husband wanted me to go cold turkey. Now he limits me to three cigarettes a day. I am a stay-at-home mom with my kids.

The participants also shared their experiences with *trying to quit or stay quit*. Only one participant was currently free of tobacco; the rest were in very different stages of readiness:

Focus Group 2 [Paraphrased]

P#3: When she was pregnant, smoking while pregnant wasn't as much of an issue. *Wants to stop smoking for the kids and herself, though she doesn't know how.*

P#3: Started smoking at age 14 because she thought it was cool; everyone was doing it. Stopped with the older 3, smoked more with the younger. Now she smokes two packs a day, doesn't drink. Cigarettes help keep her calm and she doesn't think it would be hard to quit *but hasn't put effort into stopping.*

P#4: Started smoking at 11 years old because of her peers. Stole cigarettes from her parents. In high school she smoked half a pack then to a full pack. During her pregnancy she cut back to half a pack. *Tried the patch, but no success.*

P#5: Started smoking last year. Stopped weed then turned to cigarettes. Husband wanted her to go cold turkey. *Now he limits her to 3 cigarettes a day.* She's a stay-at-home mom with her kids.

P#6: Was young when she started, used to smoke one pack a day, even through her pregnancies. *Trying to quit now.*

Focus Group 3

P#1: "I took Chantix and did not back to smoking again, it was easy to quit."

P#2: "I tried Nicorette and did not like it, husband did not smoke when we met, but now he does, smoking is a part of the routine of the day."

P#3: "I tried patches but would forget to put them on, I tried other things that didn't work."

P#4: "I have tried no smoking cessation aids—I have a stressful life now and quit for 4 months when a pill got stuck in my throat but I am now smoking again."

Participants also shared openly their experiences with their *health care providers* and their *perspectives and knowledge* about the effects of smoking.

Focus Group 3

P#1: "I know it's bad for baby and myself, we have family history of heart disease, everyone in family smokes, dad doesn't want to see me smoking, but he still smokes. Dad stole cigarettes while drunk."

P#2: "I know [it] can cause low birth weight, and I think smaller baby would feel better to push out, can heighten miscarriage, lung and asthma problems, research pregnancy on Internet. My midwife talks to me, didn't want me to quit completely, but smoke less and set goals. I smoked half a pack when first pregnant, now less than half a pack. I rip cigarettes in half and smoke them as technique to quit, sometimes feels like it's not enough. I don't want to quit because I'll gain weight."

P#3 [paraphrased]: She went to a group from 5 to 7 P.M. at County Health educators, where they talked about cigarettes (gun powder in them, rings around gun powder), secondhand smoke causes yellow teeth. Stays at mom's house, smells like smoke (she smokes outside). Midwife found out about her smoking when pregnant. Told her not to stop but to cut down. Wish she would have quit when she found out she was pregnant.

P#4 [paraphrased]: Midwife asks every month about quitting smoking. She lied, said she smoked eight, but she smoked half a pack a day. Knows risk of cleft lip, freaked her out thinking about birth defects and heart murmurs. Some days she smoked more than others, not everyday when pregnant, except when wake up puking.

These are their verbatim responses, with emphasis added in italics, to the types of support and resources they would like to see in the Coulee Region:

"*No hospital setting, community buildings are better.* Late afternoons (5 to 8 P.M.) are good. Then workers can come. *Need daycare.* Library and churches are also good."

"*No hospitals.* Have personal contact, instead of on the phone."

"*Different places to meet* the needs and interests of each person. If a Christian have it at a church, like to read have it at a library. . . ."

"I will want to quit next year . . . *have more affordable groups*, a buddy phone list."

"*Be open . . . and don't lecture.* I want what's best for my baby."

"Same. My mom and dad and husband are hypocritical. To be a good doctor, *I don't want to be talked down to, I want them to guide me.*"

"I liked this group session with health educators, only one girl who didn't smoke. It was eye-opening and I need help with routine. I want to find other hobby. *This group was open.* I just signed up for quitting smoking but it is hard to get ahead."

"No one should tell you what to do. I know what happens when I am not setting goals and meeting consistently. No time to quit when pregnant or after, it is not a high priority. Priority is working and being a mom."

"We need more solutions to quit . . . *like no smoking in restaurants, more support groups.*"

"Make it smokefree everywhere, otherwise makes you want to smoke. Support groups with the same age group as they are all going through the same things."

"*Youth center, alternate houses*, if small enough, county building (go for WIC/food stamps) making it not a comfortable atmosphere, need somewhere comfortable . . . County watches you carefully when you are there, making it not comfortable."

"Go to a restaurant, discuss field trips."

"Picnics."

"*Childcare is important.*"

"People know the hotlines but we don't always call. Health educators are good, they were to help goals. Big issue is that many people smoke, advertising for cigarettes is jumping out at kids."

"If you guys have more groups even. *Just more people who care.*"

"I don't want *no sterile group*. I just like to kick it. I would *rather have a conversation than a lecture.*"

"My doctor tells me I need to quit smoking, she just irritating me by telling me I need to quit. You can tell me anything it just go in one ear out the other. I am CNA I know this stuff. I just don't listen."

How the Needs Information Was Utilized

Dissemination of Information

All data were reported back to the funder (March of Dimes) and to the La Crosse County Health Department through a final report. The results were presented locally to the LAHI and to the University of Wisconsin Center for Tobacco Research and Intervention (CTRI). Focus group participants were invited to call back to the LCHD for further information, resources, or updates from the data collected. After completion of the focus groups, the team decided to pilot a cessation support group for pregnant and postpartum women.

Formation of Support Group

Based on the results of qualitative analyses and subsequent committee meetings, it was determined that it was important to offer the focus group participants an alternative option for tangible support in quitting tobacco. It was agreed upon to pilot three support group interventions. The researchers wanted to offer an intervention soon after the focus groups but had to deal with the barriers of extreme cold weather and the approaching holidays. A support group was established that offered three nights called "Time to Share and Breathe Fresh Air," which were offered on December 4, 11, and 18 at the Crossfire Youth Ministries (a nonprofit organization that rents out space weekdays/nights and that is centrally located in La Crosse) from 6 to 8 P.M. The site was conducive to a relaxed atmosphere. Free childcare and refreshments were offered, with the goal of providing a smokefree place where the women could relax but also learn. The focus of the intervention was threefold: tobacco education, nutrition education, and physical movement for stress management. The groups held on December 4 and 18 groups did not have any participants; the December 11 group had two participants (one from the focus group sessions and other was her friend). All participants were called 1 week before and 2 days before the group met as a reminder. The facilitators felt that there was good interest (when participants were reached via telephone) but that the timing of the offerings made it difficult for the women to commit or come (e.g., extreme cold temperatures, holidays).

Conclusion

Smoking during pregnancy and postpartum is a nationwide concern, and the reasons women smoke are as varied as the women are diverse. Thematically, in this research, it was established that a combination of life circumstances and other stressors (not just the pregnancy) precipitated and perpetuated the participants' smoking habits. Most participants had had an established smoking history prior to pregnancy. In many of the cases, the women cited the abuse of other substances (e.g., crystal meth, marijuana, alcohol); most all of them had significant others and support people who all smoked near or around them daily. All the participants had a relatively basic understanding of the risks of tobacco use (e.g., SIDS, low-birth-weight babies, lung cancer) but lacked the commitment, knowledge, and skills to stay quit. Most had tried at some point to quit through the use of quit support items or hotlines but felt that the most valuable resource would be to have a group to meet with at a nonclinical site in a format that was conducive to socializing and relaxing.

The focus group technique was successful in allowing women to fully open up regarding their pregnancies, tobacco habits, and their overall needs. The researchers felt that the data acquired would not have been as in-depth, honest, and authentic had any other methodology been used to garner the participants' insights. In the researchers' debriefings and notes, it was noted that it was essential that the setting be relaxed and noninvasive and that the women felt that they belonged and really could contribute to their community. Subsequently, the LCHD has modified and taken into account many of the findings from this project when working in the communities to provide resource materials and smoking cessation tools.

References

Crossfire Youth Ministries. (n.d.). Available at: http://www.crossfire4u.com/index2.php. Accessed August 6, 2010.

March of Dimes. (2007 March). Program grants. Available at: http://www.marchofdimes.com/professionals/685_1375.asp. Accessed May 3, 2009.

March of Dimes. (2008 April). Smoking and pregnancy: Professionals and researchers. Available at: http://www.marchofdimes.com/14332_1171.asp. Accessed May 3, 2009.

NVivo. (n.d.). Available at: http://www.qsrinternational.com/products_nvivo.aspx. Accessed August 6, 2010.

Trout Unlimited. (2005 April). "A Driftless Area: A Landscape of Opportunities." Available at: http://www.tu.org/atf/cf/%7B0D18ECB7-7347-445B-A38E-65B282BBBD8A%7D/Driftless_report_042005.pdf. Accessed May 9, 2011.

Consent to Participate in Focus Group Research

I agree to participate in the research project titled *Using Focus Groups to Assess Tobacco Usage in Pregnant and Postpartum Women* conducted by Keely Rees, Paula Silha, and Brenda Rooney, health educators/researchers from the University of Wisconsin–La Crosse, La Crosse County Health Department, and Gunderson Lutheran, respectively. I am aware that the purpose of this focus group is to learn more about my attitudes, ideas, and behaviors related to smoking before, during, or after my pregnancy and the kinds of quit and stay quit resources that would be best for me and my family. I am also aware that the researchers are interested in finding out more about why I use tobacco and how I can be stop using tobacco for the health of my baby and myself.

I have been informed that my involvement in this focus group is voluntary and that I will be given a participant number that they will use when I speak in the group and to record what I say, only identifying me through a number. My name or contact information will not be linked in any way to the information recorded. I have been informed I will be sharing information with approximately seven other women in an informal, comfortable setting regarding our demographics [age, pregnancy status, smoking habits (past/present), race/ethnicity, occupation, and family dynamics]. I also grant permission for the researchers to record me using an audio recorder and by writing down what I say on tablets by using my participant number at my table.

I have been informed that this focus group will benefit me and other pregnant women in our region who are seeking measure to quit tobacco during or after pregnancy. I understand that the focus group will take approximately 1½ to 2 hours, that all information recorded will be kept confidential, and that I am free to ask questions of the researchers at any time, and that I am free to withdraw my participation at any time without prejudice, question, or reprimand. I state that I am 18 years of age, that I have been informed the general purpose of the study, and that I agree to the procedures outlined above. I willingly consent to be a participant in this focus group study and acknowledge that I have received a copy of this consent form.

The benefits that I will receive by participating in the focus group is information regarding current resources in the community for quitting tobacco, and I will receive further information on the benefits of staying quit during and after pregnancy, support resources, and changes to services in the future.

There are no anticipated or known risks for participating in this focus group. In the unlikely event that any injury or illness occurs as a result of this research the Board of Regents of the University of Wisconsin system, and the University of Wisconsin–La Crosse, their officers, agents, and employees, do not automatically provide reimbursement for medical care or other compensation. Payment for treatment of any injury or illness must be provided by you or your third-party payor, such as your health insurer or Medicare. In any injury or illness occurs in the course of research, or for more information, please notify the researcher in charge.

I have been informed that I am not waiving any rights that I may have for injury resulting from negligence of any person or the situation.

If you have concerns or questions regarding the focus group study please contact Keely Rees at 608-785-8168. Questions regarding the protection of human subjects may be addressed to the Institutional Review Board for the Protection of Human Subjects (608-785-8124 or irb@uwlax.edu).

Participant _____   Date _____

Participant _____   Date _____

Monroe on the Go Coalition: The Use of Photovoice to Assess Perceived Opportunities for Physical Activity and Nutrition in Monroe County, Wisconsin

Bethany Kies, BS, Graduate MPH Program Preceptee, University of Wisconsin–La Crosse

Becky Campbell, RN, Monroe County Health Department, Sparta, Wisconsin

Agency Overview

This photovoice assessment was conducted by a subcommittee from the Monroe County Health Department in Sparta, Wisconsin, as part of the Health Department's participation in the Monroe On the Go Coalition (MOGO). Monroe County is a small, rural county located in western Wisconsin. According to U.S. Census data from 2000, Monroe County has a total population of 40,899 people with a median age of 36.8 years and a median family income of $37,170. The population is 50 percent male and 96.5 percent white (Hispanics comprise the largest minority group at 1.8 percent). Eighty-one percent of the population is at least a high school graduate; 12 percent of the population is below the poverty level.

The Monroe County Health Department has served its community since 1921 with a mission "to protect, promote and improve the health of county residents." It employs 12 staff, including the health officer/director, four full-time and one part-time public health nurses, three Women Infants and Children (WIC) staff, and 3 clerical support staff. The Health Department also supervises student nursing and health education interns from regional postsecondary institutions; two of whom, along with one of the public health nurses, led the photovoice assessment as a subcommittee of MOGO.

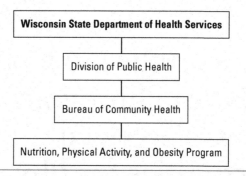

FIGURE CS5-1
Organizational chart for the Nutrition, Physical Activity and Obesity Program in Wisconsin.

The MOGO Coalition, or the Monroe County coalition for physical activity and nutrition, was formed in 2008. The coalition applied for and obtained funding from a planning grant through Wisconsin's Department of Health Services (DHS), Nutrition, Physical Activity and Obesity (NPAO) Program (see **Figure CS5-1**) to support coalition development and promote local implementation of the Wisconsin Nutrition and Physical Activity State Plan. The coalition includes members from 13 community agencies, including 3 hospitals, 3 school districts, the local health department, and a number of nonprofit organizations, all envisioning a healthier Monroe County and collectively vested in enhancing Monroe County residents' health status through physical activity and nutrition.

Target Groups and Agency Personnel Involved

MOGO conducted the photovoice assessment as one part of a formative assessment required of the coalition by the DHS NPAO Program in the planning grant cycle. Photovoice methodology was originally developed by Dr. Caroline Wang in 1992 (Wang, Burris, & Xiang, 1996). It is considered to be "an engaging photography and storytelling technique that offers community residents an opportunity to share their perceptions and impressions of their community and of the local conditions that affect their community's health" (Pies & Padmini, 2008, p. 1).

The MOGO coalition chose this methodology as an alternative assessment strategy, viewing it as a unique way to express qualitative data and give input and voice potentially to all residents living in Monroe County, regardless of age, educational level, and language. MOGO members also believed that community participation in the assessment would promote awareness, interest, and participation in MOGO activities and initiatives in future months. The coalition anticipated that the visual aspect of the photo collection would provide a succinct way to showcase the community's needs.

Because the photovoice assessment was used as one part of four total methods in the formative assessment, the coalition believed it would serve to confirm and clarify data. MOGO's original intent for the assessment was to provide the opportunity for youth adult residents of Monroe County to submit pictorial feedback to the Coalition.

For the photovoice project, MOGO selected a subcommittee of three members to take a lead coordination role. Ashley Koenig, Wisconsin Area Health Education Centers, Community Health Intern; Becky Zay, University of Wisconsin–La Crosse, Community Health Education Preceptee; and Becky Campbell, RN from the Monroe County Health Department comprised the subcommittee. They were selected due to prior knowledge of photovoice and/ or qualitative needs assessment, interest, and capacity to take on the project at the time. Other MOGO coalition members provided guidance and feedback to the subcommittee during the monthly face-to-face coalition meeting and through e-mail.

Needs Assessment Process

Preliminary Steps

Student interns, who had initial exposure to photovoice assessment procedures during coursework, developed a proposal for the MOGO coalition meeting in June 2009. With the approval of the coalition, and the formation of the subcommittee, the planning began. Although goals and objectives were not specifically identified for the assessment, the coalition discussed general outcomes and expectations to be: youth and adult resident involvement and feedback and visual representation of strengths and weaknesses of perceived opportunities relating to physical activity and nutrition in Monroe County. The subcommittee developed a time line for the assessment, which was driven by the grant time line. July 1–17 of 2009 was selected for data collection. The next step was to draft program forms and written materials, including consent and demographic forms and a press release. MOGO also purchased disposable cameras for the project and gathered donations of movie theater tickets and $10 Wal-Mart gift cards to be used as incentives.

Implementation

With the initial planning completed, the assessment implementation began. MCHD staff submitted a press release to local media outlets on July 1, 2009, describing the project and calling for participation. As explained in the press release, the MOGO coalition asked participating community members "to take 5 photos or more expressing what health means to you." Participants were instructed to "include strengths and weaknesses found in Monroe County relating to weight, physical activity, and nutrition," and to include comments with the photos. The release also was sent to MOGO members electronically, requesting that it be shared via e-mail to all MOGO member contacts. Because the subcommittee recognized the limitations of these two venues and anticipated a lower participation rate among older adults, youth, and Hispanic residents, the decision was made to specifically target those populations. This was done through in-person marketing at home visits and community locations, including a senior center, movie theater, and Hispanic community center. The goal was to reach out to key participants to explain the project, provide disposable cameras, and request participation. Residents could use digital or film cameras and submit their photos via e-mail or by dropping off photos at the Health Department. To remove cost as a barrier for participation, disposable cameras were offered to participants to complete the project; participants could receive these cameras by contacting the Health Department. Film processing was also free for the participants and was carried out after the cameras were returned to the MCHD staff. Upon return of the camera or submission of photos, participants received one of the following: two movie tickets, a disposable camera, or a $10 Wal-Mart gift card. Although the Wal-Mart gift card was the most valued incentive, some participants did not want to be included in the incentive process.

During the initial 3-week phase, MOGO received 85 photos from 7 participants. MOGO used the contributed photos and determined that the photovoice project was dynamic, with photos to be added in the future as the "picture" of Monroe County evolves. Six of the seven contributors submitted photos electronically and one used the disposable camera provided. Although captions were requested for the photos, just one of the participants provided written captions accompanying the electronic submission of the photos. Verbal comments were obtained from an additional two participants through informal subcommittee interviews conducted at the time of photo submission. The essence of these informal interviews was recorded. A consent and demographics form was signed by the individuals who were given cameras, but those persons who submitted electronic photos implied consent with their submission. Two individuals who requested disposable cameras did not take photos by the initial July 17, 2009, submission date and chose to return the cameras.

Needs Identified by the Assessment

The photovoice assessment conducted by MOGO was carried out to find both strengths and weaknesses of perceived opportunities that impact the weight, physical activity, and nutrition of Monroe County residents. The subcommittee reviewed the photos and discussed themes that emerged from the photos and any accompanying captions or verbal comments captured during the informal interviews. They did not capture the exact frequency with which each theme presented. As a result, the following list, in no priority order, of strengths and weaknesses of perceived opportunities relating to physical activity and nutrition in Monroe County was compiled by the subcommittee:

1. Monroe County has opportunities for many outdoor activities for adults and children, even in the winter season.
2. Sparta's bike trail serves as an asset to the community to promote physical activity.
3. Seniors have enhanced nutrition and social connectivity at various senior centers and meal sites around the county.
4. Monroe County has a wealth of agricultural resources; farmers' markets and farm stands with fresh produce during the summer and fall months are a result.
5. Smoking is a problem.
6. There is a lack of wheelchair and stroller accessible sidewalks and benches on some streets in population-dense areas.
7. Although the county seat is coined "the bicycle capital," many businesses lack bike racks.
8. Modern equipment may be supplanting activities that were once more physical in nature in this agricultural region (e.g., riding lawn mower versus push lawn mower).
9. Residents have access to cheap, unhealthy foods on a daily basis through fast food and convenience stores.

As previously noted, the subcommittee did not capture the exact frequencies for each theme found in the review of photos; however, MOGO did note that far more photos (greater than 90 percent) embodied the strengths of perceived opportunities impacting on weight, physical activity, and nutrition in Monroe County than on the weaknesses of these perceived opportunities to health.

How the Needs Information Was Utilized

The MOGO subcommittee compiled selected photos and theme statements into a Microsoft Office PowerPoint presentation, using those photos that best reflected the themes that occurred most often in the 85 photos. This presentation provided visual documentation of strengths and weakness of perceived opportunities to proper nutrition and physical activity within the county. It was used to inform MOGO members and member agencies on the results of the assessment. Presentations were made at a MOGO meeting, a public health staff meeting at the Monroe County Health Department, and a meeting for the Monroe County school nurses. Due to time and staff capacity issues, MOGO did not hold an open presentation for the general community.

In addition to utilizing the visual data and themes in a PowerPoint presentation, the themes were used, along with other materials, to form a strategic plan and action plan as a part of required grant deliverables and within a new grant application. The photovoice assessment, along with a secondary data analysis (e.g., 2008 Behavioral Risk Factor Surveillance System Wisconsin data, Monroe County Snapshot data from the 2009 University of Wisconsin Population County Health Rankings, Pediatric and Pregnancy Nutrition Surveillance System data), asset mapping, key-informant interviews, and a community survey, was used as one type of formative assessment. The assessment was required by DHS NPAO Program as a grant deliverable for the planning grant cycle MOGO was in at that time. Analysis of each dataset, including the photovoice project, was summarized to highlight the health needs of the community and then used to create an informed strategic plan (also a required grant deliverable) as a part of the Local Implementation of the State Physical Activity and Nutrition Plan. The MOGO strategic plan included an overall goal and four objectives. Using one of these objectives—"By 2013 MOGO Coalition will facilitate implementation of at least three strategies to improve nutrition practices in target population"—MOGO developed an intervention action plan and work plan, both of which were included in a grant application submitted to DHS NPAO Program requesting continued funding through an implementation grant cycle. MOGO received 80 percent of the requested funds and began its first ever intervention targeting increased fruit and vegetable access for students in local schools.

Recommendations

MOGO subcommittee members found that the photovoice assessment was very much a "learn by doing" project, and they identified several key findings, resulting in the following recommendations.

- Starting with clear goals, objectives, and a community message is an important step in the success of the photovoice assessment and can result in more buy-in from the target audience and more insightful data. For future photovoice assessments, MOGO concluded that one way to give the community clearer direction would be to provide an example of a photo and caption within the initial media release.
- Due to the use of personal digital cameras and electronic submission, in the future, an electronic consent/demographic form should be used.
- Getting commentary, whether through written submission or verbal interview, is crucial to understanding what the individuals' were intending to convey with each photo. MOGO recommends establishing a system to capture commentary from all participants so that the resulting assessment will truly be in their voice.

- Along with capturing commentary, a system for recording themes and the frequency of each theme is an important part of a photovoice assessment.
- Finally, although dissemination of results to coalition members and other stakeholders is important, getting the information out to the target group—those who were asked to participate in the assessment—is even more valuable. In future photovoice assessments, MOGO recommends that one or more community meetings/presentations be included in order to show the photos and discuss the assessment. Locations for such presentations could include libraries, community centers, schools, and senior meal sites.

References

Monroe County, Wisconsin. (n.d.). Health. Available at: http://www.co.monroe. wi.us/departments.php?id=7. Accessed October 20, 2010.

Pies, C., and Padmini, P. (2008). Photovoice: Giving local health departments a new perspective on community health issues. Available at: http://cchealth.org/topics/ community/photovoice. Accessed October 1, 2010.

U.S. Census Bureau. (2010 August). Monroe County QuickFacts. Available at: http://quickfacts.census.gov/qfd/states/55/55081.html. Accessed October 20, 2010.

Wang, C. C., Burris, M. A., and Xiang, Y. (1996). Chinese village women as visual anthropologists: A participatory approach to reaching policymakers. *Social Science Medicine*, 42, 1391–1400.

6

The Research Process as an Approach to Needs Assessment: A Case Study Involving Postnatal Women in England, United Kingdom

Palo Almond, PhD, Head of Primary and Public Health, Faculty of Health and Social Care, Anglia Ruskin University, Cambridgeshire, England, United Kingdom

Agency Overview: British National Health Service

This case study draws on information from a research project exploring equity in health visiting postnatal depression services and policy. It describes how research methods were used to establish needs and capacity. Health visitors are nurses with public health training who are employed in the British National Health Service (NHS) to work with families and the well population.

The NHS is provided free at the point of usage and is funded out of the taxation of the employed. It is not means tested (i.e., it is not assessed against a criteria to determine whether people should pay according to their level of income), and there is no cap on how much free health care is provided; however, less costly investigations and treatments are generally offered initially, stepping up to more costly options, as necessary. Most of the NHS funding is concerned with providing acute services, secondary care, and the management of long-term conditions, with relatively little spent on preventive care. Furthermore, despite a "free" health care service for all, inequity in health care provision and difficulties in accessing health care by some sectors of the population has resulted in inequalities in health (The Marmot Review, 2010). Though not all inequality in health is attributable to such factors, it can result from a range of determinants of health. Such determinants are well described by Dahlgren and Whitehead (1991). The term *equity* is generally used when discussing inequalities in health and health care that are avoidable and thus considered unjust (Almond, 2002, 2008).

Target Group: Postnatal Women

The population of interest were women with a 1-year-old or younger baby, with a particular focus on Bangladeshi women and lower socio-economic women. Postnatal depression is a serious condition and needs to be detected as early as possible. Briefly, it is a depression much like any other depression, with symptoms of unhappiness, pessimism, lack of hope, anxiety, and so on. It is important, because a mother's depression can affect her interaction with the baby, which can, in turn, affect the baby's health and development (Almond, 2008, 2009).

Agency Personnel Involved: Health Visiting Service

Although all employees in the NHS are concerned with the prevention and reduction of health inequalities, public health professionals hold the major responsibility. Health visitors are nurses trained in public health. They are accountable for child health surveillance; family, particularly maternal, welfare and wellbeing; and community health. All families with children younger than age 5 have an identified health visitor. Health visitors assess and monitor child health and development and take the requisite actions to promote child and family health. The setting for the project was a health visiting service in Hampshire, South England.

Needs Assessment Process

This section describes both the research methods to collect information about the needs assessment procedures as well as the health assessment approaches used by health visitors to identify needs.

Research Methods and Process

A qualitative approach to case study research as recommended by Yin (2003) was used. Following ethical approval and gaining permission to conduct the research with health visitors and their clients, all health visitors (n = 45) and their managers (n = 6) were invited to take part. Of these, 16 health visitors and all managers gave their informed consent to take part. The health visitors were asked to identify women in their case load who they planned to assess for postnatal depression or provide therapy for those diagnosed with mild to moderate postnatal depression. Twenty-one women (12 English women and 9 Bangladeshi women) agreed to be involved. In addition, a mental health practitioner who treated more complex cases and two Bengali community workers were involved in providing information.

The information gathering process involved interviews with managers using a semistructured interview guide to find out about policy relating to the detection of postnatal depression and its treatment. Health visitors were accompanied by the researcher on home visits where the needs assessment processes could be observed ($n = 21$). Following the observation, the client was interviewed about how the health visitor assessed the mother's health, what the client thought about the questions asked and the way they were asked, and her views about the treatments that were available. The health visitor also was interviewed about her thoughts about how she felt the visit went, why she asked the questions that she did, and whether she would have liked to ask other questions or carry out the assessment of health and mental health in other ways. Questions also were asked about her findings and capacity to meet the identified needs and the course of action she took or would like to take to meet the uncovered needs. The remaining participants were interviewed about their thoughts on the policy and procedures to identify women with postnatal depression and resources available and utilized to meet the need. Policies that guided health visiting practice were also obtained.

The data were analyzed using the Framework Approach (Ritchie & Spencer, 1994; Ritchie, 2003). This is a similar approach to other types of content analysis of qualitative data. It involves the development of codes, which then guide the data analysis. Charts and tables are created of the coded data, which assist the next level of analysis. From this, categories and themes are generated to summarize the key findings. This process enabled an understanding of what assessment methods were used and also what the participants felt about them, why they were used, and the resources available to meet the need. Briefly, the needs uncovered were for one-to-one or group counselling, advice about the care of the baby to allay anxiety, marital difficulties, difficulties with family members, dissatisfaction with housing, financial worries, and low self-esteem.

Findings: Needs Assessment Methods and Outcomes

Although health visitors across the UK have a responsibility for assessing women for postnatal depression, whether and how they do this is largely determined by capacity (e.g., the training they have had to screen and assess using particular tools and procedures and the time available to offer universal or targeted screening and assessment). Up until December 2007, England and Wales did not have a national policy on the assessment and management of maternal mental health during the antenatal and postnatal period. Prior to this time, health visitors largely used the Edinburgh Postnatal Depression Scale to detect the presence of postnatal depression. Other scales used are the PHQ9, Beck Depression Inventory, and the Whooley Questions, as per the National Institute of Health and Clinical Excellence Guidelines (2007).

The data revealed two key ways health visitors carried out a needs assessment. The most common way used with English-speaking clients was the administration of a 10-item questionnaire, the Edinburgh Postnatal Depression Scale (Cox, Holden, & Sagovsky, 1987). The mother is asked to respond to a range of statements. For example, one statement offered, "I have been able to laugh and see the funny side of things," to which the mother could answer, "as much as I always could," "not as quite so much now," "definitely not so much now," or "not at all." Another one is, "I have felt sad or miserable," to which the mother could answer "yes most of the time," "yes quite often," "not very often," or "no not at all." Each response is given a numerical score. At the end of the survey, the statement scores are added up to determine the level of risk to depression. Most clinicians use a score of between 10 and 12 to institute a second screening 2 weeks later or, depending on the outcome of the clinical interview, treatment is offered.

The health visitors then followed this up with a clinical interview where they asked the mother questions about her responses on the questionnaire, seeking information that would enable them to determine whether the mother was depressed and how amenable she would be to the different forms of therapy available. There is no set format to the clinical interview. The health visitor explores the reasons as to why the mother selected a particular response and finds out more detail. So for the statement "I have felt sad or miserable," if the mother has said "no not at all," the health visitor may check the accuracy of this by asking the mother when in the past she may have felt sad and miserable to determine if the statement has been interpreted correctly. Or, if the response was "yes quite often," the health visitor would inquire how often, whether there were there any triggers for the feelings, how long did the feelings last, and so on.

In this particular health visiting service, it was a mandatory requirement for health visitors to assess all women for postnatal depression at particular time points during the first postnatal year; however, this did not happen. Two key reasons for this emerged. First, health visitors' workloads and shortages in staffing resulted in them largely focusing on safeguarding (child protection) activities. Second, health visitors, although trained in the detection and management of postnatal depression, were not culturally competent to assess the needs of Bangladeshi women in relation to the detection of postnatal depression. The support therapy groups were only available in English. Women who could not speak English were not screened but were instead asked a few questions about how they felt; they were also not referred to the support therapy groups. Both the health visitors and the Bangladeshi women were dissatisfied with this situation. Several factors that encouraged health visitors to assess postnatal women's needs are summarized in **Table CS6-1**.

TABLE CS6-1
Factors that Promoted Needs Assessment

Policy	Attitudinal Shift	Resources	Knowledge
Proactive detection	Positive attitude about policy, which is a "good strategy"	District-wide training	Evidence of under detection
Early identification a priority	EPDS seen as a "good tool"	Team approach to managing postnatal depression (PND)	Incidence of PND seen as different amongst socio-economic groups
PND is part of health visitor (HV) business plan	Acknowledgment of PND	Choice in treatments available	All populations susceptible to PND
PND targeted to deprived areas	Some HVs positive about policy	Availability and use of interpreters	Skills in broaching PND
"Sure Start" targets for PND	Adoption of policy by some HVs	Bengali cohesion workers	Understanding that other cultures suffer from PND, too
All HVs will be equally skilled	PND priority for some HVs	HV doing joint visits with cohesion workers	Raising awareness of risk factors
Changes in child health surveillance	Screening visit is high priority	Support groups	Knowledge of effects on child and others
Training	Flexible adaptation of care pathway		
Detecting PND risk factors antenatally	Persistence by some HVs		

Addressing Identified Needs

Treatments health visitors could provide were nondirective counselling, solution-focused therapy, and cognitive behavioral therapy. Additionally, they facilitated support therapy groups for women who stood to benefit from a more socially orientated and peer-support approach. For more severely depressed or complex cases, pharmacological and psychiatric treatments were available. However, if the health visitors did not have training in particular treatments, they could not offer these to their clients. Therefore, some women had greater or less access to some treatments than others. However, as stated earlier, due to problems of capacity, health visitors could not devote as much time and resources to this aspect of their role because they were faced with more pressing child safeguarding priorities. Furthermore, the service was not culturally sensitive or equipped to adequately assess or meet the needs of non-English-speaking Bangladeshi women. Although health education materials on postnatal depression were available and distributed, these were only available in English. Additionally, the research found that other resources that would assist the health visitor in the assessment of needs, such as professional interpreters, were rarely used; reasons for this are provided in **Figure CS6-1.**

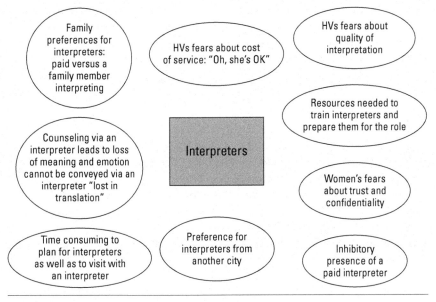

FIGURE CS6-1
Factors explaining the non-usage of interpreters.

Following completion of the research, the primary care trust was given a written report that contained a list of recommendations as to how the service could be enhanced. An oral presentation also was organized to which all participants, health visitors, and managers were invited. The senior managers were not surprised by the findings of the research and were keen to make improvements that would allow health visitors to assess need in all women. Anecdotal feedback from the primary care trust's managers suggest that some of the recommendations were indeed followed up. All health visitors underwent additional training in the assessment of postnatal depression (cognitive behavioral therapy), and resources to assist health visitors to assess the non–English-speaking women were bought and training on their effective usage was provided.

Conclusion

The case study summarized here has illustrated how research can be used to rigorously explore the "what" and "how" of needs assessment. Research can, however, be time consuming, and so is not suited to situations where needs have to be identified and responded to quickly. It can nevertheless provide robust findings of not only need, but also capacity.

Even before the research was fully completed, the health visiting service responded to the emerging findings by taking steps to make it more equitable, culturally sensitive, and capable. New resources were provided to enable health visitors to more adequately assess the needs of non-English-speaking women.

References

Almond, P. (2002). An analysis of the concept of equity and its application to health visiting. *Journal of Advanced Nursing, 37*(6), 598–606.

Almond, P. (2008). *A study of equity within health visiting postnatal depression policy and services.* Unpublished PhD Thesis. University of Southampton.

Almond, P. (2009). Postnatal depression: A global public health perspective. *Perspectives in Public Health, 129,* 221–227.

Cox, J. L., Holden, J. M., and Sagovsky, R. (1987). Detection of postnatal depression. Development of the 10-item Edinburgh Postnatal Depression Scale. *British Journal of Psychiatry, 150,* 782–786.

Dahlgren, G., and Whitehead, M. (1991). *Policies and strategies to promote social equity in health.* Stockholm: Institute of Futures Studies.

The Marmot Review. (2010). *Fair Society, Healthy Lives.* Available at: http://www.ucl.ac.uk/marmotreview. Accessed May 10, 2011.

National Institute for Clinical Excellence. (2007). *Antenatal and postnatal mental health: Clinical management and service guidelines*. London: HMSO.

Ritchie, J., and Spencer, L. (1994). Qualitative data analysis for applied policy research. In Bryman, A., and Burgess, R. G. (Eds). *Analysing qualitative data*. London: Routledge.

Ritchie, J. (2003) The application of qualitative methods to social research. In Ritchie, J., and Lewis, J. (Eds). *Qualitative research practice*. London: Sage Publications, 24–46.

Yin, R. (2003). *Case study research: Design and methods*, 3rd ed. Thousand Oaks, CA: Sage Publications.

Community Health Development in Mid Glamorgan, Wales

Elaine Jones, Former Director of Health Promotion, Mid Glamorgan Health Authority, Wales, United Kingdom

Agency Overview

Mid Glamorgan Health Authority is coterminous with the county of Mid Glamorgan, which lies at the southwestern corner of Wales, United Kingdom. The area was traditionally the focus of mining and other heavy industries, though these have largely been run down during the last 40 years. The population during the 1990s was approximately 550,000, and unemployment rates ranged between 9 and 18 percent, with 18 percent of households lacking basic amenities. The county has the highest percentage of deprived population in Wales and is one of the poorest areas of the United Kingdom. The Health Authority commissions all health care for that population, both within the community and in the hospital setting. Health Promotion is part of the Department of Public Health Medicine and operates a county-wide service. The main areas of work focus on the education of professionals, development of healthy alliances, and policy development in both the public and private sectors. All services are free or provided on a nonprofit basis.

Mid Glamorgan Health Authority and Family Health Services Authority agreed to invest in the health development approach to health promotion planning in six communities of Mid Glamorgan over a 3-year period. The first two projects were to pilot the methodologies and to test the effect that the project would have on future planning in those localities. The objectives of the project follow:

1. To select a set of data that reflects the health promotion needs and priorities of the target community

276

2. To collect soft and hard data relating to the health needs of the community
3. To determine the key individuals, groups, and organizations with the power to affect health in the community
4. To analyze the first two objectives and recommend appropriate health promotion activities that could be carried out in the locality
5. To determine the most appropriate partners in the provision of health promotion activities or services
6. To liaise with representatives from the community to monitor effectiveness and measure outcomes

Target Group

The health development project targeted six communities over a 3-year period. Each community was to be self-defining and contain approximately 20,000 to 30,000 individuals. The choice of community reflected the variety of environments within the county, from coastal holiday resorts to upper valley communities, from more affluent new industrial areas to post–Industrial Revolution deprivation.

Agency Personnel Involved

Initially, each of the two pilot communities was assigned a qualified health promotion specialist as the project coordinator. In the remaining four communities, a health promotion specialist was to be assigned to carry out the needs assessment on two communities over 1 year.

Needs Assessment Process Employed

The methods used during the project together with an indicator of effectiveness are summarized in **Table CS7-1** and **Table CS7-2**.

A vital aspect of the project was community feedback. This information was disseminated at two levels. At a formal seminar, the results were publicized and all participants and local health service managers were involved. Less formal feedback to individual groups or individuals who had contributed to the project was carried out by the project workers.

Throughout the project, use was made of local media, notably newspapers and community newsletters, to give information to all residents in the area.

TABLE CS7-1
Sources of Information

Type of Source	Nature of the Information	Purpose
Epidemiology	Death rates, SMR, disease rates, birth rates	Put local priorities against national plans
Social and economic	Employment status, transportation, social status, education, housing	
Local surveys	Planning outlines, employment, education	Identify pockets of specific need
Community members	Expressed needs, opinions, history, desires, views	Identify gatekeepers Identify opportunities for partnerships Identify the natural "flow" of a community Highlight advocates for health
NHS professional groups	Views, opinions, standards	Allow comparison with expressed needs
Cultural history	History and development of the community	Identify potential areas for action that "fit" with the community

TABLE CS7-2
Assessment Processes

Method	Description	Effectiveness
Focus group	Small groups working to a fixed agenda to reach an agreed outcome	Very
Personal interview	One-on-one to an outline set of questions	Very
Observation	Watching the community at all times of the day and night, week and weekend, over the period	Very
Life history	One-on-one with older members of the community to identify trends	Very

TABLE CS7-2
(*Continued*)

Method	Description	Effectiveness
Market research	Opportunistic questioning to a sampling frame	Did not work
Data search	Draw information from existing published data	Most data not available to the local level—of limited use
Media	News items, press releases—before, during, and after	Very

Needs Identified by the Assessment

Project findings in Bargoed and Porthcawl show that the expressed needs of the community are not reflected in the priorities set by national and local plans. A clear example is the almost complete absence of concern about smoking behavior in both communities, even though statistical evidence shows a higher rate of smoking than in the rest of Wales at 32.2 percent. The main findings are summarized in **Table CS7-3**.

TABLE CS7-3
Assessed Needs

Lifestyle Area	Community Response	Proposed Action
Smoking	No-smoking areas in public houses	Opportunities for local smoking cessation support Increased number of smoke-free places
Alcohol	Help, advice for alcohol misusers Training for professionals Local treatment services Monitor alcohol sales Server training Multi-agency approach	Develop multi-agency, multi-disciplinary substance misuse program
Nutrition	Advice of dietician available in the locality Need consistent messages on diet Local advice and support for people with diabetes	Training for NHS staff Increased availability of fresh fruit and vegetables

(*Continued*)

TABLE CS7-3
Assessed Needs (*Continued*)

Lifestyle Area	Community Response	Proposed Action
Physical exercise	Promotion of appropriate leisure and recreation services, especially for young people and older people	Creation of alliances with local services Training for leisure service staff Clean up local beaches
Stress	Coping skills training in the community, especially for cardiac rehabilitation Help for careers, unemployed and women	Increased training of NHS staff in stress management
Drug misuse	As for alcohol More advice needed on the use of prescribed medicines	As for alcohol
Healthy sexuality	Include healthy sexuality in family planning clinics	Training for all those involved in education or providing a service
Healthy environment	Dog excrement a problem Derelict buildings Noise Concern about standards of housing Safety issues	Work together with local planners to identify the health implications of actions and eliminate the detrimental effects
Parenting	Need help to deal with behavioral difficulties of children in the family	Training courses

How the Needs Were Addressed in Programming

The project reports included recommendations for future action and suggested a lead agency to take each action forward. The action following the project to date has been positive and encouraging, with agencies outside of the health care field being ready to take on board the findings.

The end of the first phase of the project has coincided with the development of the contract culture in health promotion. The findings of the projects are, therefore, addressed via contracts the Health Authority has with the local providers of health promotion. At the local level, the needs assessments are being used as increased leverage to increase funding for health promotion activity.

The Needs Assessment Simulation Game

Jay V. Schindler, PhD, MPH, CHES, Public Health Operating Unit,
Northrop Grumman Corporation, Atlanta, Georgia

Gary D. Gilmore, MPH, PhD, MCHES, Professor and Director, Graduate
Community Health/Public Health Programs, University of Wisconsin, La
Crosse, and University of Wisconsin–Extension

Introduction

For many people, the needs assessment process may seem abstract, difficult, or even a waste of time and energy. The process of collecting valid, representative information about the needs of a target group is not easy—it requires forethought and careful planning. Also, needs assessment might seem redundant for individuals who feel they already understand and empathize with the individuals in the target group. The authors have seen many individuals choose to rely on their own, possibly biased, perceptions of target group members rather than take the time and energy to interact with the actual group members and discover the true needs of the group.

This simulation was designed to give student trainees, health professionals, community organizers, and others a more direct, hands-on experience of conducting a needs assessment. The game can help them appreciate the value of performing a good needs assessment and understand how challenging it can be to get the job done efficiently and effectively. It can be a social laboratory for participants to learn about the factors that make it difficult to convene group representatives, generate helpful survey questions, collect valid data, summarize incomplete information, and more. As an experiential exercise, it provides direct experiences for the participants that a trainer, group facilitator, or educator can discuss during debriefing exercises. It has even proved beneficial to rerun the simulation so that participants can use their new insights and knowledge to improve their strategies the next time through the simulation game.

Like other simulation games, the Needs Assessment Simulation Game asks participants to take on new roles and try out new skills. It is through this practice that the process of needs assessment becomes more realistic and meaningful. The addition of gaming elements [e.g., points for correctly identifying group needs, the limited activities (moves) that each group can make, and the possibility of competition between teams in the simulation] provides additional play elements and motivation that entice group involvement.

Each of the many times the authors have run this simulation, the participants have been able to generate a valuable list of insights and important points about the proper design, implementation, and analysis of a needs assessment. For example, one group discovered that by using two different needs assessment strategies they could "triangulate" their findings and establish confidence in their answers. Sometimes, however, the insights were not always positive. For example, one group discovered that members of another group had decided to lie about their true needs when provided with a questionnaire. Only later did it come out that the trust level toward the first group was extremely low because of how the second group was treated earlier by that first group. Because human nature plays a vital role in needs assessment activities, this simulation game can be helpful in uncovering many interpersonal and cross-cultural facets of human behavior that must be considered when doing needs assessment in the real world.

For those who are interested in using this simulation game in a group setting, the authors suggest you first read through pages A, B, C, and D and examine the survey and grant application form—the handouts participants receive as they proceed through the simulation game. Once you have a basic idea of the activities participants perform and the progression through the simulation, read through the handouts for the Game Director: "Guide for Game Director" and "Guide for Debriefing the Simulation." Try to imagine your role both as a participant and as the Director for each of the Team Activities listed on page B, for each of the time periods in the simulation game, and during the debriefing.

Although the Needs Assessment Simulation Game activities can be completed in 1 hour, it can take much more time if you try to prepare the participants with too much detail or provide them too much time to conduct their needs assessment activities. You will know that you're moving at the correct pace if a small percentage of participants do need clarification on the simulation game rules and if most groups feel a bit rushed to complete their final survey form on time.

Don't forget to schedule enough time for the debriefing of the simulation game. This debriefing is your opportunity to bring clarity out of the confusion and to help your participants make explicit what they have experienced and learned. If you cannot conduct the debriefing immediately after the simulation game, have participants jot down their thoughts, feelings, and observations immediately so that they can recall their experiences later when you conduct the debriefing.

You can access additional information as a Director of the simulation activity by going to the following Web site: go.jblearning.com/gilmore4. Remember, if questions arise, you always can contact us through the publisher, Jones & Bartlett Learning. Enjoy the experience!

Introduction to Participants

Community interventions and health promotion programs rarely can proceed without first discovering the reported needs of the target population. By conducting a needs assessment, the community intervention or health promotion practitioner can ascertain which specific problems are most urgent, which factors might prevent resolution of problems, and who are the most important targets of a community-oriented activity.

This simulation will help you to understand the needs assessment process. Like most other simulations, it has simplified the real-world processes so that you can examine needs assessment within a short period of time. The simulation has, by necessity, left out many of the details that exist in actual needs assessments but has tried to keep intact the real flavor of what occurs. Please keep in mind that most participants will experience some confusion when going through the simulation—that is normal and expected—it happens in the real world of needs assessment, too.

Beginning Activities

Needs assessment activities often require the cooperation and integrated efforts of many people. To help simulate this team effort, the group should form teams of three or four people. Once a team has formed, choose or elect a Team Leader for the duration of the simulation.

[Form a team, and choose a Team Leader before reading further.]

Just as every house in a municipality has an address, for this simulation every person needs to have an address. The Game Director will come around and tell each Team Leader which street your team members live on. Each team member, including the Team Leader, should then choose a simple address number: 1, 2, 3, and so on, up to the total number of members in your group.

Every team member should have a unique address (in fact, every person in the room should have a unique address). For example, if the Game Director tells your Team Leader your four team members all live on Downing Street, your addresses could be 1 Downing Street, 2 Downing Street, 4 Downing Street, and 6 Downing Street.

[Do not read further until all team members have a unique address.]

One method of conducting a needs assessment is by developing, distributing, collecting, and then analyzing a survey composed of pertinent questions. The Game Director has such a survey that should be taken by every person in the group. Your Team Leader should get copies of this survey from the Game Director and take them back to the team. Everyone on the team, including the Team Leader, should then complete these forms (no names please!) and return them to the Team Leader.

Team Leader only: Once you have collected all of the completed team surveys (including your own), you have the additional responsibility of collating the results onto one blank form. Simply tally how many responses occurred within your team for each answer to each survey question. When you are finished tallying all of your team's answers, give the tallied survey results and all team member surveys to the Game Director.

Goal of Teams in Simulation

In brief, your team goal is to conduct a needs assessment on all the participants in the simulation—this includes your team and all the other teams in the group. Your team should attempt to find out how the whole group would tally up when examining the following topics: (1) demographics [age], (2) seatbelt use, (3) stress level, (4) physical activity, (5) blood pressure measures, (6) overall health, (7) usual sleeping habits, (8) cigarette smoking habits, and (9) body weight.

Basically, your team will work to reconstruct the survey data that the Game Director has collected from all of the teams in the room. All of the other teams are performing the same task. You are restricted as to how you can collect this information, and you have limited time and resources available to collect this information. At the end of your time limit, your team will be given an identical copy of the survey form that each of you completed at the beginning of the simulation. Your team's task will be to provide accurate estimates (or guesses) as to which answer was most frequently given for each question and how many participants gave that response for the question. Your estimates should be for the whole group, not just for your team. The team that comes the closest to matching the correct responses and counts for all the questions is the winning team.

Activities of Teams in Simulation

Your team could conduct a variety of activities to collect the information you need. However, to make this simulation more realistic, your activities are limited to the list that follows. By thinking through the needs assessment strategies listed on page D, you should be able to devise your own methods to collect information. Also, please note that you have limited resources, expressed as MET (Money, Energy, Time) points. For each activity listed your team must subtract MET points from your running total. Once you reach zero MET points, your team cannot do any other activities. (Note: There is no advantage to saving MET points. Consider your MET points to be the budget allocation for your needs assessment—you are expected to spend it all wisely.) Your team begins the game with a total of MET points (e.g., 20 METs).

Team Activities	MET Costs	Comments
Discover the address of the Team Leader of the group.	2 METs/team	Leaders know the most about their own team.
Interview one person in one team until that person says, "No more!"	5 METs/interview	Get information from members of the group.
Get information from the Game Director about one survey question (semi-random element involved).	2 METs/request	Existing records are available, but responses sometimes are not what you wanted or are not easy to use.
Quietly observe one group until the group says, "Leave!" No talking to members.	4 METs/group	Observing members of the target group provides insights.
Make a public announcement in front of the whole group.	8 METs/minute	Using "mass media" can help spread the message.
Mail out your own survey or letter to individuals in another team (return postage guaranteed).	10 METs/5 addresses	Distribute information or forms to the group. Many people use TO: (address) and FROM:.
Ask a consultant (Game Director) for advice about needs assessment.	2 METs/question	Expert consultants can save you time and money.
Rent the Community Hall to a meeting of community members.	10 METs/question	Expert consultants can save you time and money in the long run.
Submit a grant to request more MET points for your organizations.	6 METs to try for 24 METs	Writing a grant takes time, but you can get more resources.

Time Constraints for Your Team in the Simulation

You have limited time to conduct your needs assessment activities. The Game Director will keep you informed of how much time remains. Plan your strategies as efficiently as possible and collect your data using the methods explained earlier. You can use the METs Expenditure Chart to keep track of your 50 remaining METs.

Ending the Simulation

At the end of the simulation time, the Game Director will hand you a copy of the original survey. You will have exactly 10 minutes to fill in the survey as a team. You will now try to estimate what the majority responses were to each of the questions on the survey.

For each question in the survey, circle the one response that you feel was the most frequently selected response for the participants in the simulation. Also, next to the circled response, write in a number that represents the total number of participants you think chose this most popular response to the question. Your completed survey should have one answer circled for each of the questions and your estimate of the total number of people who made that response from the full group of participants. Hand in the completed survey when your team is finished with it.

Each survey will be scored as follows: For each question, if your team has circled the majority response, you will receive an initial 20 points. Then, your estimate for the number of total responses will be compared to the actual number as tallied by the Game Director from the original surveys. For each point that your estimate is off from the actual number, 1 point will be deducted from the 20 points initially received for that question. Notice that if you chose the incorrect response you will get 0 (zero) points for that question. Each question is worth a maximum of 20 points.

METs Remaining for Your Team

Strike out the number as you use up the MET point.

50 49 48 47 46 45 44 43 42 41
40 39 38 37 36 35 34 33 32 31
30 29 28 27 26 25 24 23 22 21
20 19 18 17 16 15 14 13 12 11
10 09 08 07 06 05 04 03 02 01

Activity Bought with METS	Conclusion(s) Based on Activity
1.	
2.	
3.	
4.	
5.	
6.	
7.	
8.	
9.	
10.	

Background Information

Needs assessment can involve many processes, but at a minimum, one should learn about the following major strategies: (1) a key informant strategy, (2) a community survey strategy, (3) a demographic data strategy, (4) a community forum strategy, (5) a focus group strategy, and (6) a participant observation strategy. Each strategy has its own strengths and weaknesses.

Key Informant Strategy

Key informants are individuals who know about the needs of the target group. Although key informants may include actual members of the target group, the key informant strategy often refers to individuals who are not members of the target group. For example, if a health professional wanted to learn about the health needs of college students, the professional could talk to doctors or nurses at the student medical center, counselors at the university mental health clinic, physical fitness leaders, or faculty at the university. Each key informant has a unique perspective on the needs of the target group, but the information may be seen as biased or totally subjective. The key informant strategy, however, is relatively simple to perform and can help establish a network of contacts within the community. The typical turnaround time to complete a needs assessment of this type is moderate; the typical cost to do a key informant needs assessment is moderate.

Community Survey Strategy

Go right to the people and ask them what their needs are! This process can be conducted through a mailed-out questionnaire, a telephone survey, or a door-to-door or face-to-face interview process. Nothing beats direct contact with the target group members for accuracy, but problems emerge when you are trying to determine how you will sample your group: do you really want to ask every member? Also, do you have enough money and energy to contact a large-enough sample directly? How will you reduce the complexity of collecting, storing, and analyzing your information? Surveys can have a slow turnaround time and a very high cost, but can provide the widest coverage of the target population.

Demographic Data Strategy

Data are being collected about the target group's problems and needs through existing programs and census efforts. For example, records exist on the number of arrests due to drinking and driving, the number of cases of sexually transmitted diseases in a county, and the number of female teenagers who became pregnant while in school. Although the data are often available through large data files, and the collected information can be considered fairly unbiased, the demographic data may not have been collected for your specific needs. If a database does exist for your target population, examining the database is a relatively inexpensive way to collect information if you are given access to it!

Community Forum Strategy

Sometimes it is possible to call a meeting of interested community members to have them help identify the needs within their own community. This tactic can work especially well if the community has some identified leadership, feels competent in changing its own living conditions, and has the time and energy to contribute to such activities. (Of course, many communities do not fit this description.) A local gathering of community members can discuss their needs, modes of intervention, and available resources of personnel, monies, supplies, and other items.

Focus Group Strategy

By bringing together representatives from the target group and then asking pertinent questions, a focus group can help identify the main thoughts and variations within a group. It is important to have a well-prepared set of pertinent questions for your focus group, as well as a set of ground rules so that the group process will be fair to all who are present. This method can be helpful in identifying the breadth and depth of responses to your questions and can be valuable to collect qualitative information. However, if some target group members are reluctant to participate or your group process favors one kind of responder over another, you may obtain biased results.

Participant Observation Strategy

Rather than gathering information about members of the target group as an external or outside contact, you are provided permission to quietly but directly observe and record your perceptions of the target population. As an observer, you can note various aspects of target-group behavior and activities that may be difficult to understand through surveys or other methods of needs assessment. By remaining inconspicuous, an assessor can reduce the likelihood of a false or artificial reaction within the target group. However, you must obtain permission from the target group to allow your observing to take place. Although this method can be time consuming, you may observe activities and interactions that an outsider might not normally be privileged enough to see.

Grant Application Form

Title: _____

Rationale: _____

Goals: _____

_____

_____

Method: _____

_____

_____

Potential Benefits: _____

_____

_____

Criteria for Evaluation of Grant Proposal: Outstanding = 4; Strong = 3; Adequate = 2; Weak = 1; Nonexistent = 0

1. Title is direct, descriptive, concise, and comprehensive.
2. Rationale provides solid reasoning why proposal should be funded immediately.
3. Goals clearly identify targets for achievement associated with project proposal.

4. Method clearly and completely specifies the steps needed to reach the goals and see success.
5. Potential benefits section identifies beneficial impact on intended audience and future implications.
6. Game Director's perception of the merit of the grant proposal concept.

Total Points: _____

If total of evaluation is ≥ 15, award a total of 24 MET points.

Anonymous Health Survey: The Needs Assessment Game

1. What is your age?
   _____ 20 or younger
   _____ 21 to 30
   _____ 31 to 40
   _____ 41 to 50
   _____ 51 or older

2. How often do you use a seatbelt?
   _____ 81–100 percent of the time
   _____ 61–80 percent of the time
   _____ 41–60 percent of the time
   _____ 21–40 percent of the time
   _____ 0–20 percent of the time

3. How would you describe the level of stress you have experienced during the last month?
   _____ Very high level of stress
   _____ High level of stress
   _____ Average level of stress
   _____ Low level of stress
   _____ Very low level of stress

4. On the average, how often in one week do you exercise vigorously enough to sweat?
   _____ Less than 1 time per week
   _____ 1 or 2 times per week
   _____ 3 or 4 times per week
   _____ 5 or 6 times per week
   _____ 7 or more times per week

5. Which one of the blood-pressure readings below is used as a cutoff to indicate high blood pressure?

_____ 135/80

_____ 140/80

_____ 140/90

_____ 150/90

_____ 150/95

6. How would you describe your overall health?

_____ Outstanding

_____ Excellent

_____ Good

_____ Fair

_____ Poor

7. On average, how many hours of sleep do you get each night?

_____ 9 or more hours

_____ 8 hours

_____ 7 hours

_____ 6 hours

_____ 5 hours or less

8. Which one of the following items best describes your cigarette smoking habits?

_____ Never smoked cigarettes

_____ Used to smoke, but quit

_____ Smoke less than 1 pack per day

_____ Smoke more than 1 pack, but less than 2 packs per day

_____ Smoke 2 or more packs per day

9. How would you describe your weight?

_____ More than 20 percent overweight

_____ 10–20 percent overweight

_____ Less than 10 percent overweight

_____ Less than 10 percent underweight

_____ More than 10 percent underweight

Healthstyle: A Self-Test

Everyone wants good health, but many of us don't know how to be as healthy as possible. Health experts describe lifestyle as one of the most important factors affecting our health. In fact, it is estimated that 7 of the 10 leading causes of death could be reduced through common-sense changes in lifestyle.

How to Get from Here to There . . .

The first step in a healthier lifestyle is thinking about what we are doing now. The brief self-test below, developed by the Public Health Service and adapted by Linda Bobroff, will let you know how well you are doing to stay healthy. The behaviors included in the test are recommended for most adult Americans. Some behaviors may not apply to persons with certain chronic diseases or physical challenges, or to pregnant women. Such persons may need special advice from their doctor or other health care provider.

About *Healthstyle: A Self-Test*

There are six sections:

1. Cigarette smoking
2. Alcohol and drugs
3. Eating habits
4. Exercise/fitness
5. Stress control
6. Safety and health

Source: University of Florida IFAS Extension. http://edis.ifas.ufl.edu/he778. Used with permission.

How to Use *Healthstyle: A Self-Test*

Complete one section at a time by circling the number under the answer that best describes your behavior. Then add the numbers you circled to get your score and write the score on the line provided at the end of each section.

When you are finished with all six sections, make sure to review the information under "Your Lifestyle Scores" and "What Your Scores Mean to You." You will learn what your scores mean and will get tips for living a healthier lifestyle. And that's what this self-test is all about.

For more detailed information, contact your health care provider or a registered dietitian (RD). Call your county Extension Family and Consumer Sciences (FCS) agent to see if healthy lifestyles programs are available in your county. Contact information for all county Extension offices in Florida can be found at http://solutionsforyourlife.ufl.edu/map/index.html. Written materials may be downloaded from our Extension Web site at http://SolutionsForYourLife.ufl.edu.

Cigarette Smoking	Almost Always	Sometimes	Almost Never
If you are currently a non-smoker, enter a score of ten for this section and go to the next section on Alcohol and Drugs.			
1. I avoid smoking cigarettes.	2	1	0
2. I smoke only low tar and nicotine cigarettes or I smoke a pipe.	2	1	0
Smoking Score _____			

Alcohol and Drugs	Almost Always	Sometimes	Almost Never
1. I avoid drinking alcoholic beverages or I drink no more than 1 or 2 drinks a day.	4	1	0
2. I avoid using alcohol or other drugs (especially illegal drugs) as a way of handling stressful situations or problems.	2	1	0
3. I am careful to not drink alcohol when taking certain (for example, medicine for sleeping, pain, colds, and allergies) or when pregnant.	2	1	0
4. I read and follow the label directions when using prescribed or over-the-counter drugs.	2	1	0
Alcohol and Drugs Score _____			

Eating Habits	Almost Always	Sometimes	Almost Never
1. I eat a variety of foods each day, such as fruits and vegetables; whole grain breads and cereals; lean meats; low-fat dairy products; dry peas and beans; nuts and seeds.	4	1	0
2. I limit the amount of fat, saturated fat, *trans* fat, and cholesterol I eat (including fat on meats, eggs, butter, cream, shortenings, and organ meats such as liver).	2	1	0
3. I limit the amount of salt I eat by cooking with only small amounts, not adding salt at the table, and avoiding salty snacks.	2	1	0
4. I avoid eating too much sugar (especially frequent snacks of sticky candy or soft drinks).	2	1	0
Eating Habits Score _____			

Exercise/Fitness	Almost Always	Sometimes	Almost Never
1. I do vigorous exercises for 30 minutes a day at least 5 times a week (examples include jogging, swimming, brisk walking, bicycling).	4	2	0
2. I do exercises that enhance my muscle tone for 15–30 minutes at least 3 times a week (examples include using weight machines or free weights, yoga, and calisthenics).	3	1	0
3. I use part of my leisure time partici-pating in individual, family, or team activities that increase my level of fitness (such as gardening, dancing, bowling, golf, baseball).	3	1	0
Exercise/Fitness Score _____			

Stress Control	Almost Always	Sometimes	Almost Never
1. I have a job, go to school, or do other work that I enjoy.	2	1	0
2. I find it easy to relax and express my feelings freely.	2	1	0
3. I recognize early, and prepare for, events or situations likely to be stressful for me.	2	1	0
4. I have close friends, relatives, or others whom I can talk to about personal matters and call on for help when needed.	2	1	0
5. I participate in group activities (such as religious worship and community organizations) and/or have hobbies that I enjoy.	2	1	0
Stress Control Score _____			

Safety and Health	Almost Always	Sometimes	Almost Never
1. I wear a seat belt while riding in a car.	2	1	0
2. I avoid driving while under the influence of alcohol or other drugs, or riding with someone else who is under the influence.	2	1	0
3. I obey traffic rules and avoid distractions like texting and talking on the phone when driving.	2	1	0
4. I am careful when using potentially harmful products or substances (such as household cleaners, poisons, and electrical devices).	2	1	0
5. I get at least seven hours of sleep a night.	2	1	0
Safety and Health Score _____			

Your Lifestyle Scores

After you have figured your scores for each of the six sections, circle the
number in each column that matches your score for that section of the test.

Cigarette Smoking	Alcohol and Drugs	Eating Habits	Exercise/ Fitness	Stress Control	Safety and Health
10	10	10	10	10	10
9	9	9	9	9	9
8	8	8	8	8	8
7	7	7	7	7	7
6	6	6	6	6	6
5	5	5	5	5	5
4	4	4	4	4	4
3	3	3	3	3	3
2	2	2	2	2	2
1	1	1	1	1	1
0	0	0	0	0	0

Remember: There is no total score for this self-test. Think about each section
separately. You are identifying aspects of your lifestyle that you can improve
in order to be healthier. So let's see what your scores reveal.

What Your Scores Mean to You (By Section)

Scores of 9 and 10
Excellent. Your answers show that you are aware of the importance of this
area to your health. More importantly, you are putting your knowledge to
work for you by practicing good health habits. As long as you continue to
do so, this area should not pose a serious risk. It's likely that you are setting
an example for the rest of your family and friends to follow. Since you got a
high test score on this part of the test, you may want to consider other areas
where your scores indicate room for improvement.

Scores of 6 to 8
Your health practices in this area are good, but there is *room for improvement.* Look again at the items you answered with a "Sometimes" or "Almost
Never." What changes can you make to improve your score? Even a small
change can help you achieve better health.

Scores of 3 to 5

Your health risks are showing. Would you like more information about the risks you are facing? Do you want to know why it is important for you to change these behaviors? Perhaps you need help in deciding how to make the changes you desire. In either case, help is available. You can start by contacting your health care provider, a registered dietitian, your county Extension FCS agent, or one of the Web sites provided in the "You Can Start Right Now" section of this appendix.

Scores of 0 to 2

Obviously, you were concerned enough about your health to take this test. But your answers show that *you may be taking serious risks with your health.* Perhaps you were not aware of the risks and what to do about them. You can easily get the information and help you need to reduce your health risks and have a healthier lifestyle if you wish. Are you ready to take the next step?

You Can Start Right Now

The test you just completed included many suggestions to help you reduce your risk of disease and premature death. Here are some of the most significant ones.

Avoid Cigarettes

Cigarette smoking is the single most important preventable cause of illness and early death. It is especially risky for pregnant women and their unborn babies. Persons who stop smoking reduce their risk of getting heart disease and cancer. So if you're a cigarette smoker, think twice before lighting that next cigarette. For help with smoking cessation, see the CDC Web site at http://www.cdc.gov/tobacco/quit_smoking/how_to_quit/index.htm. If you choose to continue smoking, try decreasing the number of cigarettes you smoke.

Follow Sensible Drinking Habits

Alcohol produces changes in mood and behavior. Heavy, regular use of alcohol can lead to cirrhosis of the liver, a leading cause of death. Also, statistics clearly show that mixing drinking and driving is often the cause of fatal or crippling accidents. So, if you drink, do it wisely and in moderation: no more than one drink per day for women and two drinks per day for men.

Use Care in Taking Medications

Today's greater use of drugs—both legal and illegal—is one of our most serious health risks. Even some drugs prescribed by your doctor can be dangerous if taken improperly, when drinking alcohol, or before driving. Use prescription drugs as directed and discard out-dated medications. Never share prescription medications with anyone and keep all medications out of reach of children and teens. Excessive or continued use of tranquilizers can cause physical and mental problems. Using or experimenting with illicit drugs including cocaine, heroin, "club drugs" such as Ecstasy, GHB, LSD, and other street drugs may lead to a number of damaging effects or even death. See http://clubdrugs.gov for more information on "club drugs."

Eat Sensibly

Your eating habits are related to risk for high blood pressure, heart disease, obesity, diabetes, and some forms of cancer. Eat a wide variety of plant foods like whole grain foods, dry beans (like black, red, pinto, and Great Northern beans), nuts, fruits, and vegetables every day. These foods contain a variety of nutrients as well as protective factors that may reduce your risk of chronic diseases. Also, eat an adequate amount of lean meats, fish, poultry, and fat-free or low-fat dairy foods for nutrients that they provide. Good eating habits mean limiting the amount of fat (especially saturated fat and trans fat), cholesterol, sugar, and salt in your diet. For more information on healthy eating, see http://www.choosemyplate.gov.

Exercise Regularly

Almost everyone can benefit from exercise—and there's some form of exercise almost everyone can do. (If you have any doubt, check first with your doctor.) Usually as little as 30 minutes of moderate exercise a day five times a week will help you have a healthier heart, tone up sagging muscles, and promote restful sleep. Moderate exercise includes brisk walking, ballroom or line dancing, bicycling on level ground, or water aerobics. Think about how these changes can improve the way you feel. Physical activity guidelines are available at http://www.health.gov.

Learn How to Handle Stress

Stress is a normal part of living. The causes of stress can be good (like a promotion on the job) or bad (like the death of a spouse.) Properly handled, stress does not need to cause health problems. But unhealthy responses to stress—such as driving too fast, drinking too much, or prolonged anger or grief—can cause a variety of physical and mental problems. Even on a very busy day, find a few minutes to slow down and relax. Talking over a problem with someone you trust can often help you find a satisfactory solution. Learn to distinguish between things that are "worth fighting about" and things that are less important. Get more information on stress and other health-related topics at http://www.healthfinder.gov.

Be Safety and Health Conscious

Think "safety first" at home, at work, at school, at play, and on the highway:

- Buckle seat belts and place young children in the proper type of child restraint seats for their age. Once children outgrow their forward facing car seats they should still sit in a booster seat in the back seat until they are 4'9", which is usually around age eight. All children under 13 should sit in the back seat. The National Highway Traffic Safety Administration has information on current laws and resources available related to seat belts, child restraint seats, and more, available at http://www.nhtsa.dot.gov.

- Recent research indicates that distracted driving, like driving while texting, is similar to driving while intoxicated in the danger it poses.
- The benefits of a good night's sleep include better mental and physical functioning during the day. Inadequate sleep contributes to risk for obesity, and high blood pressure, so be sure to get adequate rest. For more information, see http://www.nhlbi.nih.gov/health/public/sleep/healthysleepfs.pdf.

Health Risk Appraisals

Bob Gorsky, PhD

Health Risk Assessments (HRAs): New Technologies and Implications

Shift from Paper-Based to Technology-Based HRAs

Paper-based HRAs were the standard for about 25 years, until the late 1990s, when the electronics era began fostering technology innovations (and additional options) in the design, implementation, and application of HRAs as a population health management tool.

Around 1998, new HRA innovations began to appear (in the HRA industry) as an option for employers, health plans, and other groups. Examples include the following:

- In late 1998, HPN WorldWide (HPN) and Wellness, Inc., released a next-generation HRA using Palm computing (e.g., personal digital assistants [PDA]) technology to capture data in conjunction with or independent of health screenings and independent of Internet access.
- Between 2000 and 2005, HPN, Staywell, Inc., and other vendors released Internet versions of their conventional paper-based HRAs.
- Between 2005 and 2010, other HRA-related platforms/versions began to appear (e.g., laptop versions [for use at screenings], versions for smartphones, iPads, and other handheld devices).

Source: Courtesy of Bob Gorsky and HPN. Reprinted with permission.

Mobile Technology-Based HRAs: Early and More Recent Versions

From 1998 to 2005, over 400,000 people used early versions of mobile technology HRAs (using Palm OS and other handheld devices). These devices did not have access to the Internet and were developed for use during health screenings. The data were uploaded to a laptop (for transmission to the processing center) and/or the devices were sent to a processing center for data retrieval. These early versions of HRAs revealed some noteworthy findings:

- HRA completion time was cut by 60 percent or more (versus paper). It only took about 5 minutes to complete 40–50 questions.
- Participation rates nearly doubled.
- No questions were skipped, allowing for better data capture.
- Because paper questionnaires were not needed, money was saved through reduced paper costs, scanning time, and postage.
- Participants were attracted to the technology regardless of age, gender, education level, or ethnicity.
- Fewer than 10 people asked for a paper version.
- No mobile devices disappeared.
- Compared to paper-based questionnaires, it was easier, faster, and less costly to customize questions.
- Early handheld devices presented new issues to address (e.g., battery life, data transfer steps and risks, data loss risks, rapid evolution of device hardware and software versions).

These findings apply whether the HRA was done in conjunction with or independent of an early detection screening (e.g., blood pressure, cholesterol, other clinical tests).

When used in conjunction with worksite early detection screenings, significantly more (90 to 97 percent) screening participants completed the handheld technology-based HRA as compared to the paper-based HRA offered in previous years (47 to 55 percent).

Since 2006, these developments and findings have proven useful in adapting updates and applications for use with newer mobile technologies with more advanced features, including Internet access (e.g., laptops, smartphones, iPads). These newer mobile HRA applications are still being used at many HRA-related health screenings (with greater features and efficiencies than earlier versions). However, usage at screenings has declined, because most participants have completed the related Internet-based HRA at home, work, or elsewhere before or after the screening.

Internet-Based HRAs

Our work with groups using Internet-based HRAs has yielded trends that have shifted dramatically (180 degrees) over the past 10 years, for example:

- From about 2000–2005: Participation rates of those using Internet-based HRAs were far lower than expected. In fact, they were lower than completion rates of the same paper-based HRAs done in previous years. It was not uncommon for users completing the online HRA to stop and not finish it for any of a multitude of reasons—slow computer, slow dial-up modem, Internet service providers (ISPs) terminating the session, or interruptions at work or home. Employee communications regarding the Internet-based HRA were much more involved than anticipated and still yielded less than desirable participation rates. When done in conjunction with worksite early detection screenings, significantly fewer screening participants completed the Internet-based HRA (as compared to the paper-based HRA in previous years).
- From 2006 to date: Since 2006, virtually all of the earlier trends have reversed 180 degrees. Now, over 95 percent of HRA participants use Internet-based options to complete them. These trends can be attributable to improvements in the design of HRA applications and migration to higher-speed Internet services and computers (by service providers and end users). Today, only 0 to 3 percent of each employer-based group (employees and covered spouses) request a paper-based option, with fewer participants than projected actually using paper—to the pleasant surprise of all.

Discussion

Since 2005, Internet-based HRAs have been shown to have superior participation rates, shorter completion times, data capture and other efficiencies, and cost-effectiveness over all other options. The current form and/or implementation methods of Internet-based HRAs appear to have many of the aforementioned and other advantages.

Regardless of the technology platform, a number of variables can influence HRA participation rates and results, such as the following:

- *HRA languages available.* If needed, is the HRA available in Spanish or other languages? Can it be translated to other languages if funding is available?
- *Promotional efforts and communications.* How will the HRA be promoted and communicated to the targeted population?

- *Design of personal reports.* Are they available online and in print? Are they easy to understand? How are online reports different from printed reports? What is the basis of the design (e.g., goals, research)?
- *Completion incentives.* What are the incentives to complete the HRA? It is not uncommon for effective incentives to result in 100 percent of targeted populations completing the HRA!
- *Completion protocols.* What questions *must* be answered and which are optional? What must be done before completing the HRA? Is HRA completion required before being able to sign-up for the related health screening? How many days does a person have to complete an HRA once the first question has been answered?
- *User interface.* Does the HRA have a user-friendly design, layout, functionality, etc., regarding online, mobile, and paper versions?
- *Convenience.* Will eligible participants have 24/7 access to complete the HRA before, during, or after screening at work, home, or elsewhere? How? What else do participants have online access to (e.g., archived reports, content tools for follow-up and to improve) and for how long?
- *Access.* Access can be affected by the use of older, slow computers; the browser used (certain browsers and browser versions have more problems than others); firewall issues (if accessing at work); and the availability of high-speed Internet (e.g., cable).

As always with any HRA, no HRA (regardless of platform) should be done without serious commitment to linking to existing resources (e.g., health screenings, follow-up information and resources, training, health coaching) and/or adding and integrating other appropriate support resources to help participants begin to reduce and better manage identified risks.

Conclusions and Best Practice Recommendations

Based on research and field experience over the past 27 years, our conclusions (assuming all other variables are equal) are as follows:

1. Internet-based HRAs are associated with the highest participation rates, greatest efficiencies (completion times and other), and lowest costs.
2. Laptop and other handheld devices offer better efficiencies and cost-effectiveness at worksite screenings than paper-based options.
3. Paper-based HRA options may still be needed in some cases, but are rarely used for many reasons—mainly the pervasiveness of Internet access by the general population (at home, work, and/or public libraries); the ability of users to skip questions; and higher costs associated with paper, postage, and data capture.

Based on findings to date, we recommend the following as HRA best practices:

1. Be sure the right HRA is elected based on meeting key selection criteria (those important to key decision makers); for example, research basis and usefulness of questions, analytics, and reports; vendor experience and references; group reports; customization options (questions, interface, reports); available technical support; integration abilities (e.g., with screening data, incentive programs); HIPAA/HITECH compliance; turnaround times (e.g., setup, uploads, reports); other meaningful platform features (for participant, administrative, and clinical users); costs; and other factors.
2. Internet-based HRAs are the preferred option for completing HRAs and accessing results and related support, ideally in conjunction with HRA-related health screenings. As a general rule, allow 3 days to complete an HRA once the first question has been answered.
3. Consider using laptop or other mobile device HRA versions for completion of the HRA at screenings where Internet-based HRAs are not feasible and/or for those individuals who did not complete the HRA online prior to the screening.
4. Have a paper-based and/or phone-based option available for use, as needed.
5. Carefully review Internet accessibility and languages of the targeted population to optimize effective planning and related success.
6. To maximize interrelated participation rates, efficiencies, and population health related results: (a) implement HRAs and related core health screenings during the same 4- to 6-week time period (using Internet-based HRAs as the primary HRA method, plus mobile devices and paper, as appropriate) with assurances of confidentiality, and (b) include an effective incentive for completing both the HRA and the related screening by a specified deadline.

For More Information

See the following resources for additional information:

- U.S. Preventive Services Task Force (http://www.uspreventiveservicestaskforce.org)
- Gorsky, B. (2010). *Best practices: Health risk management and loss control*, version 4.1. Elmhurst, IL: HPN WorldWide.
- HPN WorldWide (http://www.hpn.com/screenings.html)
- Bob Gorsky, PhD (bobgorsky@hpn.com; 630-941-9030 ext. 101)

Note: This update considered more than 300 employers and/or health plans (e.g., businesses, government, schools, unions) using the technology platforms discussed with more than 1,000,000 employees and spouses spanning more than 600 worksites throughout the United States.

La Crosse Wellness Project

For background and context, the message below is provided to those who are going through the Wellness Development Process of the La Crosse Wellness Project.

Preface

Welcome to the Wellness Development Process of the La Crosse Wellness Project (LWP). Earlier you completed the La Crosse Wellness Inventory, which was the Assessment stage. Now you have the opportunity to go through the *Intervention* and *Reinforcement* stages of wellness. In these stages, you will examine your current level of wellness and establish a process for wellness enhancement in your life.

There are several points that we would like to make before you continue. Please notice that we have made every effort in this project to stay away from establishing the kind of scoring system that forces you to compare yourself with others. While we believe that "comparing ourselves to others" is one way of valuing our lives, we also believe that people should learn how to value themselves. This means comparing yourself with yourself, rather than constantly comparing yourself to the expectations of society. As a result, we have designed an inventory that encourages you to assess yourself and then to make decisions based on your assessment. This provides you with the basis to make some plans for your lifestyle choices.

Your potential for an improved lifestyle corresponds to your investment in reading the Wellness Development Process booklet and your investment in understanding the process. We recognize that this booklet is lengthy. Its structure provides you with educational and conceptual information on the left side and a worksheet to the right. We highly recommend that you take the time to read the information on the left before completing the worksheet to the right.

The Wellness Development Process, contained in this booklet, consists of four sections:

1. Establishing a Wellness Area for Enhancement
2. Identifying Wellness Outcomes
3. Establishing Wellness Activities
4. Working Toward Personal Enhancement

Their order and content are designed to foster specific understanding of how to make changes in your life. The purpose of the LWP is to help you learn how to:

1. Assess your life patterns at this time
2. Select areas for enhancement
3. Establish activities for enhancement
4. Establish rewards for enhancement

Wellness involves a lifelong learning process in which health-related decisions are made to maximize your health promotion potential. Health promotion involves a way of life, and the responsibility belongs to each of us to enhance our lifestyles.

You will get out of this development process what you choose to put into it.

Margaret F. Dosch, Gary D. Gilmore, and Thomas L. Hood
Steering Committee Members for the La Crosse Wellness Project

Introduction

What Do You Most Want from Life?

If someone were to ask you this question, how would you respond? Obviously, the answers that people give to this question are numerous and diverse; yet, there appears to be a common theme that underlies the answer by most people. At a more basic level, it appears that what most people want from life is "to be happy." Most of the things that we work for in life—"to get an education," "develop relationships," "earn money," "be important," and the like—are all achieved to create some form of happiness.

How Do We Attain Happiness?

The answers to this question are quite distinct. How or what creates happiness is different for different people. Yet, once again, we find common factors that help to create happiness. Two such factors are (1) achieving some level of success in what we attempt, and (2) feeling like we are able to have an impact on our lives so as not to feel overwhelmed.

Consider: "How will you learn how to increase your chance of success, to feel good about yourself, and to make choices that will have an impact on your life?" This question relates to the heart of the La Crosse Wellness Project, which is to help you as an individual to (1) understand how you can become more aware of your present lifestyle, (2) design a plan for your own lifestyle changes, and (3) overall, improve your feelings about yourself.

Wellness is not sitting around waiting for the world to provide you with what you want, and lamenting when it does not happen. Wellness is an active process. The process includes:

1. Accepting yourself as human, identifying your strengths and weaknesses, learning to accept those that you cannot change, and establishing a process for changing those for which you can be more responsible.
2. Reducing your world into workable activities and outcomes.
3. Taking ownership and responsibility for what you believe in and for your own decisions.
4. Perceiving yourself as able to make changes and not allowing yourself to be overwhelmed by the many small problems of life or the major problems of life to the point of becoming frustrated.
5. Seeing the big picture of life.
6. Learning how to strive for excellence in life rather than trying to be perfect.
7. Establishing expectations, outcomes, and activities that are achievable, yet challenging, and doing this in such a way that you do not set yourself up for failure.
8. Not letting yourself rationalize the difficulties of life.
9. Seeing yourself as human, being made up of many parts that include feelings, beliefs, and behaviors, and recognizing that you cannot be perfect in all of these areas, and that this is OK.
10. Taking areas of your life you have identified for change and developing activities to achieve that change.
11. Addressing positive and negative issues in your life.

Wellness is all of these and more. You are probably able to add more statements to this list. The purpose of the La Crosse Wellness Project is to get you thinking about wellness and to recognize that you, as an individual, have a great amount of potential to improve your own life and to affect your own sense of happiness.

The process that follows is a method to reduce large areas into workable units. Three factors are used in reducing a large area: need, ability, and desire. These interrelated factors are vital to success, and they are assessed as each participant goes through the Wellness Development Process (WDP) in developing an individualized plan of action based on the findings from the La Crosse Wellness Inventory (LWI).

Establishing a Wellness Area for Enhancement

Educational Module

A worksheet is provided to guide you through a process that enables you to narrow down the nine areas of wellness to the one that you now wish to attempt to change. (A common error that prevents our effectively changing our lives is that we see problems as "too big" because we don't know how to narrow them down.)

Enhancement means reducing or eliminating unhealthy actions and/or maintaining or improving healthy actions in each wellness area.

A unique educational concept in the La Crosse Wellness Project (LWP) is:

> We too frequently compare ourselves to others and do not look into ourselves. We do this by comparing our "scores" with others' "scores" or by comparing ourselves with what is "normal." Too frequently, this does not allow us to find value in the positive things we do because they seem to be "not enough." This project encourages you to focus on yourself and to give yourself credit for all the positives you create in your lifestyle, even when you may see a need to do more. Your ability to feel good about yourself and to see yourself as being able to change is related to your ability to acknowledge positive behaviors, even when you recognize you have improvements to make.

Contact information for the La Crosse Wellness Project is found in Appendix D.

Available Health Risk Appraisals and Wellness Inventories

All of these appraisals can be completed and scored on a computer with Internet access.

La Crosse Wellness Project

Contact
La Crosse Wellness Project
203 Mitchell Hall
University of Wisconsin–La Crosse
La Crosse, WI 54601
608-785-8162
gilmore.gary@uwlax.edu

Description
Emphasizes current levels of wellness with follow-up materials for planned change and reinforcement.

LifeScan

Contact
Lifestyle Improvement Systems
718 Linwood Avenue
Stevens Point, WI 54481
715-345-1735
http://wellness.uwsp.edu/other/lifescan/lifescan.asp

Description
Emphasizes physical activity, drug usage, driving habits, cholesterol level, medical history, and women's health issues.

LiveWell

Contact
Lifestyle Improvement Systems
718 Linwood Avenue
Stevens Point, WI 54481
715-345-1735
http://wellness.uwsp.edu/other/livewell

Description
Emphasizes one's social environment, emotional awareness, emotional control, and intellectual, occupation, and spiritual health.

Stress Symptoms Input Form

Contact
Lifestyle Improvement Systems
718 Linwood Avenue
Stevens Point, WI 54481
715-345-1735
http://wellness.uwsp.edu/other/stress/symptoms.asp

Description
Emphasizes the signs and symptoms of stress.

Stress Sources Input Form

Contact
Lifestyle Improvement Systems
718 Linwood Avenue
Stevens Point, WI 54481
715-345-1735
http://wellness.uwsp.edu/other/stress/sources.asp

Description
Emphasizes the sources of stress.

Stress Balancing Strategies Input Form

Contact
Lifestyle Improvement Systems
718 Linwood Avenue
Stevens Point, WI 54481
715-345-1735
http://wellness.uwsp.edu/other/stress/balancing.asp

Description
Emphasizes strategies for balancing stress.

Personal Wellness Profile

Wellsource
P.O. Box 15431
Clackamas, OR 97015
503-656-7446
http://www.wellsource.com

Description
Addresses worksite wellness through assessments of coronary and cancer risk, fitness, lung function, body composition, nutrition, tobacco and alcohol use, and blood pressure.

Testwell (HLQ or HRA)

Contact
National Wellness Institute
1300 College Court
P.O. Box 827
Stevens Point, WI 54481
715-342-2969
http://www.testwell.org

Description
Measures strength in social, occupational, spiritual, physical, intellectual, and emotional dimensions of wellness.

IHRA Online

Contact
CPM Corporate Offices and Technology Center
6720 Frank Lloyd Wright Avenue
Suite 200
Middleton, WI 53562
608-831-7880 or 800-332-2631
608-831-7889 (fax)
http://www.hraonline.com

Description
Analyzes medical factors and lifestyle choices. It is a customized, programmed, mortality-based instrument that can estimate participants' longevity.

Community Capacity Assessment Inventory

United Neighbors Capacity Survey

What would you say are some of the best things about our neighborhood?

_____

_____

_____

Why did you choose to live here?

_____

_____

_____

What are some things that you would like to do to improve the neighborhood?

_____

_____

_____

Have you ever participated in any of the following activities?

_____ Boy Scouts/Girl Scouts

_____ Church fundraisers

_____

Source: From Kretzmann, J., McKnight, J., and Sheehan, G. (1997). *A Guide to Capacity Inventories: Mobilizing the Community Skills of Local Residents.* Chicago: ACTA Publications; ABCD Institute. Davenport, IA: United Neighbors, Inc. Used with permission.

_____ Bingo

_____ Parent/Teacher Association (PTA) or school associations

_____ Sports teams

_____ Camp trips or field trips

_____ Political campaigns

_____ Neighborhood associations

_____ Rummage sales or yard sales

_____ Church suppers

_____ Tutoring

_____ 4-H or gardening

_____ Arts or crafts

_____ Chess or game clubs

_____ Music

_____ Other

What could we do at the school that could benefit the neighborhood?

_____

_____

_____

When you think about your own skills, what are three things that you think you do best?

_____

_____

_____

What are three skills you would most like to learn?

_____

_____

_____

Are there any skills you would like to teach or show others?

_____

_____

_____

Are there some hobbies or special interests of yours that we have not covered?

_____

_____

_____

How often do you go outside the neighborhood to have fun (in a week)?

_____ Once a week or less

_____ 2 to 4 times

_____ Every day

Where do you go?

_____

_____

_____

What kinds of new places or activities would you like to see in the neighborhood?

_____

_____

_____

Are you part of any groups that gets together on a regular basis?

_____

_____

_____

Are you currently employed? Which shift?

_____

_____

_____

Is there any product or service related to your work that could be sold in the neighborhood?

_____

_____

_____

Should we let you know about our next meeting or activity? _____

Would you be interested in interviewing others? _____

Name: _____

Address: _____

Phone: _____

Interviewer's Name: _____

_____

Date: _____

United Neighbors, Inc.
Paul Fessler
808 Harrison Street
Davenport, IA 52803
536-322-7363

Early Detection Tips and Tools: Health Screening Guidelines and Resources

Put Your Plan in Motion

Daily, Monthly, and Yearly Checks

Learn what is normal for you, and to recognize important changes. There are many things you can do to detect problems early. These actions involve some "detective work" on your part—detective work called self-inspection. Self-inspection means that you monitor your own body and the way it's working. This helps you to learn what is normal for you, and to recognize important changes.

Your detective work involves three different types of self-inspection:

- *Every day.* Do quick checks of the way your body looks and feels and the way it's functioning.
- *Monthly.* Perform more thorough, overall self-exams. If you have a spouse or significant other, you can do some of these for each other.
- *Every 1 to 5 years.* Talk to your doctor about medical exams and screenings recommended every 1 to 5 years, based on your age and other risk factors.

You'll need to see the doctor for some of these tests. However, some may be available at low or no cost through early detection screenings at the worksite, community health fairs, or public health departments.

Do It for Life!

Remember, it's important that you play an active role in your early detection plan. Your doctor is very knowledgeable about diagnosing diseases and recommending treatments. But you will most likely be the first to recognize any changes. After all, only you know what's normal for your body.

Putting these three strategies into practice can ensure the earliest detection and fastest treatment of serious health problems. Doing them could save your life!

Source: Courtesy of Bob Gorsky and HPN. Reprinted with permission.

Use Reminders: Don't Forget!

Use this list to jog your memory. If you have a reminder card or copy of this list, hang it in the shower or on the bathroom door. Write reminders in your calendar. Seeing and acting on these reminders may save your life—or someone else's!

- Monitor yourself in the ways listed on these pages daily, monthly, and every 1 to 5 years.
- Use one or more self-care books to follow up on any symptoms.
- Consider your common sense or "gut" feelings when making medical decisions.
- Work with your doctor on early detection strategies and handling of problems.

Every Day

After you wake up, look in the mirror.

- Does your skin look healthy?
- Do your eyes look clear and alert?
- Look inside your mouth. Use your finger to feel around your gums and tongue for any sores. Note how your mouth and tongue look and feel.

Keep track of your bowel and bladder habits.

- Do you go more or less than normal?
- Any unusual color or appearance to your urine or stools?

Examine your feelings, energy level, and your body overall.

- If you don't feel your best, how long have you felt this way?
- Is there any pattern?

Examine your lifestyle choices.

- Are you eating foods high in nutrients and fiber, and low in fat and sodium most of the time?
- Are you getting 30 minutes of vigorous walking or some other aerobic activity at least 3 times each week?
- Are you getting 7–8 hours of sleep each night?
- Do you always wear your seatbelt when traveling?
- Do you limit alcohol intake to fewer than 2 drinks per day?
- Are you safety conscious?

- Does your sexual conduct help you to avoid communicable diseases and unwanted pregnancy?
- Do you avoid the use of tobacco and other dangerous substances?
- Do you wash your hands regularly to avoid getting and spreading infections?

Every Month

Once per month, undress and observe your body in the mirror. Look at your skin color and texture from head to toe. Don't forget to check hidden areas (e.g., scalp, back, behind legs).

Look for areas of:

- Bruising or unusual colors
- Abnormal growths
- Changes in freckles or moles
- Unusual lumps

Reflect on how you've felt over the past month.

- Any unusual patterns in feelings, thoughts, relationships, and/or actions?

Weigh yourself and pinch your skin at the chest, waist, and thigh. Record and keep track of your results.

- Did you pinch more than 1 inch anywhere?
- Any unusual fluctuations in weight?

Women:

- Do a breast self-examination.
- Keep a record of the dates of your menstrual cycle and any associated problems.

Men (ages 15–40):

- Do a testicular self-examination.

You can learn how to do self-exams of the breasts, testicles, and skin from self-care books, training programs, your doctor, and other health professionals.

Every 1 to 5 Years

Work with your doctor and use all available resources to create a schedule of recommended screenings and exams. Be sure to take into consideration your gender, age, current health status, and any other relevant risk factors. These tests and exams should be performed every 1 to 5 years and may include the following.

History and physical exam:

- Health risk assessment
- Blood pressure, body mass index (BMI), and body fat
- Cholesterol, glucose, and other blood tests
- Urinalysis
- Vision and hearing

Anyone 50 years and older: Screenings for colon cancer—fecal occult blood test (FOBT) and colonoscopy (or sigmoidoscopy).

Females 18 years and older: Pap tests, clinical breast exams, and mammograms.

Males 50 years and older: Screenings for prostate cancer—digital rectal exam and prostate-specific antigen (PSA) test.

Males 65–75 years: An abdominal aortic aneurysm screening.

Anyone with other risks due to travel, work, lifestyle choices or other exposures: Screenings for hepatitis, tuberculosis, HIV/AIDS, sexually transmitted and other communicable diseases.

Remember

You may be at increased risk for certain conditions if:

- You have a personal or family history of certain health problems
- Your travel and/or work expose you to other risks (e.g., diseases in other countries, certain careers in health care, working with or around certain animals).
- Lifestyle and other choices expose you to risks (e.g., hepatitis, HIV/AIDS, other communicable diseases including pet-related diseases).

If you are considered high risk, you may need certain tests earlier and/or more often. Talk with your doctor about the tests you need and how often, based on your risks. Be sure to ask about immunizations you may need, too.

Community Risk Estimation

Harriet H. Imrey, PhD*

Community risk estimation is a natural outgrowth of individual health appraisal. It depends on the same basic sciences of public health—epidemiology and biostatistics—and can be done with more or less attention to the basic rules of evidence and statistical rigor. Barring serious biases in the selection of risk factors and relative risks for the model, a community risk appraisal is likely to be more accurate than an individual appraisal because one can use the law of large numbers as a security blanket.

We are hearing more about community risk estimation in public health circles than we used to. Risk reduction programs in the public sector must demonstrate an effect upon public health to justify public support. Community risk estimation is exactly what it says: an estimate. It is a way of projecting efficacy of risk reduction without waiting for years to demonstrate efficacy (or lack of it).

Appraising the health of a community also can be a source of civic pride if the appraisal is good, or a spur to action if it is not. It is easy to imagine: communities bidding for new industries on the grounds of a demonstrably healthy workforce. It is also easy to imagine the new industry listening to the argument, because we already know that a healthier workforce is a cheaper workforce.

Risk estimation can also be a useful means of needs assessment for program development, public relations, or policy decisions. It provides a tool

* Occupational Health Strategies, Inc., Charlottesville, VA, and Greenstone Healthcare Solutions, Kalamazoo, MI. Reprinted with permission of Harriet H. Imrey, PhD, and the Society of Prospective Medicine. This paper appeared in the *Proceedings of the 21st Annual Meeting of the Society of Prospective Medicine*, 1986, pp. 8–11. Revised version, 1995.

for simulating the results of any number of health policy options in terms of deaths postponed or diseases prevented.

Community risk estimation can be used for business purposes. Private vendors of health risk appraisal instruments have already discovered the marketing potential for cost-effectiveness projections following worksite wellness programs—in this case, the individual company is the community of interest.

Before giving you a choice of several methods for estimating community risk, I would like to review some of the reasons for approaching this issue carefully. The bottom line for risk estimation in the community is calculating the population attributable risk proportion (PARP)—the percentage of deaths due to a particular risk factor—and then multiplying this percentage by the number of deaths in the community. The only parameters you need to calculate this figure are the proportion of the population with the risk factor and the relative risk of death or disease for people who have the factor compared to those who do not:

$$\mathrm{PARP} = \frac{p(\mathrm{RR}-1)}{1+p(\mathrm{RR}-1)}$$

This is very straightforward when you are working with one binary risk factor (people have it or they don't). The only complications arise when you want to use more than one risk factor or a risk factor with several gradients of risk, such as heavy smoking, light smoking, and nonsmoking. Unfortunately, we almost always want to do it this way and have to cope with the complexities.

The simplest example is a dataset based on two risk factors, where the data show no confounding and no interaction. For our purposes, "no confounding" means that people who have or do not have risk factor A have equal probabilities of having risk factor B; that is, A and B are not associated. "No interaction" means that the relative risk of B is the same whether the person has risk factor A (see **Table G-1**).

TABLE G-1
PARP Example of Two Risk Factors with No Confounding and No Interaction

	N	p	r	d	RR
AB	1000	0.10	0.04	40	4.0
A$\bar{\mathrm{B}}$	3000	0.30	0.02	60	2.0
$\bar{\mathrm{A}}$B	1500	0.15	0.02	30	2.0
$\bar{\mathrm{A}}\bar{\mathrm{B}}$	4500	0.45	0.01	45	1.0
Total	10,000		0.0175	175	

(*Continued*)

TABLE G-1
(Continued)

Population Attributable Risk Proportion (PARP)

$$= r \frac{(Total) - r(\overline{A}\,\overline{B})}{r(Total)} = \frac{0.0175 - 0.01}{0.0175} \times 100 = 42.86\%$$

or

$$1 - \frac{1}{\sum pRR} = 1 - \frac{1}{0.10(4) + 0.30(2) = 0.15(2) = 0.45(1)}$$

$$= 1 - \frac{1}{1.75} = 42.86\%$$

One variable at a time:

	N	p	r	d	RR
A	4000	0.40	0.025	100	2.0
$\overline{A}$	6000	0.60	0.0125	75	1.0
	10,000 I		0.0175	175	

$$PARP(A) = 28.57\%$$

	N	p	r	d	RR
B	2500——0.25		0.028	70	2.0
$\overline{B}$	7500	0.75	0.014	105	1.0
	10,000		0.0175	175	

$$PARP(B) = 20.0\%$$

Total Population Attributable Risk Proportion

$$=1- \pi[1-PARP(X)] = 1 - (1 - 2\,7\%)(1 - 20.0\%) = 42.86\%$$

The easiest way to look at population attributable risk, when you have a complete set of data such as this, is to look at the death rate among the group that has neither risk factor, and see by what proportion the total death rate would go down if everyone were at that low risk level. In this case, it would be 42.86 percent. In the real world, we don't have this information for the community we are working with, so we have to make the first great leap of faith: We assume that a relative risk represents some sort of biological truth that applies to the world at large, and that unknown risk factors are not busily confounding our data source. Then we can go ahead and use these relative risk figures with prevalence data from our own community.

Again, back in the real world, we might not know anything about the joint distribution of the risk factors and know only what proportion of people have factor A and what proportion have factor B. In this case only, we have the option of working with one variable at a time. The total PARP, calculated by combining the PARP figures for the two variables and using the last formula for Table G-1, is the same as that calculated with the first formula. One important thing to notice here is that the PARP figures cannot be added together, because the same death would be accounted for more than once: Your community risk estimate would look odd if you promised to reduce the death rate by 150 percent.

The next example shows the effects of confounding: What happens when your risk factors are not distributed independently in the original data sources (see **Table G-2**)? The important thing here is that the relative risks you would be using are not the true (unconfounded) relative risks: Part of the effect measured for factor A is due to the larger proportion of B people in the A category, and vice versa. Both relative risks are overestimates of the true relative risk; that is, the risk after adjustment for confounding. The result in this case is an overestimate of the community attributable risk by 18 percent.

TABLE G-2
PARP Example of Two Risk Factors with Confounding and No Interaction [$P(B|A) = 0.15$, not 0.10]

Confounding: The likelihood of possessing risk factor B is different depending on whether or not the person possesses factor A (e.g., a sedentary person may be somewhat more likely to smoke than a jogger).

	N	p	r	d	RR
AB	1500	0.15	0.04	60	4.0
A$\bar{\text{B}}$	2500	0.25	0.02	50	2.0
$\bar{\text{A}}$B	1000	0.10	0.02	20	2.0
$\bar{\text{A}}\bar{\text{B}}$	5000	0.50	0.01	50	1.0
Total	10,000		0.018	180	

(Continued)

TABLE G-2
(*Continued*)

$$PARP = \frac{0.018 - 0.01}{0.018} \times 100 = 44.44\%$$

One variable at a time:

	N	p	r	d	RR
A	4000	0.40	0.0275	110	2.36
$\overline{A}$	6000	0.60	0.0117	70	1.0
	10,000		0.018	180	

$$PARP(A) = 35.0\%$$

	N	p	r	d	RR
B	2500	0.25	0.320	80	2.41
$\overline{B}$	7500	0.75	0.0133	100	1.0
	10,000		0.0180	180	

$$PARP(B) = 26.06\%$$

$$1 - (1 - 0.35)(1 - 0.2606) = 51.94\% \textbf{ (not right)}$$

Table G-3 shows confounding and interaction at the same time. If the only information you have is two separate relative risks and the population prevalence for each, your community attributable risk estimate will be inaccurate.

The point of this somewhat tedious review is to demonstrate that you will almost never have enough information to estimate community risk correctly for more than a very few variables at a time because you need to be sure that the relative risks have been adjusted for confounding, that interactions have been accounted for, and that you know the joint distribution of all risk factors in your population. The latter procedure becomes especially tedious when more than very few risk factors are involved.

The catch to this methodological warning is that these conditions cannot be met with relative risk data available at this point in time. The choices are to do nothing, even though many of us have a real need for estimates of community risk, or to proceed very carefully with the best data we can get, but make no

TABLE G-3
PARP Example of Two Risk Factors with Confounding and Interaction [*RR*(AB) = 5, not 4]

Interaction: The effect on mortality of risk factor B is greater if the person also possesses risk factor A (e.g., a sedentary lifestyle may be more hazardous among smokers than among nonsmokers).

	N	p	r	d	RR
AB	1500	0.15	0.05	75	5.0
A$\overline{\text{B}}$	2500	0.25	0.02	50	2.0
$\overline{\text{A}}$B	1000	0.10	0.02	20	2.0
$\overline{\text{A}}\overline{\text{B}}$	5000	0.50	0.01	50	1.0
Total	10,000		0.0195	195	

$$PARP = \frac{0.0195 - 0.01}{0.0195} \times 100 = 48.72\%$$

One variable at a time:

	N	p	r	d	RR
A	4000	0.40	0.03125	125	2.68
$\overline{\text{A}}$	6000	0.60	0.0117	70	1.0
	10,000		0.0195	195	

$$PARP(A) = 40.2\%$$

	N	p	r	d	RR
B	2500	0.25	0.038	95	2.85
$\overline{\text{B}}$	7500	0.75	0.0133	100	1.0
	10,000		0.0195	195	

$$PARP(B) = 31.62\%$$

$$1 - (1 - 0.402)(1 - 0.3162) = 59.11\% \text{ (not right)}$$

unwarranted claims about the precision of the estimates. By supporting the use of individual health risk appraisals, we have already decided to take the latter course. All of us are barefoot empiricists who jump into applications based on epidemiologic evidence that usually falls far short of proof. What we do is make decisions on the weight of the evidence, as a jury in a civil court must do. If we waited for "beyond a reasonable doubt," we would still hesitate about advocating any form of health education or health promotion activities.

We have just reviewed the methodological reasons why community risk estimation should not be attempted. However, here are some directions to accomplish such an estimation. **Table G-4** shows what to do if the only facts you know are the proportion of the population with each of several risk factors, and the relative risks that apply to that factor. You have to have faith that the risk factors are distributed independently in the study population that the relative risks came from and in your own community, and faith will be less strenuous if you don't try to account for factors you know to be related, such as relative weight, blood pressure, and exercise, in the same model. No one can force you to be sensible about it, because the equations don't care one way or the other.

TABLE G-4
Risk Estimation Process with Community Prevalence Rates for Individual Risk Factors

What You Know:
1. Number (or rate) of deaths
2. Relative risks (RR) for one or more risk factors
3. Community prevalence rates (p) for one or more risk factors
What You Believe:
Risk factors are distributed independently in the population and there are no interactions among the relative risks.
What You Do:
1. For *one* risk factor:

$$PARP = \frac{p(RR - 1)}{1 + p(RR - 1)}$$

Deaths that may be postponable = number of deaths $\times$ $PARP$

2. For *one or more* risk factors:

$$PARP = 1 - \pi[1 - PARP(X)]$$

For example, if the $PARP$ for smoking is 30% and the $PARP$ for inactivity is 20%, the total attributable risk proportion is $1 - (1 - 0.30)(1 - 0.20) = 44\%$.

You can do a much better job of community risk estimation if you know the joint prevalence distribution of all the risk factors in your model, and if you have faith that the relative risks you use are "pure" ones; that is, relative risks adjusted for confounding or derived from a multivariate model. You might even have relative risks for interactions. In practice, if you know the joint prevalence of risk factors, you probably know the composite relative risk of each member of your community sample. You have a choice of equations. Table G-5 shows the computation of the population attributable risk proportion for grouped data. If you have a computerized data set with risk factor prevalence survey data, it is more efficient to use this formula.

The composite relative risk for a community (relative to what the community would be like if every resident reduced all reducible risk factors) is always the inverse of the population unattributable risk proportion, just as the composite relative risk for an individual is the inverse of his or her own unattributable risk proportion. Given this fact, it is easy to compare two states or communities directly, and make inappropriate comparisons. One can imagine health educators arguing indefinitely over a model that asserted that Montana is exactly 37.5 percent healthier than Arkansas. A large lawsuit over a suspected environmental contaminant centered on the argument, based

TABLE G-5
Risk Estimation Process with Community Prevalence Rates for Combination of Risk Factors

What You Know:
1. Number (or rate) of deaths
2. Relative risks (RR) for one or more risk factors
3. Community prevalence rate (p) for each combination of risk factors, from a population survey or from risk appraisals
What You Believe:
The risk factors are not distributed independently, but you believe that the relative risks in your model do not interact with one another except in those cases where you have identified a separate relative risk for the categories where interactions take place.
What You Do:
$$PARP = 1 - \frac{1}{\sum pCRR}$$ where p is the proportion of the population with a particular combination of risk factors, and CRR is the composite relative risk for that particular combination (i.e., the product of all relative risks for each separate risk factor).

on this methodology, that the cancer rate in the affected community, after accounting for other known risk factors, was even lower than the cancer rate in the control community, proving that no excess cases could be blamed on a carcinogen in the water supply.

In the future, we will see a growing number of examples of this sort, and we can expect to see more people estimating community risk based on more accurate models. In the meantime, it is necessary to be very cautious about creating synthetic models from very crude data, but that doesn't mean it can't be done. We haven't even touched on questions of selecting all-cause mortality models versus summing over individual causes of death, although the former is generally more conservative. We also haven't considered inaccuracies based upon different risk factor prevalence distributions in different age groups: The safest procedure is to use proportions and relative risks for the narrowest age groups for which data are available. We haven't talked about additive versus multiplicative models, although similar techniques have been derived for additive models. Failing to consider any one of these issues can make your community risk estimates less accurate. However, if you back off because the procedure is complicated, you will miss the opportunity to get some very interesting and useful information that may be only a little bit in error.

In summary, take whatever information you have, add any information you can reasonably get, and take full advantage of every single piece of it. If you have access to your state's Risk Factor Prevalence Survey database or to a file of computerized health risk appraisals, you are ready to do community risk appraisal with a fair degree of accuracy for a very small investment.

Technical Notation: How to Read the Tables

The probability notation used in the examples may be unfamiliar to many readers, but it is not nearly as complicated as it looks. The A and B stand for two different risk factors, such as smoking and obesity. A bar over the top is a negative symbol: It means that the risk factor is not present. In Table G-1, the second row that starts out with $A\bar{B}$ stands for that part of the population of 10,000 people who have risk factor A (they smoke), but do not have risk factor B (they are not overweight). The number (N) of people in that category is 3000; the category's proportion (p) of the total is 0.30.

The rate (r) of death is 0.02, meaning that $3000 \times 0.02 = 60$ people in the category will die (d). The relative risk (RR) is the death rate in that category compared to the death rate among people who do not have either of the risk factors (the row that starts with $\bar{A}\bar{B}$), so the relative risk for category $A\bar{B}$ is $0.02 \div 0.01 = 2$. It takes a little bit of time to figure out any new notation, but using this one can be very time-saving when communicating complex numerical examples.

Assessment in Health Promotion: Deconstruction and Metaphoric Considerations in a Nutshell

Richard B. Hovey, PhD, Adjunct Assistant Professor, Department of Community Health Sciences, Faculty of Medicine, University of Calgary, Alberta

Preamble

The complexity of health is undeniable, and health promotion practitioners find themselves working within this complexity to provide positive health outcomes for individuals, families, and communities. This article provides an alternate perspective to understanding the complexities of health promotion through a philosophical exploration of learning, connecting, and engaging one another. The means through which we will accomplish this is learning from the philosophical thinking of Derrida about deconstruction (Caputo, 2010, 1997; Rolfe, 2004). In health promotion, turning to a philosophical approach as a model for assessment in health promotion may be considered unusual. However, through this journey the ideas of health and the traditionally recognized dimensions of health composed of the *physical* (ability of human body structure to function properly), *social* (ability to interact with other individuals), *mental* (ability to process information and act properly), *emotional* (ability to cope, adjust, and adapt), *spiritual* (belief in some force or dynamic other than humans), *environmental* (composed of the external environment, which includes one's surroundings [e.g., habitat, occupation]), and *internal environment* (an individual's internal structure [e.g., genetics]) (Donatelle, Munroe, Munroe, & Thompson, 2007) dimensions are deconstructed to reveal absences and gaps that invite deeper consideration from the health promotion practitioner.

Even with the aid of deconstruction to help read beyond the recognizable health dimensions, there is the acknowledgment that the dimensions

Source: Article written by Richard B. Hovey exclusively for this book.

of health are influenced by cultural, personal, social–relational, and other situational contexts that contribute to an understanding of health. Also, to acknowledge that within each dimension of health are its elements, which collectively comprise each of the larger dimensions described previously. The elements comprising the larger dimension of health reveal other subcontexts and content and, when deconstructed, offer other factors that may influence a person's health and offer significant contributions to understanding health promotion in practice.

For example, a person diagnosed with diabetes as an adult is deemed unhealthy based on biomedical assessments that are connected to that person's physical attributes, being overweight, unhealthy nutritional choices, and physical inactivity with other detrimental health behaviors can be prescribed an appropriate health promotion intervention. The implementation of best practices to achieve a positive health outcome includes a strategy for weight reduction, increased physical activity, and successful pharmacological management for the person living with diabetes. As a health promotion practitioner, the design of an appropriate model for an effective intervention is based on best practices with current theoretical frameworks. From a thorough assessment of a person living with diabetes, an intervention comprised of the appropriate aspects for potential success is developed, implemented, and assessed. However, if the person living with diabetes consults with a physician, an exercise physiologist, a nutritionist, and a personal trainer with access to facilities and fails to achieve his or her health outcome, then what? Researchers, educators, and health promotion practitioners need to ask the question, "What else is going on here?" This question opens our thinking to consider other possible reasons for this person's health condition; he or she may be depressed, injured, unmotivated, or living a life that seems hopeless and without meaning due to a previous traumatic experience or find the intervention culturally inappropriate. Deconstruction provides the means to explore the deeper concerns found within through expanding our assessment of the dimensions of health. We need to explore what influences one's physical health and what social, emotional, intellectual, environmental, occupational, and spiritual aspects are possible contributors to one's ill health. Once we find which dimension or dimensions are affecting the health of the person living with diabetes, we can deconstruct further to uncover which element or elements require specific attention (Donatelle et al., 2007).

My position in this article is to forward that deconstruction, as part of the health promotion assessment process, provides a means to gain a multifaceted understanding of the determinants of health and illness. To guide us through this discussion I will provide a brief overview of the philosophy and application of Derrida's conceptualization of deconstruction for health promotion assessment and practice as well as an understanding of how we, as health promotion collaborators, consider the assessment of multiple dimensions of health supported through the use and utility of metaphor (Lakoff & Johnsen 2003; McCrickerd, 2000). By proceeding with specific deconstructions, we are continually opening up other possibilities and considerations of understanding health by learning from alternate interpretations provided by other health professionals. The process of health promotion means to regard health in its totality, in addition to its parts, and to be aware that each time we consider one dimension, others may influence a person's overall health. We will endeavor to work though this with the assistance of deconstruction and metaphor to engage our understanding of how this assessment works in education and health promotion practice.

Introduction to Learning with Deconstruction and Metaphor

Learning should be transformational. As such, new or different understandings, even seemingly insignificant ones, may lead to other more substantial and profound understandings of a topic, person, or thing as we become open to other possibilities, conceptualizations, and interconnections of knowledge (Gadamer, 1992). As reflective health promotion practitioners and students, we need to question ourselves as we conduct assessments to whether "something else is going on here." Deconstruction and metaphor provide an opportunity to explore the complexity of health, and more specifically the dimensions of health, to further our insight about a person and/or community's health-related experiences. The opportunity to learn with and from other students, professionals, disciplines, and communities offers alternative ways to understand the complexity of living in health.

This is an invitation for the reader to consider health, in ways other than his or her own discipline-specific and sometimes encultured understandings of health theories, practice, and modes of assessment. It is also important to be reminded that when our discipline-specific knowledge and understandings of practice, research, and learning are challenged, this experience may initially be one of negation; that is, to dismiss new information as unfamiliar to one's foundational paradigm specific understanding, "because something is not what it was supposed to be" (Gadamer, 1989, p. 354). A holistic assessment of health requires different considerations and discussion, which may be stimulated by deconstruction and metaphor. If we view health promotion theories, practices, and assessments as a field of interprofessional conversations, then how we measure and evaluate health outcomes becomes more holistic and inclusive of the experience of health. Whenever people are conversing, they are co-constructing meaning while learning with and from knowledgeable others (Gergen, 2009; Hovey, Dvorak, Hatlie, Burton, Padilla, Worsham, & Morck, 2011).

Accordingly, it is through the reader's own interpretation and subsequent conversations with others not from their health perspective, and subsequent knowledge that new learning may lead to other unique understandings referred to as transformational understanding, which is when one's way of understanding something changes due to learning from another through a reconceptualization of knowledge into new understandings of the same topic. In this way, health promotion practice and assessment embraces the idea that the greater number of voices who enter into the conversation about health promotion and its assessment, the greater the sophistication of the outcome and the greater possibility of health promotion and its assessment becoming person-centered, collaborative, and innovative (Gergen, 2009; Hovey et al., 2011).

A useful literary device to support a broader understanding of health is metaphor (McCrickerd, 2000). Metaphors invite conversations about a topic, person or thing. In the text to follow, you will be introduced to the use of metaphor to help health care practitioners, promoters, and students to engage with health care consumers. In this case, the metaphor of plate spinning, with a juggler who is the health care consumer who spins plates on top of poles, is offered as a way to consider the interconnectedness of the dimensions of health and how effective health promotion necessitates interdisciplinary approaches. To further address this understanding, the concept of deconstruction needs to be addressed. The reader will be provided with an exploration of health through Jacques Derrida's conceptualization of the process of deconstruction. I will guide you through this activity using an inquiring approach to connect seemingly unrelated concepts in order to borrow from one paradigm/philosophy to gain a unique understanding of health in another. The deconstruction of health offers a reconsideration of what health means, with the use of metaphor to bring it back into the real world of health promotion and assessment.

Making Connections from an Interdisciplinary Approach

Creating new understandings to enhance health promotion and assessment necessitates inquiry; where *inquiry* refers to a way of learning that requires learners to actively question, to conduct research, and to interpret a wide range of materials in order to draw new connections among theories, particular experiences, and realities.

For the author, this inquiry was the result of participating in two separate learning opportunities during the summer of 2010. The first at the Canadian Hermeneutic Institute (CHI) in Toronto, with guest philosopher Dr. John Caputo, and the other at the 2010 International Union of Health Promotion and Education (IUHPE) World Conference in Geneva, Switzerland. The CHI brought together approximately 40 people with diverse professional backgrounds, including nursing, education, social work, medical anthropology, psychology, and physiology to learn with and from Dr. Caputo and each other. The focus of this 3-day event was to explore Derrida's philosophical analysis of several topics, including deconstruction, as a means to analyze complex systems, with the opportunity to investigate what is known, supposed, or theorized. French philosopher Jacques Derrida's conceptualization of deconstruction is an approach to rigorously question, interpret, and reinvent the meanings of texts, institutions, traditions, societies, and beliefs to reveal the contradictions and internal oppositions upon which they were established. In its most specific understanding, deconstruction is about gaining insight and new understandings.

In an exploration of the utility of deconstruction, Derrida (1997) offered:

> Whenever deconstruction finds a nutshell—a secure axiom or a pithy maxim— the very idea is to crack it open and disturb this tranquility. Indeed, that is a good rule of thumb in deconstruction. That is what deconstruction is all about, its very meaning and mission, if it has one. One might even say that cracking nutshells is what deconstruction is. In a nutshell. (p. 32)

Three weeks later during the IUHPE conference, I participated in a series of sessions that invited reflection from participants about the conference and health promotion in general. This reflective group comprised an eclectic collection of people engaged in health promotion from grass roots community-based organizations, institutions, researchers, educators, and medical health practitioners. The dynamic, impassioned discussions led to an emerging discontent with several aspects of health promotion. A need was voiced to reconsider, reinvent, and reconceptualise current thought, because something else was going on in real-world health promotion. Throughout the week, the reflective group began to describe an evolution of new directions for health promotion that included enhanced participant engagement, inclusivity, changes to what constituted research evidence, authentic learning (i.e., where learning is the product of theoretical considerations as well through its contextual situation), and viewing health and health promotion in its complexity and dimensions. As I sat listening, it became apparent to me that as a group we were engaged in an organic process of deconstructing health promotion *in a nutshell.*

Overall, I became more curious as to the utility of deconstruction in health promotion practice and decided to inquire, interpret, and to further connect these two experiences through Derrida's analytical deconstruction of justice and laws and apply this analogy to health and the dimensions of health. I began to notice a disconnection between this idea of "health" and the dimensions that comprise health, because "health," as it is utilized within health promotion, is all encompassing, as is "justice," and the dimensions, our points of intervention and understanding are very specific, as are laws to "justice." Deconstruction in a nutshell (Caputo, 1997) and the analogy of "justice" and "health" provided an opportunity to consider the possibility of the impossible. The impossible in this context is the formidable task of undertaking a complex analysis of "health." Here is where conversations with others with different backgrounds in education, health care, philosophy, and research created the opportunity to understand how "health" and "its dimensions" can be deconstructed in a way to understand interprofessional collaboration in health promotion.

Derrida's Deconstruction of Justice and Law

Derrida's analysis and deconstruction of justice and law surmised that the concept of justice is undeconstructable because "justice" is representative of an all-encompassing concept that is a product of its laws. "Justice is always on the horizon and just out of our reach" (Caputo, 2010). In other words justice is something with which most of us live; we sense its meaning and presence, but justice as a conceptualization is too expansive, too endless, and too complex to be deconstructed—to define its meaning. Thus, "justice" like "health," is undeconstructable. However, "laws," like the "dimensions of health," are deconstructable. Laws constitute justice just as the dimensions of health constitute health. Deconstruction, or reconsideration, of laws, or in this case, the dimensions of health, is possible and necessary in order for justice, as with health, to evolve and remain relevant in content and context to the specifics of this person, this health care team.

During the CHI, John Caputo conveyed Derrida's analysis of deconstruction as a means and opportunity for reinvention or reconceptualization of things through a disruption of our habitual and paradigm-specific discourse about a topic. Deconstruction is about opening up, expanding, and dismantling what has already been described to be resistant to a definable unified meaning, such as texts, institutions, traditions, societies, beliefs, and health promotion practices of whatever size and sort (Caputo, 1997; Rolfe, 2004). The idea is that every time there is an attempt to compartmentalize the meaning of a thing and to frame it by definition, the thing itself stagnates. Meaning and understanding, in this context, becomes fixed, and thus is presumed to be resistant to challenge and remains unchallenged. Deconstruction invites us to ask questions like "What is really going on here?" and "What is really happening?" In this mode of thinking, as health care practitioners we open ourselves to learning with and from others as part of an interprofessional team when we challenge that which seemed to be unchallengeable. Core to effective health promotion is the ability for practitioners to engage efficiently with the multiple considerations to accommodate the complexity of their work. It is an engagement that animates relations and mobilizes people to action while understanding the role of each member of the team, including the patient and/ or community member (Gergen, 2009; Waring, 2009).

Undeconstructable Health

Health resists being universally defined because it can only be interpreted, constituted, and reconstituted through specific professional, promotional, educational, cultural, and governmental lenses and perspectives. There is difficulty implicit in defining health precisely and adequately because health is an overarching conceptualization of human experience. Nevertheless, this does not negate the value of discipline-specific definitions that provide direction, focus, and professional enculturation for health care practitioners, health promoters, and educators. Rather, what is important to recognize is that through the activity of uncovering (defining) one aspect or engagement of health we inadvertently cover up others. Consequently, we simultaneously expand and limit our perspective and understanding of health. This brings to our awareness that the complexity of health rests in trying to understand health as a universally definable construct. Derrida's (1997) conceptualization of deconstruction in a nutshell offers health promotion researchers, educators, and practitioners a way to interpret the complexity of health through its dimensions.

Dimensions of Health: Deconstructable

The dimensions of health, which comprise the substance and the focus of health promotion, are separate but interconnected components of health, but like laws they are deconstructable. Promoting health through multiple perspectives and dimensions such as physical, occupational, environmental, spiritual, emotional, intellectual, social, sexual, mental health, and so on begins with a deconstruction, as one would reinvent and reconsider laws (Caputo, 2010, 1997).

There is a note here, however, to proceed with caution, because health is expansive, diverse, endless, and infinitely transcendent and cannot be fully understood as only a matter of theoretical determinations. Deconstruction, as a process of analysis, also directs us to the contextual nature of health promotion. The human context of living in and with one's dimensions of health serves as it own nutshell to momentarily contain deconstruction by providing a sense of boundary, which prevents endless interpretation; nutshells that can be cracked open another time in a different context for a different purpose.

Let us recall our example of the person living with diabetes. In this instance we may need to shift our attention from the prescriptive elements of health promotion to regard an illness such as diabetes as a function of the social conditions in which this person lives. The context of where and how someone lives is considered with an understanding of who they are. This is achieved by looking at other dimensions of health influencing the person's development of diabetes and those factors remaining persistent within her life preventing her from effectively managing her illness. In this way, as we deconstruct health we are led to consider the contextual nature of the conditions that created the conditions for becoming ill. In a sense, we move from one aspect of understanding diabetes, a biomedical one, to one of the social-relational aspects of environmental (personal, family, and community), occupational (how does one view themselves in the workplace or being unemployed), social (what are the social realities and expectations within their life), or their spiritual connections (if any) and the importance the person places on these. These inquires represent an approach to assessment that is working to help answer the question of "What else is going on in this person's life?" The intention of asking this question is to ensure that in our assessment of a health promotion intervention that should have worked but did not that we keep exploring why it did not match our expectations.

Deconstruction and Metaphor in Health Promotion and Practice

Deconstruction of the dimensions of health is achieved through an interpretive recontextualization of the dimensions of health, which is dynamic, person-centered, and unreducible. Deconstruction is about reverence for the "other" (the "other" being the people we encounter in our personal and professional lives) as we attempt to understand our world and create new possibilities for understanding health. Derrida (1997) reminds us that the "other" is irreducible and is more than someone who is not me or who lives in the world like me.

Deconstruction offers a mindful reconceptualization and realization that health is open to multiple interpretations and multiple truths. "It is between different things that one can think difference" (Derrida, 1997, p. 223). In the real world, health promotion has a presence in which deconstruction needs to be delivered with others through practice, relationship, context, and theory. The discussion about deconstruction and what it has to offer for health promotion is a substantial undertaking. Deconstruction of the dimensions of health requires knowledgeable others and necessitates interdisciplinarity to provide multiple considerations of theories, context, and health promotion. Learning how to achieve interdisciplinarity requires more than theoretical conceptualizations, because collaboration is the interconnection of professional enculturation as something that is lived and experienced.

Reinvention of Health Promotion Through Deconstruction and Metaphor

The use of metaphor is helpful to assist students, health promoters, and educators to envision how their paradigm-specific perspectives can interconnect with others and be inclusive of the person, family, or community. Interdisciplinary consideration of health promotion promises a holistic representation and subsequent understanding of health deconstructed into its dimensions and guiding practices. In practice, finding ways to engage people to consider how their professional and personal perspective on health promotion interconnects meaningfully with others reinforces interdisciplinarity in theory and practice (Waring 2009; Hovey et al., 2010).

As health professionals, students or others are confined within their own discipline-specific knowledge and practice; the work of deconstruction is to crack that nutshell. This task requires that our professionally encultured epistemological thinking, the possibility of learning something one already knows in a different way, or from another health professional's perspective can be supported by the use of metaphor. Caputo speaks about the use of metaphor, saying "Metaphors break the rule of language from its habitual contextual representation and disrupt discourse in an *odd* way, but it must not be *too odd*" (Caputo, personal communication, 2010). In creating a metaphoric relationship—one thing to another—the goal is to get the attention of the intended person (creating a somewhat odd metaphor) to ensure that the chosen metaphor is relevant but not too obscure as to detract from its purpose (not too odd). Metaphors operate to help reinterpret understandings for specific audiences that are mindful of culture, gender, age, illness, professional/interprofessional, person/patient-centered care (Gadamer, 1996).

Fundamentally, metaphor is a widely used figure of speech in both literary and everyday language. Metaphor characterizes an action, concept, or object in terms usually used to denote something else, often quite different. Metaphor implies a comparison between the thing being described and the thing used to describe it, but is not articulated as comparison. The act of creating metaphors may work to enhance an understanding of a topic, as Gadamer (1989) stated:

> If a person transfers an expression from one thing to the other, he has in mind something that is common to both of them; but in this in no way needs generic universality. Rather, he is following his widening experience, which looks for similarities, whether in their appearance or in their significance to use. . . . This is its fundamental metaphoric nature. (p. 429)

Metaphors also provide opportunities to stop and reflect on their meaning within which we appreciate, think, and act in relation to an issue of interest and other possible solutions (McCrickerd, 2000). Deconstruction alongside metaphor provides an opportunity to explore the complexity of health, more specifically the dimensions of health with one's colleagues within an interprofessional collaborative framework and the person or persons who are the intended recipient of our health promotion activities.

Deconstructing the Dimensions of Health with Metaphor

In teaching an undergraduate university course for Community Rehabilitation and Disability Studies, I have used the metaphor of a juggler spinning plates to engage students to think and practice health promotion differently. Imagine a juggler balancing multiple poles. On the top of each of these poles is a spinning plate. Each plate represents a dimension of health—physical, psychological, occupational, environmental, spiritual, emotional, intellectual, social, sexual, and so on—the list grows because it is dependent on what needs to be understood from the person of interest. While envisioning the juggler's attempts to balance the spinning plates, the students are asked to reflect on their own health and the health of others. Through the students' reflections with one another the complexity and interconnectedness of health and its dimensions emerge. The metaphor of juggling multiple spinning plates highlights both the theory and the art of achieving this feat. Because there is a need to carefully monitor each plate or one or another will begin to wobble, there are also times when all the plates are spinning simultaneously and harmoniously, and the juggler experiences his or her health without concern. In those moments, the plates and the task of spinning each plate disappears (we are in good health). The juggler is free to experience the world without conscious concern for a specific spinning plate or plates (dimensions of health are intact). The juggler only realizes the drama and concern of attending to the spinning plates when one or more falter and require attention to reestablish equilibrium.

Let us bring in deconstruction alongside the use of metaphor to consider the dimensions of health—physical, psychological, occupational, environmental, spiritual, emotional, intellectual, social, sexual, and mental health—as spinning the plates we all have. Each of us stands in the middle of our world with all of these dimensional plates spinning, unaware that at any time our health can be disrupted. When we are healthy, as with the juggler, all of our plates spin without concern; our health is invisible. When our health is invisible, we are able to engage our world, physically and socially without concern. When one or more of our dimension(s) of health begin to waver through illness, disease, or trauma, health is revealed as a wobbly plate.

Deconstruction brings to our awareness the dimensions of health that were previously encapsulated in the expansive undeconstructable nature that is health. Deconstruction offers a way to view the dimensions of a person's health and how within that complexity the dimensions of health are interconnected and simultaneously influence the other. This is the possibility of the impossible found through deconstruction. A deconstruction of the dimensions of health provides an opportunity to make known the interconnectedness of the dimensions of health. Deconstruction invites conversation, collaboration, and interdisciplinarity because no single health promotion professional can hold expert knowledge in all the dimensions of health. Therefore, successful health promotion requires bringing together the right people with the right knowledge to enable the person to rebalance their metaphorical wobbly plate(s). If we consider the relevance of deconstruction and metaphor for the example of the person living with diabetes, we might re-envision a holistic approach to helping that person regain a sense of well-being, or even introduce them to a new sense of health, one not previously experienced. The key to deconstruction lies not in its complexity, but in the process of working to understand the person, family, and community of interest through multiple perspectives. In this way, we shift our focus to being concerned with the holistic aspect of the person, which is inclusive of the medical science of the biomedical model, best practices, and interventions as well as an ongoing consideration for the well-being of that person. Reconsideration of the dimensions of health thus cannot be uniquely confined into professional paradigms of practices. Health promotion is both its theories and an interpretive art that enables multiple considerations of the meaning of health and how to assist one another in the pursuit of health promotion.

For the students, this approach became an invitation for collaboration because, as they assessed their client, patient, or community member, they came to realize that holistic health promotion needed other perspectives about the dimensions of health that resided outside of their discipline-specific knowledge and understanding. In this context, an acknowledgment that health promotion was enhanced through interprofessional collaboration meant that it was necessary to seek out others to build a person/patient-centered approach for health promotion. The idea of the person who is ill being a juggler provided a space for conversation for inclusion of other aspects related to understanding health promotion from multiple interconnected dimensions.

Conclusion

A common topic of conversation at the IUHPE conference was to find new, innovative, and dynamic approaches for health promotion. This suggests there is a need for and interest in other kinds of thinking, approaches, and missing elements in health promotion. Interestingly, I had been simultaneously exposed to deconstruction in a nutshell and the impossible possibility of health and the dimensions of health. Innovation, missing elements, and new approaches in health promotion may arise and come to us from other paradigms of study and used in ways not originally intended. This requires of us to inquire, to connect, and to reconceptualize our understanding of how we deal with and engage in the complexity of health.

An understanding of health through its dimensions has valuable implications for research, education, and assessment where we, as health promotion practitioners, view health as a field of conversations, which are inclusive of diversity of knowledge, experience, and practice.

References

Caputo, J. (2010). Personal communication. Canadian Hermeneutic Institute, Toronto, Ontario, June 23–25.

Caputo, J. (1997). *Deconstruction in a nutshell. A conversation with Jacques Derrida.* New York: Fordham University Press.

Clark, A. M., Lissel S. L., and Davis, C. (2008). Complex critical realism: Tenets and application in nursing research. *Advances in Nursing Science, 31*(4), E67–E79.

Derrida, J. (1997). *Deconstruction in a nutshell.* Bronx, NY: Fordham University Press.

Donatelle, R., Munroe, A., Munroe, A. J., and Thompson, A. (2007). *Health: The basics.* San Francisco: Benjamin Cummings.

Gadamer, H. G. (1996). *The enigma of health: The art of healing in a scientific age.* Gaiger, J., and Walker, N. (Trans.). Stanford: Stanford University Press.

Gadamer, H. G. (1992). *Hans-Georg Gadamer on education, poetry and history.* Misgeld, D., and Nicholson, G. (Eds.), Schmidt, L., and Reuss, M. (Trans.). Albany: State University of New York Press.

Gadamer, H. G. (1989). *Truth and method,* 2nd rev. ed. Weinsheimer, J., and Marshall, D. G. (Trans.). New York: The Continuum International Publishing Group Ltd.

Gergen, J. K. (2009). *An invitation to social construction,* 2nd ed. London: Sage Publications.

Hovey, R., Dvorak, M., Hatlie, M., Burton, T., Padilla, J., Worsham, S., and Morck, A. (2011). Patient safety: A consumer's perspective. *Qualitative Health Research, 21,* 662–672.

Hovey, R., and Paul, J. (2007). Healing, the patient narrative-story and the medical practitioner: A relationship to enhance care for the chronically ill patient. *International Journal of Qualitative Methods, 6*(4), 53–66.

Lakoff, G., and Johnsen, M. (2003). *Metaphors we live by.* London: The University of Chicago Press.

McCrickerd, J. (2000). Metaphors, models and organizational ethics in health care. *Journal of Medical Ethics, 26*(5), 340–345.

Rolfe, G. (2004). Deconstruction in a nutshell. *Nursing Philosophy, 5,* 274–276.

Waring, J. (2009). Constructing and re-constructing narratives of patient safety. *Social Science & Medicine, 69,* 1722–1731.

Zbikowski, L. M. (1998). Metaphor and music theory: Reflections from cognitive science. *The Online Journal of the Society for Music Theory.* Available at: http://mto.societymusictheory.org/issues/mto.98.4.1/mto.98.4.1.zbikowski.html. Accessed May 26, 2011.

Index